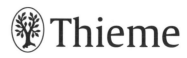

Medical Histology and Embryology Q&A

Manas Das, MD, MS
Associate Professor
Basic Biomedical Sciences
University of South Dakota
Vermillion, South Dakota

134 illustrations

Thieme
New York • Stuttgart • Delhi • Rio de Janeiro

Acquisitions Editor: Delia DeTurris
Managing Editor: Elizabeth Palumbo
Developmental Editor: Julia Nollen
Director, Editorial Services: Mary Jo Casey
Production Editor: Kenneth L. Chumbley
International Production Director: Andreas Schabert
Editorial Director: Sue Hodgson
International Marketing Director: Fiona Henderson
International Sales Director: Louisa Turrell
Director of Institutional Sales: Adam Bernacki
Senior Vice President and Chief Operating Officer: Sarah Vanderbilt
President: Brian D. Scanlan

Library of Congress Cataloging-in-Publication Data
Names: Das, Manas, author.
Title: Medical histology and embryology Q&A / Manas Das.
Description: New York : Thieme, [2018] | Includes index.
Identifiers: LCCN 2017023727 | ISBN 9781626233348 (softcover) |
ISBN 9781626233355 (eISBN)
Subjects: | MESH: Histological Techniques | Embryology |
Examination Questions
Classification: LCC QM601 | NLM QS 518.2 | DDC 612.6/4076—dc23
LC record available at https://lccn.loc.gov/2017023727

© 2018 Thieme Medical Publishers, Inc.
Thieme Publishers New York
333 Seventh Avenue, New York, NY 10001 USA
+1 800 782 3488, customerservice@thieme.com

Thieme Publishers Stuttgart
Rüdigerstrasse 14, 70469 Stuttgart, Germany
+49 [0]711 8931 421, customerservice@thieme.de

Thieme Publishers Delhi
A-12, Second Floor, Sector-2, Noida-201301
Uttar Pradesh, India
+91 120 45 566 00, customerservice@thieme.in

Thieme Publishers Rio de Janeiro, Thieme Publicações Ltda.
Edifício Rodolpho de Paoli, 25º andar
Av. Nilo Peçanha, 50 – Sala 2508
Rio de Janeiro 20020-906, Brasil
+55 21 3172 2297

Cover design: Steve Debenport
Typesetting by Prairie Papers

Printed in China by Everbest Printing Co.   5 4 3 2 1

ISBN 978-1-62623-334-8

Also available as an e-book:
eISBN 978-1-62623-335-5

Important note: Medicine is an ever-changing science undergoing continual development. Research and clinical experience are continually expanding our knowledge, in particular our knowledge of proper treatment and drug therapy. Insofar as this book mentions any dosage or application, readers may rest assured that the authors, editors, and publishers have made every effort to ensure that such references are in accordance with **the state of knowledge at the time of production of the book.**

Nevertheless, this does not involve, imply, or express any guarantee or responsibility on the part of the publishers in respect to any dosage instructions and forms of applications stated in the book. **Every user is requested to examine carefully** the manufacturers' leaflets accompanying each drug and to check, if necessary in consultation with a physician or specialist, whether the dosage schedules mentioned therein or the contraindications stated by the manufacturers differ from the statements made in the present book. Such examination is particularly important with drugs that are either rarely used or have been newly released on the market. Every dosage schedule or every form of application used is entirely at the user's own risk and responsibility. The authors and publishers request every user to report to the publishers any discrepancies or inaccuracies noticed. If errors in this work are found after publication, errata will be posted at www.thieme.com on the product description page.

Some of the product names, patents, and registered designs referred to in this book are in fact registered trademarks or proprietary names even though specific reference to this fact is not always made in the text. Therefore, the appearance of a name without designation as proprietary is not to be construed as a representation by the publisher that it is in the public domain. The knowledge base for medicine is always changing and expanding, especially regarding new methods for diagnosing diseases and proposed therapies or treatment regimens for those diseases. The author and publisher of this book have used reliable resources to provide the information in this book; however, given both the possibility for human error and the changing nature of medicine, neither the author nor the publisher warrants that the material contained in this book is completely accurate or complete in coverage and they disclaim all responsibility for any errors or omissions. Users of this book are encouraged to independently confirm any information contained herein believed to be in error. Although the contents of this book provide example patient vignettes and, through the explanations for the questions, offer diagnoses for medical conditions, the reader should not use the information contained herein for self-diagnosis, and should always seek the opinion of a health care provider if they suspect themselves to have an illness.

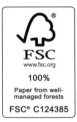

To Swapna and Parimal, my parents
for everything that made me who I am today

To Mimi, my wife
for her unconditional love and support

To Ryan, my son
for understanding my long absences at his age of less than three years

Contents

Preface

Histology and Embryology are two pillars for Anatomical Sciences. This book presents a collection of multiple choice questions that test histological and embryological concepts that are integrated across disciplines to the desired levels of competencies, consistent with testing standards of the Unites States Medical Licensing Examination Step 1.

Most of these clinically oriented questions are presented in a patient-centered vignette style that is used by the National Board of Medical Examiners (NBME). These questions link various basic science concepts and should be helpful for the student to synthesize information that might be obtained from a wide range of disciplines. The questions should also help the student to understand the direct relevance of a basic science concept in clinical practice.

All questions belong to type A, which means there is one best answer for each. Each question is provided with a difficulty level of easy, moderate, or hard. While "easy" questions require, for the most part, simple recall of information, harder questions require analysis and application of information. A brief explanation follows each question, indicating why the author-indicated correct answer outmatches the distractors.

The book is organized into four sections. The first section tests application of knowledge related to cell biology. The second section encompasses analysis of the microstructure of basic tissue and body systems. The third section highlights concepts from general embryology that include placentation and development of fetal membranes, and development of major body systems. The final section presents miscellaneous questions that are intended for practice tests.

High quality images have been incorporated throughout the text. These should add to integration, challenge the ability to analyze and interpret, and meet appropriate standards.

The book is also available on Thieme's online platform. Searchable tags (symptoms, organs, structures, etc.) have been provided with each question for ease of navigation.

Finally, this book is not a substitute for textbooks. Neither is it intended to be used as the primary resource for the subjects. As with any other question bank, use of this book should follow an initial understanding of the concepts gained from reading textbooks and lecture notes. Information used in this book has been drawn from a pool of standard textbooks used in medical schools. It is highly advisable to return to the pool for concept clarification.

Manas Das, MD

Acknowledgments

I would like to express my gratitude to everyone who saw me through this book.

First, I would like to thank all my past and present students who have inspired me to write this book. I would like to extend special thanks to Jed Assam, Ethan Young, Hannah Statz, Christopher Lucido, and Ashley Schmidt, for their valuable suggestions.

I would like to thank Steve Waller, the Associate Dean of Basic Biomedical Sciences at the University of South Dakota, for being my friend, philosopher, and guide. This work would not be possible without his constant support and encouragement. I also thank him for lending me permission to use the University of South Dakota's virtual image database.

I am grateful to the Dean of Basic Biomedical Sciences at the University of South Dakota, William Mayhan, and the former Dean, Ron Lindahl, for their support.

I would like to thank my colleagues in Basic Biomedical Sciences at the University of South Dakota for their support. Special thanks go to William Percy, Kathy Eyster, and Pat Manzerra for their endless support and good wishes.

Kelsey Stevens and Denise Arrick, my colleagues and fellow Anatomists, have made writing this book easy for me. They have taken up additional responsibilities without blinking an eye, provided me with nontiring ears whenever I needed to bounce off an idea, and have served as the primary driving forces for me to meet deadlines.

I would like to thank my fellow Anatomists/Histologists/Embryologists Donald Lowrie Jr., Lisa Lee, and John Fredieu, for their valuable opinions and support.

Michael Hortsch, my friend and fellow Histologist from the University of Michigan, has been kind enough to share several images from his school's virtual image database. His support and encouragement are greatly appreciated.

Finally, this book would be a distant dream without the support of Delia DeTurris (Associate Acquisitions Editor, Thieme Publishers) and Julia Nollen (Developmental Editor, Thieme Publishers). This book is a result of countless hours of conversations, meetings, and exchanging of ideas with them. I also sincerely thank them for lending me permission to use the image database of Thieme Publishers, which accounts for a large proportion of images used in the book.

For their thoughtful and careful review of the proposal and manuscript, thanks to:

Student Reviewers:

Ryan Norman, Lincoln Memorial University

Joseph Johnson, Lincoln Memorial University–DeBusk College of Osteopathic Medicine

Ton La Jr., Baylor College of Medicine

Daniel Gomez Ramos, Ohio University Heritage College of Osteopathic Medicine

Beverly Wong, Rutgers Robert Wood Johnson Medical School

Haley Zlomke, Rutgers Robert Wood Johnson Medical School

Neil Vallabh, Northeast Ohio Medical University

Dhaarak Desai, All Saints University School of Medicine

Ashley Schmidt, Sanford School of Medicine–University of South Dakota

Ethan Young, Sanford School of Medicine–University of South Dakota

Deborah Chen, Rutgers Robert Wood Johnson Medical School

Instructor Reviewers:

Matthew Velkey, Duke University School of Medicine

Lisa Lee, University of Colorado School of Medicine

Sheila Nunn, Ross University School of Medicine

Nancy Halliday, PhD, University of Oklahoma College of Medicine

Dr. Roger A. Dashner, The Ohio State University

John Fredieu, Case Western Reserve University

Judith Litvin (Daniels), Temple Medical School

How to Use This Series

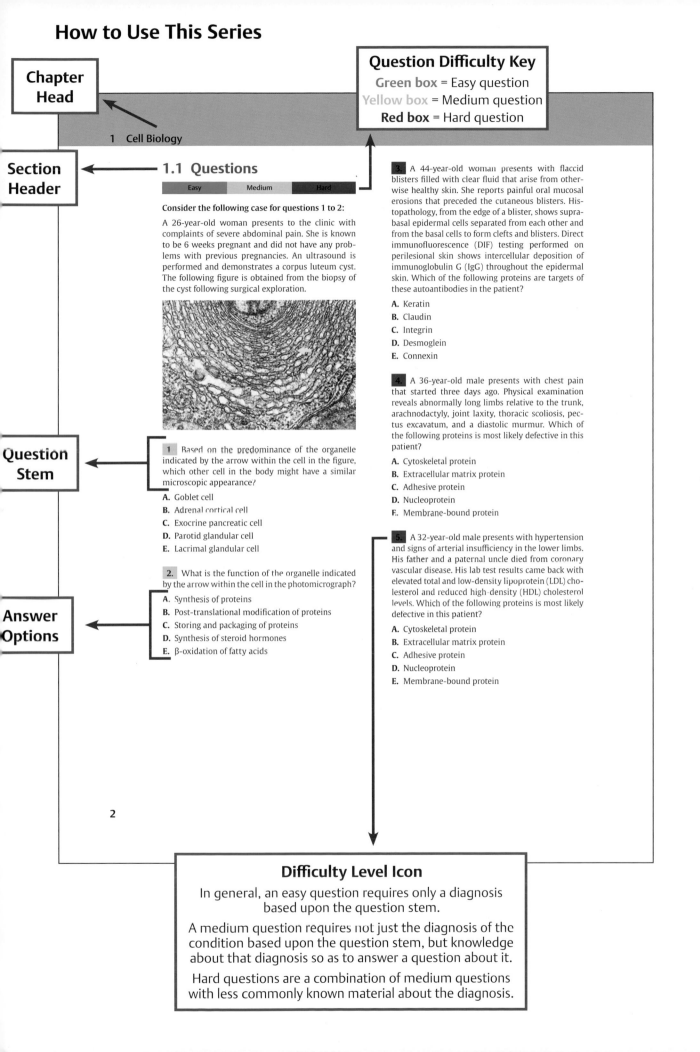

Chapter Head

Question Difficulty Key
Green box = Easy question
Yellow box = Medium question
Red box = Hard question

1 Cell Biology

Section Header

1.1 Questions

| Easy | Medium | Hard |

Consider the following case for questions 1 to 2:

A 26-year-old woman presents to the clinic with complaints of severe abdominal pain. She is known to be 6 weeks pregnant and did not have any problems with previous pregnancies. An ultrasound is performed and demonstrates a corpus luteum cyst. The following figure is obtained from the biopsy of the cyst following surgical exploration.

Question Stem

1 Based on the predominance of the organelle indicated by the arrow within the cell in the figure, which other cell in the body might have a similar microscopic appearance?

A. Goblet cell
B. Adrenal cortical cell
C. Exocrine pancreatic cell
D. Parotid glandular cell
E. Lacrimal glandular cell

Answer Options

2 What is the function of the organelle indicated by the arrow within the cell in the photomicrograph?

A. Synthesis of proteins
B. Post-translational modification of proteins
C. Storing and packaging of proteins
D. Synthesis of steroid hormones
E. β-oxidation of fatty acids

3 A 44-year-old woman presents with flaccid blisters filled with clear fluid that arise from otherwise healthy skin. She reports painful oral mucosal erosions that preceded the cutaneous blisters. Histopathology, from the edge of a blister, shows suprabasal epidermal cells separated from each other and from the basal cells to form clefts and blisters. Direct immunofluorescence (DIF) testing performed on perilesional skin shows intercellular deposition of immunoglobulin G (IgG) throughout the epidermal skin. Which of the following proteins are targets of these autoantibodies in the patient?

A. Keratin
B. Claudin
C. Integrin
D. Desmoglein
E. Connexin

4 A 36-year-old male presents with chest pain that started three days ago. Physical examination reveals abnormally long limbs relative to the trunk, arachnodactyly, joint laxity, thoracic scoliosis, pectus excavatum, and a diastolic murmur. Which of the following proteins is most likely defective in this patient?

A. Cytoskeletal protein
B. Extracellular matrix protein
C. Adhesive protein
D. Nucleoprotein
E. Membrane-bound protein

5 A 32-year-old male presents with hypertension and signs of arterial insufficiency in the lower limbs. His father and a paternal uncle died from coronary vascular disease. His lab test results came back with elevated total and low-density lipoprotein (LDL) cholesterol and reduced high-density (HDL) cholesterol levels. Which of the following proteins is most likely defective in this patient?

A. Cytoskeletal protein
B. Extracellular matrix protein
C. Adhesive protein
D. Nucleoprotein
E. Membrane-bound protein

2

Difficulty Level Icon

In general, an easy question requires only a diagnosis based upon the question stem.

A medium question requires not just the diagnosis of the condition based upon the question stem, but knowledge about that diagnosis so as to answer a question about it.

Hard questions are a combination of medium questions with less commonly known material about the diagnosis.

Chapter Head

Question Difficulty Key
Green box = Easy question
Yellow box = Medium question
Red box = Hard question

1.2 Answers and Explanations

| Easy | Medium | Hard |

1.   Correct: Adrenal cortical cell (B)

The arrow indicates smooth or agranular endoplasmic reticulum (SER). This usually takes the form of a tightly woven network of branched tubules with no ribosomes attached [point of difference with the rough endoplasmic reticulum (RER)]. RER proliferates to SER, where the synthesis of lipid and steroid molecules occurs. Therefore, there is pronounced expansion of SER in steroid hormone–producing cells, such as the one in the figure, obtained from corpus luteum (progesterone-secreting granulosa lutein cells).

Cells of the adrenal cortex have a characteristic steroid-synthesizing cell structure. These cells produce mineralocorticoids, glucocorticoids, and androgens.

Goblet cell (**A**) is a mucus-producing cell with pronounced RER and perinuclear Golgi complex, with typical apical secretory granules containing mucinogen. Exocrine pancreatic cell (**C**), parotid glandular cell (**D**), and lacrimal glandular cell (**E**) are protein (enzyme)-secreting cells characterized by abundant RER and pronounced perinuclear Golgi complex. These cells also feature apical secretory granules.

2.   Correct: Synthesis of steroid hormones (D)

Synthesis of steroid hormones is an important function of SER. It also plays major roles in lipid synthesis (including cholesterol) and metabolism of xenobiotics (drugs, carcinogens, etc.).

Synthesis of proteins (**A**) is the function of RER. Post-translational modification (**B**) and storing and packaging (**C**) of proteins are functions of the Golgi apparatus. β-oxidation of fatty acids (**E**) occurs in the mitochondria, although those with very long chains are oxidized in the peroxisomes.

3.   Correct: Desmoglein (D)

The facts that the suprabasal epidermal cells are separated from each other and from the basal cells and that there is intercellular deposition of antibodies (IgG) throughout the epidermis point toward disruption of epithelial cell junctions in the lateral domain. The patient is suffering from pemphigus vulgaris (PV), which is a mucocutaneous blistering disease that predominantly affects patients > 40 years of age. Patients with PV have IgG autoantibodies to desmogleins, transmembrane desmosomal proteins that belong to the cadherin family of calcium-dependent adhesion molecules.

Keratin (**A**) is an intermediate filament present in epithelial cells, and mutations of keratin genes cause epidermolysis bullosa simplex (EBS), a disease group characterized by intraepidermal blistering. The common EBS types are dominantly inherited and present at birth, in infancy, or at the latest during early childhood. Claudin (**B**) is a transmembrane protein that forms occluding junctions (zonula occludens) in epithelial cells. These confer tightness or leakiness and help establish functional domains (apical versus lateral) in epithelia. Integrin (**C**) is a transmembrane protein that forms hemidesmosomes, anchoring junctions that affect the basal domain of epithelial cells. A disruption in these junctions would result in a dermal-epidermal dissociation, as occurs in bullous pemphigold. Connexin (**E**) is a unit protein that forms nexus or gap junctions. These are communicating junctions involved in molecular transport between adjacent cells that need to be highly coordinated. These do not directly participate in cell anchorage.

4.   Correct: Extracellular matrix protein (B)

The patient presents with classical features of Marfan's syndrome. The defect is due to a mutation of the *FBN1* gene that codes for the protein fibrillin. Fibrillin is an essential extracellular matrix protein that forms microfibrils and plays a role in subsequent assembly of elastic fibers. Abnormalities in this protein cause distinct clinical problems involving multiple systems, of which the musculoskeletal, cardiac, and ocular predominate.

Cytoskeletal proteins (actin, etc.) (**A**), adhesive proteins (desmosomal and hemidesmosomal proteins, etc.) (**C**), nucleoproteins (histones, transcription factors, etc.) (**D**), or membrane-bound proteins (ion channels, receptors, etc.) (**E**) are not involved in the pathophysiology of Marfan's syndrome.

5.   Correct: Membrane-bound protein (E)

Familial hypercholesterolemia (FH) is an autosomal dominant disorder that causes severe elevations in total and LDL cholesterol, with decreased HDL. It is associated with a high risk for premature coronary artery disease. It is a disorder of absent or defective LDL receptors, the gene for which is located on the short arm of chromosome 19. The LDL receptor (LDLR) gene family consists of cell surface proteins involved in receptor-mediated endocytosis of specific ligands. LDL is normally bound at the cell membrane and taken into the cell, ending up in lysosomes, where the protein is degraded and the cholesterol is made available for repression of microsomal enzyme HMG CoA reductase, the rate-limiting step in cholesterol synthesis.

Cytoskeletal proteins (actin, etc.) (**A**), extracellular matrix proteins (collagen, elastin, etc.) (**B**), adhesive proteins (desmosomal and hemidesmosomal proteins, etc.) (**C**), or nucleoproteins (histones, transcription factors, etc.) (**D**) are not involved in the pathophysiology of FH.

Indicates Question Difficulty

Correct Answer

Correct Answer Explanation

Incorrect Answer Explanation

6

Chapter 1
Cell Biology

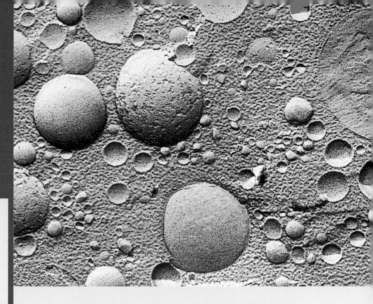

LEARNING OBJECTIVES

▶ Describe the organization of smooth endoplasmic reticulum. Critique its ultrastructure in histologic sections. Analyze its role in steroid synthesis, drug metabolism, and detoxification.

▶ Describe the organization of desmosomes. Critique their ultrastructure in histologic sections. Analyze their role in cell anchorage.

▶ Describe the etiopathogenesis of Marfan's syndrome. Correlate this with its clinical features.

▶ Classify membrane-associated proteins. Evaluate their physiologic roles.

▶ Describe the etiopathogenesis of familial hypercholesterolemia. Correlate this with its clinical features.

▶ Define the role of molecular motors in axonal transport.

▶ Describe the organization of ribosomes. Critique their ultrastructure in histologic sections. Analyze their role in protein synthesis.

▶ Describe the etiopathogenesis of hereditary spherocytosis. Correlate this with its clinical features.

▶ Describe the organization of cilia. Critique their ultrastructure in histologic sections. Analyze their role in mucociliary clearance.

▶ Describe the organization of a zonula adherens. Critique its ultrastructure in histologic sections. Analyze its role in cell anchorage during embryogenesis.

▶ Describe the organization of peroxisomes. Critique their ultrastructure in histologic sections. Analyze their role in oxidation of very-long-chain fatty acids.

▶ Describe the organization of microvilli. Critique their ultrastructure in histologic sections. Analyze their role in absorption of luminal content.

▶ Describe the organization of the epithelial basement membrane zone. Critique its ultrastructure in histologic sections. Analyze its role in mediating cellular interaction with the extracellular matrix.

▶ Describe the organization of rough endoplasmic reticulum. Critique its ultrastructure in histologic sections. Analyze its role in protein synthesis.

▶ Describe the organization of intermediate filaments. Critique their ultrastructure in histologic sections. Analyze their role in mechanical support for the cell.

▶ Describe the organization of the Golgi apparatus. Critique its ultrastructure in histologic sections. Analyze its role in post-translational modification.

▶ Describe the organization of hemidesmosomes. Critique their ultrastructure in histologic sections. Analyze their role in anchoring the cell to the extracellular matrix.

▶ Describe the etiopathogenesis of Kartagener's syndrome. Correlate this with its clinical features.

1.1 Questions

Easy | Medium | Hard

Consider the following case for questions 1 to 2:

A 26-year-old woman presents to the clinic with complaints of severe abdominal pain. She is known to be 6 weeks pregnant and did not have any problems with previous pregnancies. An ultrasound is performed and demonstrates a corpus luteum cyst. The following figure is obtained from the biopsy of the cyst following surgical exploration.

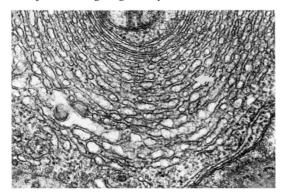

1. Based on the predominance of the organelle indicated by the arrow within the cell in the figure, which other cell in the body might have a similar microscopic appearance?

A. Goblet cell

B. Adrenal cortical cell

C. Exocrine pancreatic cell

D. Parotid glandular cell

E. Lacrimal glandular cell

2. What is the function of the organelle indicated by the arrow within the cell in the photomicrograph?

A. Synthesis of proteins

B. Post-translational modification of proteins

C. Storing and packaging of proteins

D. Synthesis of steroid hormones

E. β-oxidation of fatty acids

3. A 44-year-old woman presents with flaccid blisters filled with clear fluid that arise from otherwise healthy skin. She reports painful oral mucosal erosions that preceded the cutaneous blisters. Histopathology, from the edge of a blister, shows suprabasal epidermal cells separated from each other and from the basal cells to form clefts and blisters. Direct immunofluorescence (DIF) testing performed on perilesional skin shows intercellular deposition of immunoglobulin G (IgG) throughout the epidermal skin. Which of the following proteins are targets of these autoantibodies in the patient?

A. Keratin

B. Claudin

C. Integrin

D. Desmoglein

E. Connexin

4. A 36-year-old male presents with chest pain that started three days ago. Physical examination reveals abnormally long limbs relative to the trunk, arachnodactyly, joint laxity, thoracic scoliosis, pectus excavatum, and a diastolic murmur. Which of the following proteins is most likely defective in this patient?

A. Cytoskeletal protein

B. Extracellular matrix protein

C. Adhesive protein

D. Nucleoprotein

E. Membrane-bound protein

5. A 32-year-old male presents with hypertension and signs of arterial insufficiency in the lower limbs. His father and a paternal uncle died from coronary vascular disease. His lab test results came back with elevated total and low-density lipoprotein (LDL) cholesterol and reduced high-density (HDL) cholesterol levels. Which of the following proteins is most likely defective in this patient?

A. Cytoskeletal protein

B. Extracellular matrix protein

C. Adhesive protein

D. Nucleoprotein

E. Membrane-bound protein

6. A 56-year-old man presents with leg spasticity and gradually develops clinical signs suggestive of amyotrophic lateral sclerosis, which is supported by neurophysiologic and radiologic findings. Defective anterograde axonal transport of mitochondria is suggested as the possible pathologic mechanism, and impaired transport is confirmed by perikaryal aggregations of neurofilament and other proteins. Mutation in the gene encoding which of the following proteins is the most probable cause of his symptoms?

A. Actin

B. Dynein

C. Kinesin

D. Connexin

E. Nexin

7. A 16-year-old girl presents with status epilepticus and is treated aggressively with phenobarbital. The drug is known to be metabolized by the cytochrome p450 electron transfer chain within the hepatocytes. Which of the following would exhibit an expansion of its surface area in response to the drug?

A. Peroxisomes

B. Lysosomes

C. Rough endoplasmic reticulum

D. Smooth endoplasmic reticulum

E. Mitochondria

8. A 6-year-old girl presents with mild pallor, intermittent jaundice, and splenomegaly. Her lab test results came back with moderate anemia, reticulocytosis, hyperbilirubinemia, and spherocytes in the peripheral blood smear. An abnormal osmotic fragility test confirms the diagnosis. Which of the following cellular organelles might be malfunctioning in her, given the deficient synthesis of the protein most commonly associated with her disease?

A. Free (non-membrane-bound) ribosomes

B. Membrane-bound ribosomes

C. Peroxisomes

D. Lysosomes

E. Mitochondria

9. Which of the following would be a presenting symptom in an infant born with dysfunction of the structures in the accompanying photomicrograph?

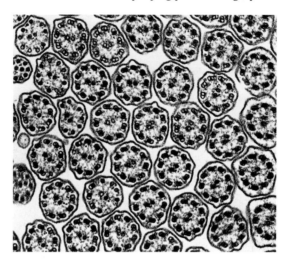

A. Peptic ulcer

B. Intestinal malabsorption

C. Jaundice

D. Recurrent respiratory infection

E. Hearing impairment

10. A 2-day-old neonate presents with gradually worsening ventilation defects since birth. An asymmetric branching pattern of his lower respiratory tract was observed, and was assumed to have occurred due to defective morphogenesis of epithelial tubes during development. Which of the following proteins might have been defective in him?

A. Claudin

B. Occludin

C. Desmoglein

D. Desmocollin

E. E-cadherin

11. A male neonate presents with profound hypotonia, poor feeding, and frequent seizures. He is noted to have a large anterior fontanelle, large forehead, and broad nasal bridge. A physical examination reveals hepatomegaly. Laboratory studies reveal hyperbilirubinemia with a mild elevation in liver transaminases, and elevated levels of very-long-chain fatty acids in the blood. Neuroimaging reveals ventriculomegaly, microgyria, and diffuse brain atrophy. Which of the following cellular organelles is dysfunctional in the newborn?

A. Mitochondria

B. Ribosomes

C. Lysosomes

D. Peroxisomes

E. Rough endoplasmic reticulum

12. A 72-hour-old male neonate presents with intractable watery diarrhea. Biopsy samples from his small intestine reveal severe villous atrophy with crypt hypoplasia, and inclusions containing microvilli within the apical cytoplasm of the enterocyte. The surface microvilli are short, scanty, and disorganized. Which of the following proteins might be responsible for his symptoms?

A. Tubulin

B. Myosin

C. Nexin

D. Desmin

E. Vimentin

13. A female neonate was born with large areas of skin damage and erosion and was admitted to the hospital several hours after birth. She eventually developed multiple bullae followed by skin peeling and erosion, mostly in areas of the body subject to friction. Bacterial cultures obtained from the skin lesions were negative. Electron micrograph of the histopathology specimen obtained from the lesions shows disruption of the dermoepidermal basement membrane zone. Immunomapping studies with antibodies to a hemidesmosomal protein and an antibody to a lamina densa protein reveal both localizing at the roof of the blister. Which of the following proteins is most likely defective or absent in her case?

A. Keratin 5

B. Integrin β4

C. Laminin 5

D. Collagen type XVII

E. Collagen type VII

14. A 56-year-old man presents with sharp, shooting pain and vesicular eruptions confined to his chest and back. The eruptions are in the form of grouped vesicles developing on an erythematous base. Both the pain and the eruptions follow a dermatomal pattern and do not cross midline. He is febrile and reports both the fever and the pain started 3 days prior to the cutaneous manifestations. Which of the following molecular motors is responsible for moving the responsible organism to the site of his skin eruptions?

A. Myelin

B. Dynein

C. Kinesin

D. Connexin

E. Desmin

Consider the following case for questions 15 to 16:

A 56-year-old man presents with gradual onset of mid-epigastric pain and significant weight loss. A physical examination reveals moderate jaundice and skin excoriations from unrelenting pruritus. Imaging studies confirm carcinoma affecting the head of the pancreas, and an endoscopic ultrasound-guided fine-needle aspiration is performed. The figure below was obtained from an exocrine pancreatic cell.

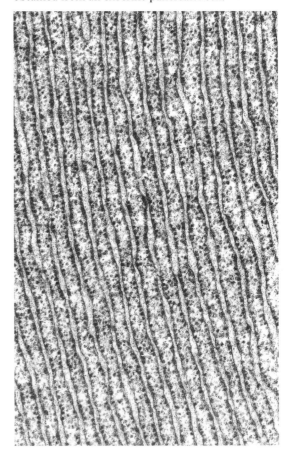

15. Based on the predominance of the organelle within the cell, which other cell in the body might have a similar microscopic appearance?

A. Corpus luteum

B. Adrenal cortical cell

C. Interstitial cell in testis

D. Interstitial cell in ovary

E. Parotid glandular cell

16. What is the function of the predominant organelle within the cell?

A. Synthesis of proteins

B. Post-translational modification of proteins

C. Storing and packaging of proteins

D. Synthesis of steroid hormones

E. β-oxidation of fatty acids

17. An undifferentiated tumor mass obtained from the skin of a 6-month-old infant revealed desmin as the intermediate filament. Which of the following cells is most likely the source of the tumor tissue?

A. Keratinocytes

B. Fibroblasts

C. Smooth muscles

D. Neurons

E. Schwann cells

18. A newborn presents with coarse facial features, hip dislocation, and hepatomegaly. Cultured fibroblasts from the neonate show reduced activities of lysosomal enzymes. The serum levels of these enzymes, however, are markedly elevated. Which of the following cell organelles might be the site of defect in the neonate?

A. Lysosome

B. Golgi apparatus

C. Rough endoplasmic reticulum

D. Smooth endoplasmic reticulum

E. Mitochondria

19. A 24-year-old woman presents with generalized tense blisters, which are particularly widespread in the axilla, the groin, and the inframammary region. There is no involvement of the oral mucosa. Histopathology, from the edge of a blister, shows subepidermal blisters. The inflammatory infiltrate is typically polymorphous, with an eosinophil predominance. Direct immunofluorescence (DIF) tests demonstrate immunoglobulin G (IgG) deposition in a linear band at the dermal-epidermal junction. Which of the following proteins are targets of these autoantibodies in the patient?

A. Keratin

B. Claudin

C. Integrin

D. Desmoglein

E. Connexin

20. A 6-day-old boy presents with a chronic wet cough with unexplained respiratory distress. His heart sounds are better heard in the right side of the chest. A cross section of a biopsied structure obtained from his respiratory tract is shown in image (**b**), and (**a**) demonstrates the same from a normal individual. Which of the following proteins might be deficient in the child?

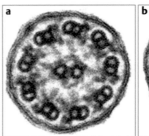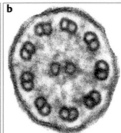

A. Actin

B. Dynein

C. Kinesin

D. Connexin

E. Nexin

1.2 Answers and Explanations

Easy	Medium	Hard

1. Correct: Adrenal cortical cell (B)

The arrow indicates smooth or agranular endoplasmic reticulum (SER). This usually takes the form of a tightly woven network of branched tubules with no ribosomes attached [point of difference with the rough endoplasmic reticulum (RER)]. RER proliferates to SER, where the synthesis of lipid and steroid molecules occurs. Therefore, there is pronounced expansion of SER in steroid hormone–producing cells, such as the one in the figure, obtained from corpus luteum (progesterone-secreting granulosa lutein cells).

Cells of the adrenal cortex have a characteristic steroid-synthesizing cell structure. These cells produce mineralocorticoids, glucocorticoids, and androgens.

Goblet cell (**A**) is a mucus-producing cell with pronounced RER and perinuclear Golgi complex, with typical apical secretory granules containing mucinogen. Exocrine pancreatic cell (**C**), parotid glandular cell (**D**), and lacrimal glandular cell (**E**) are protein (enzyme)-secreting cells characterized by abundant RER and pronounced perinuclear Golgi complex. These cells also feature apical secretory granules.

2. Correct: Synthesis of steroid hormones (D)

Synthesis of steroid hormones is an important function of SER. It also plays major roles in lipid synthesis (including cholesterol) and metabolism of xenobiotics (drugs, carcinogens, etc.).

Synthesis of proteins (**A**) is the function of RER. Post-translational modification (**B**) and storing and packaging (**C**) of proteins are functions of the Golgi apparatus. β-oxidation of fatty acids (**E**) occurs in the mitochondria, although those with very long chains are oxidized in the peroxisomes.

3. Correct: Desmoglein (D)

The facts that the suprabasal epidermal cells are separated from each other and from the basal cells and that there is intercellular deposition of antibodies (IgG) throughout the epidermis point toward disruption of epithelial cell junctions in the lateral domain. The patient is suffering from pemphigus vulgaris (PV), which is a mucocutaneous blistering disease that predominantly affects patients > 40 years of age. Patients with PV have IgG autoantibodies to desmogleins, transmembrane desmosomal proteins that belong to the cadherin family of calcium-dependent adhesion molecules.

Keratin (**A**) is an intermediate filament present in epithelial cells, and mutations of keratin genes cause epidermolysis bullosa simplex (EBS), a disease group characterized by intraepidermal blistering. The common EBS types are dominantly inherited and present at birth, in infancy, or at the latest during early childhood. Claudin (**B**) is a transmembrane protein that forms occluding junctions (zonula occludens) in epithelial cells. These confer tightness or leakiness and help establish functional domains (apical versus lateral) in epithelia. Integrin (**C**) is a transmembrane protein that forms hemidesmosomes, anchoring junctions that affect the basal domain of epithelial cells. A disruption in these junctions would result in a dermal-epidermal dissociation, as occurs in bullous pemphigold. Connexin (**E**) is a unit protein that forms nexus or gap junctions. These are communicating junctions involved in molecular transport between adjacent cells that need to be highly coordinated. These do not directly participate in cell anchorage.

4. Correct: Extracellular matrix protein (B)

The patient presents with classical features of Marfan's syndrome. The defect is due to a mutation of the *FBN1* gene that codes for the protein fibrillin. Fibrillin is an essential extracellular matrix protein that forms microfibrils and plays a role in subsequent assembly of elastic fibers. Abnormalities in this protein cause distinct clinical problems involving multiple systems, of which the musculoskeletal, cardiac, and ocular predominate.

Cytoskeletal proteins (actin, etc.) (**A**), adhesive proteins (desmosomal and hemidesmosomal proteins, etc.) (**C**), nucleoproteins (histones, transcription factors, etc.) (**D**), or membrane-bound proteins (ion channels, receptors, etc.) (**E**) are not involved in the pathophysiology of Marfan's syndrome.

5. Correct: Membrane-bound protein (E)

Familial hypercholesterolemia (FH) is an autosomal dominant disorder that causes severe elevations in total and LDL cholesterol, with decreased HDL. It is associated with a high risk for premature coronary artery disease. It is a disorder of absent or defective LDL receptors, the gene for which is located on the short arm of chromosome 19. The LDL receptor (LDLR) gene family consists of cell surface proteins involved in receptor-mediated endocytosis of specific ligands. LDL is normally bound at the cell membrane and taken into the cell, ending up in lysosomes, where the protein is degraded and the cholesterol is made available for repression of microsomal enzyme HMG CoA reductase, the rate-limiting step in cholesterol synthesis.

Cytoskeletal proteins (actin, etc.) (**A**), extracellular matrix proteins (collagen, elastin, etc.) (**B**), adhesive proteins (desmosomal and hemidesmosomal proteins, etc.) (**C**), or nucleoproteins (histones, transcription factors, etc.) (**D**) are not involved in the pathophysiology of FH.

6. Correct: Kinesin (C)

Kinesin is the molecular motor for anterograde axonal transport. This occurs from the cell body (-ve terminal) to the periphery (+ve terminal).

Actin (**A**) is a cytoskeletal protein that provides structural support for cells. Dynein (**B**) is a motor protein that moves along microtubules and is involved in retrograde axonal transport. This occurs from the periphery (+ve terminal) to the cell body (-ve terminal). Connexin (**D**) is a protein that forms gap junctions. It permits ions and small molecules to move between adjacent cells. The primary function of the nexin links (**E**) is to connect the peripheral doublet microtubules and maintain the structural integrity of the cilium.

7. Correct: Smooth endoplasmic reticulum (D)

Smooth endoplasmic reticulum plays a major role in metabolism of xenobiotics (drugs, carcinogens, etc.). It also functions in synthesis of steroid hormones and lipids (including cholesterol).

Peroxisomes (**A**) are responsible for β-oxidation of very-long-chain fatty acids, the α-oxidation of phytanic acid, pipecolic acid oxidation, and early plasmalogen synthesis. Lysosomes (**B**) are involved in intracellular digestion of endogenous substances (autophagy) and phagocytosed substances (heterophagy). Rough endoplasmic reticulum (**C**) is involved in protein synthesis. Mitochondria (**E**) are responsible for β-oxidation of fatty acids with smaller carbon chains.

8. Correct: Free (non-membrane-bound) ribosomes (A)

The girl is suffering from hereditary spherocytosis (HS), an inherited hemolytic disorder associated with a variety of mutations that lead to defects in red blood cell (RBC) membrane skeleton, which render RBCs less deformable and vulnerable to splenic sequestration and destruction. The morphologic hallmark of HS is the microspherocyte, which is caused by the loss of RBC membrane surface area and has abnormal osmotic fragility in vitro. Spectrin deficiency is the most common defect in HS. Spectrin is a cytoskeletal protein that lies closely opposed to the internal surface of the plasma membrane. It connects to and stabilizes the membrane by interacting with ankyrin, band 4.2, and protein 4.1. Free ribosomes are responsible for synthesizing cytosolic (cytoskeletal—spectrin, in this case) proteins, peripheral membrane proteins, or some proteins destined for the nucleus, mitochondria, and peroxisomes.

Proteins synthesized on membrane-associated ribosomes (**B**) include integral transmembrane plasma membrane proteins, ER, Golgi complex, endosomal, and lysosomal proteins, and proteins to be secreted from the cell. Peroxisomes (**C**), lysosomes (**D**), and mitochondria (**E**) are not associated with protein synthesis.

9. Correct: Recurrent respiratory infection (D)

The micrograph shows cross sections of cilia. These are long, slender extensions of apical plasma membrane that contain an axonemal core, which in turn consists of 9 peripheral microtubules uniformly spaced around 2 central microtubules (9+2 arrangement). Ciliary movements propel fluid or particulate matter in one direction over the epithelial surface. Dysfunctional cilia would lead to impaired mucociliary clearance with subsequent recurrent respiratory tract infections.

Peptic ulcer (**A**) is caused by hypersecretion of HCl by gastric parietal cells and is not related to ciliary motility. Intestinal malabsorption (**B**) might be related to dysfunctional microvilli. The core of a microvillus comprises actin microfilaments and not microtubules in 9+2 arrangement. Jaundice (**C**) is due to abnormal bilirubin production, metabolism, or excretion, and is not related to ciliary dysfunction. Hearing impairment (**E**) could be due to dysfunctional stereocilia. Stereocilia, like microvilli, comprises a core of actin microfilaments and not microtubules in a 9+2 arrangement.

10. Correct: E-cadherin (E)

Zonula adherens are anchoring junctions that play a pivotal role in epithelial morphogenesis during development. Transmembrane proteins (E-cadherins) are the major cohesive factors for epithelial cell groups when they fold into different shapes (tubes, etc.) during embryogenesis.

Claudin (**A**) and occludin (**B**) are transmembrane proteins that form occluding junctions (zonula occludens) in epithelial cells. These confer tightness or leakiness and help establish functional domains (apical versus lateral) in epithelia. Desmoglein (**C**) and desmocollin (**D**) are cadherins (transmembrane proteins) that form macula adherens (desmosomes). These also are anchoring junctions that form spot welds and provide high tensile strength to epithelia.

11. Correct: Peroxisomes (D)

β-oxidation of very-long-chain fatty acids (VLCFA) occurs in peroxisomes.

The clinical scenario is that of Zellweger's syndrome (ZS), an autosomal recessive inherited disorder of the peroxisome, an intracellular organelle composed of a single membrane containing a matrix embedded with enzymes for metabolism of very-long-chain fatty acids. The proper assembly of a peroxisome requires a unique set of proteins termed "peroxin." A mutation in the PEX gene coding for peroxin yields peroxisomes that fail to perform their metabolic duties, including the β-oxidation of fatty acids with a chain length of more than 22 carbons, the α-oxidation of phytanic acid, pipecolic acid oxidation, and early plasmalogen synthesis. The intracellular accumulation of VLCFA damages developing organs (e.g., liver, bone, kidneys) and is especially deleterious to the organizing brain.

Mitochondria (**A**) are responsible for β-oxidation of fatty acids with smaller carbon chains. Ribosomes (**B**) and rough endoplasmic reticulum (**E**) are involved in protein synthesis. Lysosomes (**C**) are involved in intracellular digestion of endogenous substances (autophagy) and phagocytosed substances (heterophagy).

12. Correct: Myosin (B)

The clinical features and biopsy findings are consistent with microvillus inclusion disease (also referred to as congenital microvillus atrophy). Diarrhea starts in the first few hours of life and is immediately life threatening. The pathogenesis of the disease is associated with mutations in the *MYO5B* gene, encoding the actin-based motor protein myosin Vb. These mutations lead to severe disruption of the microvillar cytoskeleton caused by abnormal binding of myosin to actin (remember actin and myosin are microfilaments that form the core of microvilli).

Tubulin (**A**) is a protein that forms microtubules and not microvilli. Nexin (**C**), found in cilia, interconnects the outer doublet microtubules and prevents their relative movements with respect to each other during ciliary motion. Desmin (**D**) is an intermediate filament found in skeletal, cardiac, and smooth muscle cells. Vimentin (**E**) is an intermediate filament found in cells of mesenchymal origin (fibroblasts, etc.).

13. Correct: Collagen type VII (E)

The key to answering this question is the findings that both antibodies to a hemidesmosomal protein and to a lamina densa protein localizes at the roof of the blister. This can be best explained with the figure below.

Immunomapping with antibodies to a hemidesmosomal protein and an antibody to a lamina densa protein can distinguish epidermolysis bullosa simplex (EBS), junctional epidermolysis bullosa (JEB), and dystrophic epidermolysis bullosa (DEB). As is evident from the figure:

- In case of mutations in genes coding for keratin 5 (**A**), as in EBS, both antibodies localize to the floor of the blister.
- In case of mutations in genes coding for β4 integrin (**B**), laminin 5 (**C**), collagen XVII (**D**), as in JEB antibody to BP230 localizes to the roof of the blister, while antibody to type IV collagen localizes to the floor.
- In case of mutations in genes coding for collagen type VII (**E**) as in DEB, both antibodies localize to the roof of the blister.

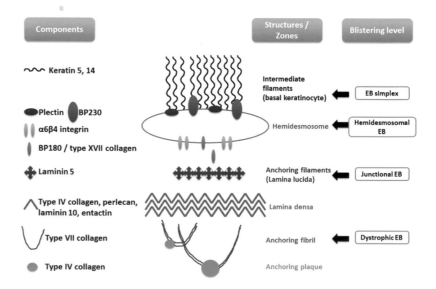

14. Correct: Kinesin (C)

The patient is suffering from herpes zoster (shingles), the diagnosis of which is largely based on history and physical findings. Reactivation of varicella-zoster virus (VZV) that has remained dormant within dorsal root ganglia, often for decades after the patient's initial exposure to the virus in the form of varicella (chickenpox), results in herpes zoster. The reactivated virus is carried from the dorsal root ganglia (neuronal cell bodies) toward the skin via the peripheral neuronal processes (axons). This is an example of an anterograde axonal transport mediated by kinesin. The prodromal symptoms (pain and fever) prior to onset of cutaneous findings are believed to represent the spread of varicella-zoster virus (VZV) particles along sensory nerves (axons).

Myelin (**A**) insulates the axons and allows fast and efficient transmission of neural impulses. Dynein (**B**) is a molecular motor responsible for retrograde axonal transport, i.e., transport of substances from the periphery toward the nerve cell body. After primary infection, the virus migrates along sensory nerve fibers to the satellite cells of dorsal root ganglia where it becomes dormant. It is interesting to note that this takes place by retrograde axonal transport mediated by dynein. Connexin (**D**) is a protein that forms gap junctions. It permits ions and small molecules to move between adjacent cells. Desmin (**E**) is an intermediate filament found in skeletal, cardiac, and smooth muscle cells.

15. Correct: Parotid glandular cell (E)

The predominant organelle is rough endoplasmic reticulum (RER). The RER double membranes have granules (membrane-bound ribosomes) attached to their outer surfaces. Dependent on cell specialization and activity, RER may occur in different forms, such as stacks or tubules. Elaborate systems of RER membranes are found predominantly in cells that biosynthesize proteins.

Cells from the parotid gland (exclusively serous cells) have a characteristic protein (enzyme) synthesizing cell structure. These are characterized by abundant RER and pronounced perinuclear Golgi complex. These cells also feature apical secretory granules.

Corpus luteum (**A**), adrenal cortical cell (**B**), interstitial cells in testis (**C**) and ovary (**D**) are steroid hormone–secreting cells characterized by abundant smooth endoplasmic reticulum (SER). These cells also feature several cytoplasmic lipid droplets and abundant mitochondria with tubular cristae.

16. Correct: Synthesis of proteins (A)

Synthesis of proteins is an important function of the RER. Post-translational modification (**B**) and storing and packaging (**C**) of proteins are functions of the Golgi apparatus. Synthesis of steroid hormones (**D**) is a function of smooth endoplasmic reticulum (SER). β-oxidation of fatty acids (**E**) occurs in the mitochondria, although those with very long chains are oxidized in the peroxisomes.

17. Correct: Smooth muscles (C)

Desmin is a muscle-specific protein and a key subunit of the intermediate filament in cardiac, skeletal, and smooth muscles. These filaments are mainly located at the periphery of the Z-disk of striated muscles and at the dense bodies of smooth muscle cells. They play a critical role in the maintenance of structural and mechanical integrity of the contractile apparatus in muscle tissue.

Keratin, the hallmark protein in epithelial cells, is expressed in keratinocytes (**A**). Fibroblasts (**B**) and other mesenchyme-derived cells exhibit vimentin as the intermediate filament. Neurons (**D**) express neurofilament as the major intermediate filament.

The intermediate filament glial fibrillary acidic protein (GFAP) is the marker for astrocytes and Schwann cells (**E**). The intermediate filament subunit of undifferentiated Schwann cells, however, is vimentin.

18. Correct: Golgi apparatus (B)

The neonate is most likely suffering from I-cell disease. It is an autosomal-recessive disorder caused by a deficiency of the enzyme UDP-N-acetylglucosamine-1-phosphotransferase. Deficiency of this phosphotransferase prevents the addition of the mannose-6-phosphate recognition marker to lysosomal enzymes, which occurs in the Golgi apparatus. Lysosomal enzymes, therefore, cannot be endocytosed into the lysosome for normal processing and use. The patients' plasma contains very high activities of lysosomal enzymes, suggesting that the enzymes are synthesized but fail to reach their proper intracellular destination and are instead secreted. Developmental delay is severe and is often the presenting symptom. Coarse facial features, severe skeletal dysplasia, corneal clouding, and hepatomegaly are commonly found at birth. Lysosomes (**A**) fail to receive the enzymes without the marker, and are therefore not the site of the underlying defect. Rough endoplasmic reticulum (**C**) is where the enzyme is synthesized, but not where the marker is attached. Mitochondria (**E**) provide energy for the process, while smooth endoplasmic reticulum (**D**) is not directly associated with the defect.

19. Correct: Integrin (C)

The facts that the blisters are subepidermal and that intercellular deposition of antibodies (IgG) is at the dermal-epidermal junction point toward disruption of epithelial cell junctions in the basal domain. From the list provided, integrin is the only transmembrane protein that forms hemidesmosomes, which are anchor-

9

ing junctions that affect the basal domain of epithelial cells. Disruptions in these junctions result in dermal-epidermal dissociation. The clinical scenario is that of bullous pemphigoid, a chronic, inflammatory, subepidermal, blistering disease.

Keratin (**A**) is an intermediate filament present in epithelial cells. Antibodies directed against it will not selectively deposit in the dermoepidermal junction. Claudin (**B**) is a transmembrane protein that forms occluding junctions (zonula occludens) in epithelial cells. These junctions affect the most apical part of the lateral domain and confer tightness or leakiness in epithelia. Desmoglein (**D**) is a transmembrane protein that forms desmosomes, which are anchoring junctions that affect the lateral domain of epithelial cells. A disruption in these junctions would result in separation of suprabasal cells from each other and from the basal epidermal cells. Connexin (**E**) is a unit protein that forms nexus or gap junctions. These are communicating junctions that affect lateral domains and are involved in molecular transport between adjacent cells that need to be highly coordinated.

20. Correct: Dynein (B)

The child is suffering from Kartagener's syndrome. This is an autosomal recessive disorder that comprises a characteristic triad of chronic sinusitis, bronchiectasis, and situs inversus. The electron micrograph in panel B clearly demonstrates absence of outer dynein arms. These arms are seats of dynein ATPase activity, which split ATP to provide energy for ciliary movement. Absence of these arms renders the patient with primary ciliary dyskinesia and the resultant respiratory infections. Also, note that ciliary movement is essential during embryogenesis to establish right-left asymmetry of internal organs. Hence, situs inversus is observed in patients with dysfunctional cilia.

Actin (**A**) is a cytoskeletal protein which forms the core of microvilli but not cilia. Kinesin (**C**) is a motor protein that moves along microtubules and is involved in ciliogenesis. It is not involved in Kartagener's syndrome. Connexin (**D**) is a protein that forms gap junctions. It permits ions and small molecules to move between adjacent cells. The primary function of the nexin links (**E**) is to maintain the structural integrity of the cilium.

The following labeled illustration is of a cross-section of the cilium.

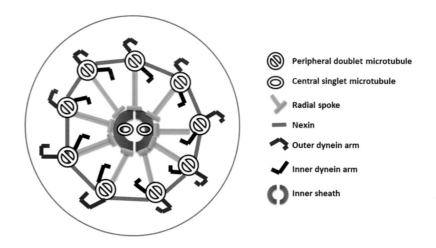

Peripheral doublet microtubule

Central singlet microtubule

Radial spoke

Nexin

Outer dynein arm

Inner dynein arm

Inner sheath

Chapter 2

Epithelial Tissue Histology

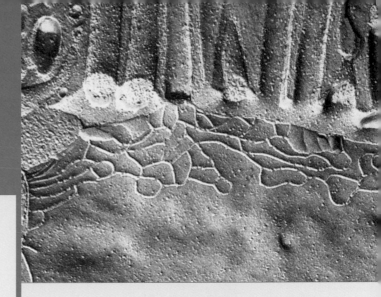

LEARNING OBJECTIVES

▶ Describe the organization of microvilli. Critique their ultrastructure in histologic sections. Analyze their role in absorption of luminal content.

▶ Describe histological characteristics of steroid-secreting cells. Critique their ultrastructure in histologic sections. Predict their distribution in the human body.

▶ Describe the organization of gap junctions. Critique their ultrastructure in histologic sections. Analyze their role in intercellular communication.

▶ Classify epithelial tissues according to structure. Analyze their distribution according to their functions.

▶ Describe the etiopathogenesis of acute appendicitis. Correlate this with its clinical features.

▶ Describe the organization of cilia. Critique their ultrastructure in histologic sections. Analyze their role in mucociliary clearance.

▶ Describe the organization of desmosomes. Critique their ultrastructure in histologic sections. Analyze their role in cell anchorage.

▶ Describe the organization of occluding junctions Critique their ultrastructure in histological sections. Analyze their role in regulating paracellular transport.

▶ Describe the etiopathogenesis of ruptured ectopic pregnancy. Correlate this with its clinical features.

▶ Describe the organization of epithelial basement membrane zone. Critique its ultrastructure in histologic sections. Analyze its role in mediating cellular interaction with extracellular matrix.

▶ Describe the etiopathogenesis of Kartagener's syndrome. Correlate this with its clinical features.

▶ Describe the etiopathogenesis of pemphigus vulgaris. Correlate this with its clinical features.

▶ Describe the organization of stereocilia. Critique their ultrastructure in histologic sections. Analyze their role in absorption.

2.1 Questions

Easy	Medium	Hard

1. A tissue biopsy was obtained from a 36-year-old man presenting with multiple organ failure. Which of the following statements regarding the indicated structures in the figure is true?

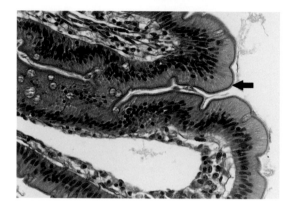

A. These are anchored to the cell by a basal body.

B. These contain a core of microtubules.

C. These facilitate absorption.

D. These are localized on the basal surface of epithelial cells.

E. These facilitate adhesion of the cell with the extracellular matrix.

2. A 26-year-old man presents with an abscess in a primary retroperitoneal organ related to the left posterior abdominal wall. At surgery, clamping the left renal artery partially, but not completely, interrupted blood flow to the organ. Also, veins from the inflamed organ were found to drain in the left renal vein. Cortical tissue from the organ (which was surgically removed and biopsied) was examined under the electron microscope. An abundance of which of the following organelles is most likely in the cytoplasm of the cells?

A. Rough endoplasmic reticulum

B. Smooth endoplasmic reticulum

C. Secretory vesicles

D. Lysosomes

E. Golgi bodies

3. You decide to review electron micrographs of intercellular junctions before histology finals. Which of the following statements is correct about the type of junction indicated by key 3 in the figure?

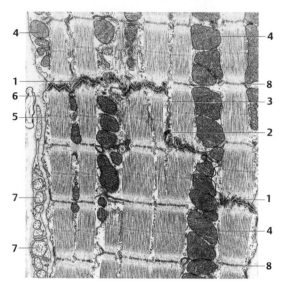

A. It extends as a zone around the apical perimeter of adjacent cells.

B. It possesses dense plaques that are anchored to intermediate filaments.

C. It permits the passage of ions from one cell to another.

D. It requires calcium to bind adjacent cells.

E. It mediates adhesion of cells to an underlying basal lamina.

4. A 25-year-old female reported to the ER with severe pain localized to the right lower abdominal quadrant. The pain started off in the periumbilical area 3 days before and was accompanied by severe nausea. Physical examination reveals maximum tenderness at a point that is a third of the distance from the right anterior superior iliac spine to the umbilicus. Which of the following is true for the inflamed organ in her?

A. It is lined by nonkeratinized stratified squamous epithelium.

B. It is lined by keratinized stratified squamous epithelium.

C. It is lined by simple cuboidal epithelium.

D. It is lined by simple squamous epithelium.

E. It is lined by simple columnar epithelium.

5. Irritation due to cigarette smoke results in squamous metaplasia within the respiratory tract. Why would it have negative consequences?

A. Ineffective clearance of mucus and particles

B. Ineffective secretion of mucus

C. Ineffective protection against frictional damage of mucosa

D. A and B

E. A, B, and C

Consider the following case for questions 6 to 8:

A male child presents with refractory diarrhea. An intestinal biopsy (see figure) was ordered and examined under the electron microscope to confirm the structural detail.

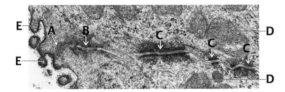

6. What would be the primary function for structure C?

A. Forms spot welds between adjacent cells

B. Interacts with actin in the apical cytoplasm of cells

C. Facilitates communication between adjacent cells by ion exchange

D. Seals membranes between adjacent cells

E. Extends as a zone around the apical perimeter of adjacent cells

7. Which of the following structures might be affected if an antibody directed against claudin were applied?

A. A

B. B

C. C

D. D

E. E

8. Which of the following would be a possible consequence if the antibody referred to in question 7 were actually applied?

A. Cardiac arrhythmia

B. Defective absorption by the enterocytes

C. Increased leakiness of enterocytes

D. Defective morphogenesis of epithelial cells

E. Vesicular skin eruptions affecting the oral mucosa

9. A 23-year-old female presents with vaginal bleeding, lower abdominal pain, and severe hypotension. She has a previous history of pelvic inflammatory disease and admits to having unprotected sexual intercourse during the past 2 months. Which of the following is true of the organ that, most probably, has ruptured in her?

A. It is lined by pseudostratified columnar epithelium with goblet cells.

B. It is lined by ciliated pseudostratified columnar epithelium.

C. It is lined by ciliated simple columnar epithelium.

D. It is lined by simple columnar epithelium with numerous microvilli.

E. It is lined by simple squamous epithelium.

10. A neonate rapidly developed extensive blistering of the skin shortly after birth. A physical examination revealed painful erosions of the oral mucosa. Immunomapping studies with antibodies to a hemidesmosomal antigen (BP230) and an antibody to a lamina densa protein (collagen type IV) was done. BP230 localized to the roof, while type IV collagen localized to the floor of the blister. In which of the following zones would you expect to see the disruption?

A. Apical zone, within the epithelial cell

B. Lateral zone, within the epithelial cell

C. Basal zone, within the epithelial cell

D. Lamina lucida, basal lamina

E. Reticular lamina, extracellular matrix

11. A 58-year-old man presents with abdominal pain, constipation, and nausea of 3 days' duration. On examination, the abdomen is distended and tender with auscultation of high-pitched bowel sounds in the epigastric region. Imaging reveals a growth affecting the head of the pancreas. Which of the following is true for the compressed structure that is most likely responsible for the patient's symptoms?

A. It is lined by pseudostratified columnar epithelium with goblet cells.

B. It is lined by ciliated pseudostratified columnar epithelium.

C. It is lined by ciliated simple columnar epithelium.

D. It is lined by simple columnar epithelium with microvilli.

E. It is lined by simple squamous epithelium.

12. An 11-year-old boy presents with chronic sinusitis and bronchiectasis. He has had persistent infections and otitis media since birth. A PA radiograph shows dextrocardia. Which of the following is true for the structures defective in him?

A. These are surface specializations that affect the permeability of cells.

B. These are surface specializations that affect the apical domains of cells.

C. These are surface specializations that affect the basal domains of cells.

D. These are surface specializations that affect the lateral domains of cells.

E. These are surface specializations that affect the tensile strength of cells.

13. A 48-year-old woman presents with blisters on her trunk that have been there for 3 days. The blisters are large, turbid, and flaccid, and are located within the superficial epidermis. She reports of painful oral blisters preceding the cutaneous lesions by a week. Which of the following would be targets for autoantibodies in her serum?

A. Hemidesmosome

B. Anchoring fibrils

C. Macula adherens

D. Gap junctions

E. Lamina densa

14. A male neonate presents with a mutation of the gene encoding actin within his epithelial stem cells. Which of the following structures might be affected in him due to such mutation?

A. Microvilli

B. Cilia

C. Stereocilia

D. A and C

E. A, B, and C

15. The glomerular basement membrane repels negatively charged proteins, including albumin, and prevents their filtration (charge-selective barrier). Which of the following components, conferring negative electrostatic charge to the basal lamina, is most crucial for this role?

A. Laminin

B. Entactin

C. Type IV collagen fibers

D. Heparan sulfate

E. Type VII collagen fibers

16. During a near-peer review session, a first-year medical student is being quizzed about structure and functions of epithelial tissue and its specializations. Which of the following is a correct statement for epithelial cells?

A. Function of desmosomes is dependent on Ca^{2+} ions.

B. Epithelia are classified by the shape of the cells in the basal layer.

C. Desmin is the intermediate filament in the epithelial cells.

D. A defect in the zonula adherens might lead to a defective paracellular transport.

E. Stereocilia are absorptive structures abundant in the respiratory tract.

17. Biopsies from several organs were obtained from a 22-year-old human subject suffering from disorders of sexual differentiation. Which of the following organs might be a probable source for the figure?

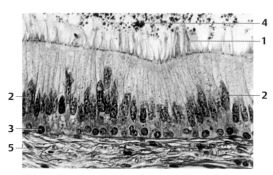

A. Trachea

B. Vagina

C. Epididymis

D. Duodenum

E. Urinary bladder

18. A cell isolated from the testis of a 26-year-old was found to contain numerous stacks of smooth endoplasmic reticulum. What additional feature is most likely to be present in the cell?

A. Numerous stacks of rough endoplasmic reticulum

B. Numerous free ribosomes

C. Numerous apical secretory vesicles

D. Numerous mitochondria with tubular cristae

E. Extensively developed Golgi apparatus

19. A female child is born with an absence of the normal structures indicated by the blue arrow in the figure. What is the primary function of such structures?

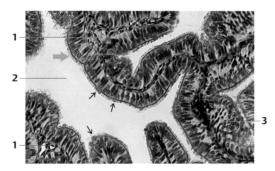

A. Increase in surface area for absorption

B. Extensive movement of substances over cell surfaces

C. Formation of anchoring junctions between adjacent cells

D. Linkage of intermediate filaments between adjacent cells

E. Linkage of intermediate filaments in the cell to the extracellular matrix

20. During a routine busy day in the laboratory, the technician forgets to label the accompanying figure. From your knowledge of histology, you understand it might have been obtained from which of the following organs/structures?

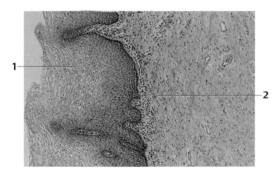

A. Epidermis

B. Trachea

C. Vagina

D. Urinary bladder

E. Lung alveoli

2.2 Answers and Explanations

Easy	Medium	Hard

1. Correct: These facilitate absorption. (C)

The indicated structures are microvilli, and the biopsy is from the small intestine. Microvilli are identified in the light micrograph by a brush-border appearance. The diagnosis is further established by simple columnar lining cells of intestinal epithelium, cellular lamina propria in the indicated villus, and a large lacteal in the adjacent villus.

Cilia contain a core of microtubules (**B**) and are anchored to apical cytoplasm by basal bodies (**A**). Microvilli are apical modifications (**D**) of the epithelial cell, while integrins facilitate adhesion of the cell with extracellular matrix (**E**).

2. Correct: Smooth endoplasmic reticulum (B)

The patient had an inflamed left adrenal gland. This can be deduced from its primary retroperitoneal location, multiple source of arterial blood (abdominal aorta, inferior phrenic artery, and renal artery), and its veins draining into the left renal vein. The adrenal cortex is composed of three distinct layers of endocrine cells that produce critical steroid hormones. Steroid-secreting cells are characterized by the presence of acidophilic cytoplasm that contains abundant smooth endoplasmic reticulum, excess mitochondria with tubular cristae, and lipid droplets.

An abundance of rough endoplasmic reticulum (**A**), secretory vesicles (**C**), and Golgi bodies (**E**) are usually found in protein-secreting cells. An abundance of lysosomes (**D**) is found within cells active in intracellular digestion (e.g., macrophages).

3. Correct: It permits the passage of ions from one cell to another. (C)

The electron micrograph shows heart muscle cells, and key 3 indicates gap junctions. Three different types of cell contacts [fascia adherens, maculae adherentes (desmosomes), and nexus (gap junctions)] occur within the struts between the cardiac myocytes. Fascia adherens (key 1) exists as the contact plate in the transverse sectors. A desmosome (macula adherens, key 2), in this image, is present in the longitudinal sector of the struts. Nexus occur usually in the longitudinal sectors. They facilitate passage of ions and coordinate electrical coupling between cardiac muscle cells.

Zonula occludens and zonula adherens extend as zones around the apical perimeter of adjacent cells (**A**). Desmosomes and hemidesmosomes possess dense plaques that are anchored to intermediate filaments (**B**). Desmosomes utilize calcium-dependent proteins to bind adjacent cells (**D**). Hemidesmosomes mediate adhesion of cells to the underlying basal lamina and extracellular matrix (**E**).

15

4. Correct: It is lined by simple columnar epithelium. (E)

The patient is suffering from acute appendicitis, the diagnosis suspected by the clinical presentation, and confirmed by localization of maximum tenderness at McBurney's point. The vermiform appendix is lined by simple columnar epithelium. Intestinal crypts and lymphatic nodules extending through variable thickness of the mucosa are other notable features.

5. Correct: A and B (D)

In squamous metaplasia, normal pseudostratified ciliated columnar epithelia of the respiratory tract change into stratified squamous. Clearance of mucus and particles would be disrupted due to loss of cilia, while secretion of mucus is interrupted when the cells change from columnar to squamous. The only advantage of a stratified squamous epithelium over a ciliated columnar is better protection against frictional damage. Please remember this is hypothetical and not the real case for cigarette smokers.

Consider the following for questions 6 to 8:

Image key: **A**, zonula occludens; **B**, zonula adherens; **C**, macula adherens (desmosome); **D**, mitochondria; **E**, microvilli.

6. Correct: Forms spot welds between adjacent cells (A)

Desmosomes link cytokeratin filaments between adjacent cells. These occur at small discrete sites and form spot welds that provide high tensile strength.

Microvilli interact with actin (terminal web) in the apical cytoplasm (**B**). Occluding junctions seal the apical membranes of adjacent cells (**D**). These, together with zonula adherens, extend as zones around the apical perimeter of adjacent cells (**E**). Gap junctions facilitate communication by ion exchange (**C**).

7. Correct: A (A)

Claudin and occludin are transmembrane proteins that form occluding junctions (zonula occludens).

8. Correct: Increased leakiness of enterocytes (C)

Occluding junctions seal the apical membranes of adjacent cells and regulate paracellular transport. A defect in these increases epithelial permeability.

Cardiac arrhythmias (**A**) might be caused by defective communication through gap junctions. Defective absorption by enterocytes (**B**) is likely due to microvilli dysfunction. Defective morphogenesis of epithelial cells (**D**) is due to defects in anchoring junctions (zonula adherens). Vesicular skin eruptions affecting the oral mucosa (**E**) could be due to dysfunctional desmosomes (as found in pemphigus vulgaris).

9. Correct: It is lined by ciliated simple columnar epithelium. (C)

The patient, most probably, is suffering from ruptured tubal pregnancy. It should be suspected in any woman of child-bearing age who presents with abdominal pain, vaginal bleeding following a period of amenorrhea, and hypotension. Pelvic inflammatory disease is a strong risk factor for such occurrences. The uterine tubes are lined by ciliated simple columnar epithelium.

10. Correct: Lamina lucida, basal lamina (D)

The key to answering this question is the finding that antibodies to a hemidesmosomal protein localizes to the roof, while antibodies to a lamina densa protein localizes at the floor of the blister. This can be best explained with the accompanying figure.

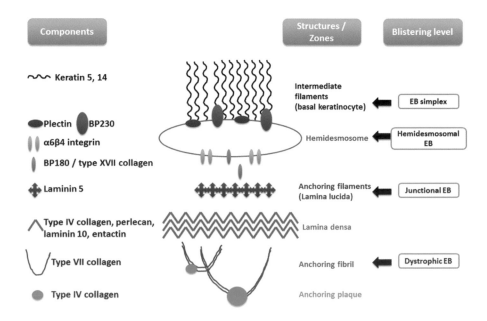

As is evident from the figure, in the case of mutations in genes coding for laminin 5 (lamina lucida of basal lamina), as in junctional epidermolysis bullosa, BP230 localizes to the roof of the blister, while type IV collagen localizes to the floor. In the case of mutations in genes coding for keratin (as in epidermolysis bullosa simplex) or any intraepithelial protein (**A–C**), both antibodies localize to the floor of the blister. In the case of mutations in genes coding for collagen type VII (reticular lamina, extracellular matrix; **E**) as in dystrophic epidermolysis bullosa, both antibodies localize to the roof of the blister.

11. Correct: It is lined by simple columnar epithelium with microvilli. (D)

The patient has clinical features suggestive of intestinal obstruction. This is characterized by intermittent, poorly localized, and crampy abdominal pain that tends to be associated with altered bowel function. Hyperperistalsis is typical proximal to the obstruction.

A growth affecting the head of the pancreas will most likely compress the second part of the duodenum, to which it is intimately related. The duodenum is lined by simple columnar epithelium with numerous microvilli.

12. Correct: These are surface specializations that affect the apical domains of cells. (B)

The child is suffering from Kartagener's syndrome. This is an autosomal recessive disorder that comprises a characteristic triad of chronic sinusitis, bronchiectasis, and situs inversus. The pathogenesis of the disease is marked by absence of dynein arms in the peripheral microtubules within the core of cilia. These arms are seats of dynein ATPase activity that split ATP to provide energy for ciliary movement. Absence of these arms renders the patient with primary ciliary dyskinesia and the resultant respiratory infections. Also, note that ciliary movement is essential during embryogenesis to establish right-left asymmetry of the internal organs. Therefore, situs inversus is observed in patients with dysfunctional cilia.

Cilia are hairlike projections of the apical plasma membrane. These are not related to the lateral (**D**) or basal (**C**) domains, nor do they affect permeability (**A**) or tensile strength (**E**) of cells.

13. Correct: Macula adherens (C)

The patient is suffering from pemphigus vulgaris. It is a generalized, mucocutaneous, autoimmune, and blistering eruption with grave prognosis. It typically begins on mucosal surfaces and often progresses to involve the skin. This disease is characterized by fragile, flaccid blisters that rupture to produce extensive denudation of mucous membranes and skin. Patients have autoantibodies to desmogleins, which are transmembrane desmosomal proteins that belong to the cadherin family of calcium-dependent

adhesion molecules. Intraepidermal vesicle formation secondary to loss of cohesion between epidermal cells is commonly found.

Basal keratinocytes remain attached to the epidermal basement membrane, and there is no disruption of the dermal-epidermal basement membrane zone since hemidesmosomes (**A**), anchoring fibrils (**B**), or the proteins in the basal laminae (**E**) are unaffected. Gap junctions (**D**) are not formed by desmogleins and therefore are not affected in pemphigus vulgaris.

14. Correct: A and C (D)

Actin microfilaments form the core of microvilli and stereocilia. A defect in actin would lead to disruption of both. Cores of cilia (**B**), on the other hand, comprise microtubules in a 9+2 arrangement.

15. Correct: Heparan sulfate (D)

Heparan sulfate is a glycosaminoglycan present in the basal lamina that confers a strong negative charge to it.

Laminin (**A**) present in the basal lamina forms a bridge between the integrin receptors and type IV collagen. Entactin (**B**) is a glycoprotein that forms a bridge between laminin and type IV collagen. Type IV collagen (**C**) forms the major scaffold in lamina densa, while type VII collagen fibers (**E**) form anchoring fibrils that link the basal lamina to underlying reticular lamina.

16. Correct: Function of desmosomes is dependent on Ca²⁺ ions. (A)

Desmogleins and desmocollins are transmembrane desmosomal proteins that belong to the cadherin family of calcium-dependent adhesion molecules. These link cytokeratin filaments between adjacent cells.

Epithelia are classified by the shape of the cells in the apical (most superficial) layer (**B**). Keratin is the intermediate filament in the epithelial cells (**C**). A defect in the zonula occludens leads to defective paracellular transport (**D**). While stereocilia are absorptive structures, they are not found in the respiratory tract (**E**).

17. Correct: Epididymis (C)

The key is to identify stereocilia, which are unusually long, immotile microvilli (structure 1). These are present in the epididymis and the inner ear, not in any of the other locations listed in the choices. Also, note the pseudostratified columnar epithelium (structure 2) and spermatozoa in the lumen (structure 4).

18. Correct: Numerous mitochondria with tubular cristae (D)

The cell seems to be involved in steroidogenesis (because of the presence of numerous stacks of smooth endoplasmic reticulum), and is most likely the Leydig cell (secretes testosterone). The mitochondria of steroid-producing cells are integrally involved with steroidogenesis. Cristae are lamellar in typical mitochondria and tubular in steroid cell mitochondria.

Numerous stacks of rough endoplasmic reticulum (**A**), free ribosomes (**B**), apical secretory vesicles (**C**), and extensive Golgi apparatus (**E**) are found in protein-secreting cells.

19.   Correct: Extensive movement of substances over cell surfaces (B)

The structure indicated by the blue arrow is cilia, identified by hairlike projections taller than microvilli, along apical epithelial surfaces. The slide is from the uterine tube, which can be identified by the lining single-layered columnar cells interrupted by secretory or peg cells (black arrows). Cilia generate a streaming motion of fluid toward the uterus that supports movement of the oocyte.

Microvilli increase the surface area for absorption (**A**). Zonula adherens and macula adherens (desmosomes) form anchoring junctions between adjacent cells (**C**). Desmosomes link intermediate filaments between adjacent cells (**D**). Hemidesmosomes link intermediate filaments in the cell to extracellular matrix (**E**).

20.   Correct: Vagina (C)

The photomicrograph shows nonkeratinized stratified squamous epithelium, identified by flattened surface cells in the multilayered epithelium (structure 1). This type of epithelium lines moist surfaces exposed to the exterior, such as the oral cavity, tongue, pharynx, esophagus, anal canal, and vagina.

The lining cells of the epidermis (**A**) are stratified squamous keratinized, the trachea (**B**) are pseudostratified ciliated columnar, the urinary bladder (**D**) are transitional (multi-layered with surface umbrella cells), and the lung alveoli (**E**) are simple squamous.

Chapter 3

Connective Tissue Histology

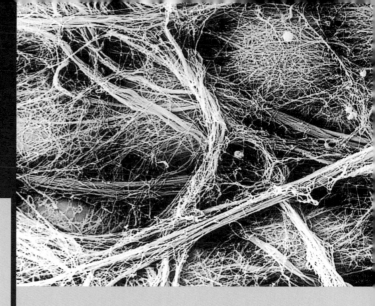

LEARNING OBJECTIVES

► Describe the organization of basal lamina. Critique its ultrastructure in histologic sections. Analyze its role as selectively permeable barrier in the renal glomerulus.

► Describe the etiopathogenesis of Alport's syndrome. Correlate this with its clinical features.

► Describe the organization of a mast cell. Critique its ultrastructure in histologic sections. Analyze its role in type I hypersensitivity reactions.

► Describe the etiopathogenesis of anaphylaxis (type I hypersensitivity reactions). Correlate this with its clinical features.

► Describe the organization of a plasma cell. Critique its ultrastructure in histologic sections. Analyze its role in synthesis of immunoglobulins.

► Describe the etiopathogenesis of multiple myeloma. Correlate this with its clinical features.

► Classify general types of connective tissue according to structure. Identify these in histologic sections. Analyze their distribution according to their functions.

► Describe the organization of a macrophage. Critique its ultrastructure in histologic sections. Analyze its role in synthesis of matrix metalloproteinases.

► Describe the synthesis of elastic fibers. Analyze their distribution according to their functions.

► Describe the etiopathogenesis of pulmonary emphysema. Correlate this with its clinical features.

► Describe the synthesis of collagen fibers. Analyze their distribution according to their functions.

► Describe the etiopathogenesis of osteogenesis imperfecta. Correlate this with its clinical features.

► Describe the organization of a fibroblast. Critique its ultrastructure in histologic sections. Analyze its role in synthesis of connective tissue matrix.

► Describe the etiopathogenesis of Marfan's syndrome. Correlate this with its clinical features.

► Describe the synthesis of reticular fibers. Analyze their distribution according to their functions.

► Describe the etiopathogenesis of Ehlers-Danlos syndrome. Correlate this with its clinical features.

► Describe the etiopathogenesis of scurvy. Correlate this with its clinical features.

► Describe the organization of glycosaminoglycans. Analyze their role within the connective tissue matrix.

► Predict functional outcomes of defective turnover of glycosaminoglycans as occurs in mucopolysaccharidoses.

► Describe the etiopathogenesis of Hurler's syndrome. Correlate this with its clinical features.

3.1 Questions

Easy	Medium	Hard

1. A 30-year-old man presents with hematuria and deafness. Electron microscopy reveals an irregularly thickened glomerular basement membrane with splitting of the central lamina densa. Defects in biosynthesis of which of the following proteins might be responsible for his symptoms?

A. Type I collagen

B. Type II collagen

C. Type III collagen

D. Type IV collagen

E. Fibrillin

2. A 9-year-old female presents with flushing, urticaria, pruritus, dizziness, and shortness of breath following an insect bite. In the ER, she was treated with high-flow oxygen, fluids, and corticosteroids. Activation of which of the following cells (indicated by arrows in the figure) was responsible for her presenting symptoms?

A. a

B. b

C. c

D. d

E. e

3. A 56-year-old man presents with bone pain, pathologic fractures, weakness, and anemia. A bone marrow aspirate obtained from him shows an excess of cells of the type indicated in the figure. Which of the following might be an important function of the cell?

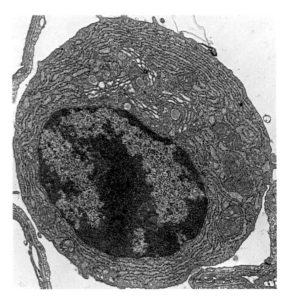

A. Synthesizes collagen

B. Synthesizes histamine

C. Synthesizes proteoglycans

D. Synthesizes antibodies

E. Synthesizes lipoprotein lipase

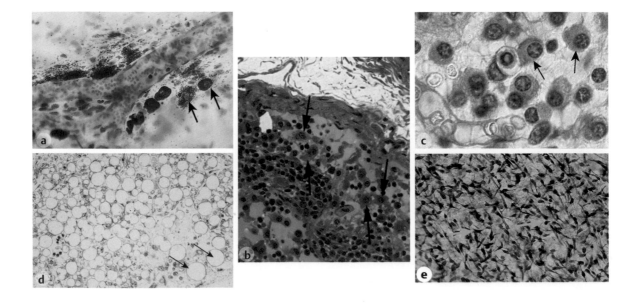

4. A pathology intern is reviewing how connective tissue structure correlates to function of an organ. Which of the following might be the source of the tissue shown in the figure below?

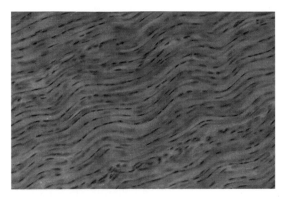

A. Lamina propria of jejunum

B. Paranephric fat

C. Umbilical cord of neonate

D. Dermis of skin covering the anterior chest wall

E. Achilles tendon

5. A 56-year-old man presents with symmetric polyarthritis with major involvement of the distal interphalangeal joints. Skin overlying the affected joints has translucent reddish-brown nodules of 1 to 2 mm in size. A biopsy obtained from perilesional skin shows an excess of cells indicated in the accompanying figure. Which of the following might be an important function of the cell?

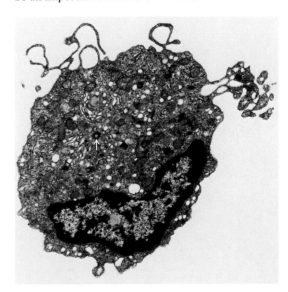

A. Synthesizes type I collagen

B. Synthesizes histamine

C. Synthesizes matrix metalloproteinases

D. Synthesizes IgG

E. Synthesizes lipoprotein lipase

6. A 63-year-old man presents with dyspnea and a productive cough of 2 weeks' duration. The cough, typically worse in the morning, is associated with production of white sputum. His urinary and blood desmosine levels, measured by mass spectrometry methods, were elevated. Degradation of which of the following might be responsible for his symptoms?

A. Skeletal muscle fiber

B. Nerve fiber

C. Collagen type I fiber

D. Elastic fiber

E. Reticular fiber

7. A male neonate was diagnosed with osteogenesis imperfecta, which is characterized by a defect in biosynthesis of type I collagen. During the process of formation of stable type I collagen fibrils, where within the cell do pro-α chains wind together to form procollagen triple helices?

A. Nucleus

B. Rough endoplasmic reticulum

C. Mitochondria

D. Golgi apparatus

E. Cell exterior

8. A 23-year-old woman is brought to the ER in respiratory distress, minutes after she was stung on the arm by a wasp. Physical examination reveals tachycardia, tachypnea, labored breathing, and hypotension. There is generalized urticaria. Which of the following is likely responsible for the patient's symptoms?

A. Activation of IgA

B. Activation of IgG

C. Activation of IgM

D. Activation of T lymphocytes

E. Activation of mast cells

9. A biopsy obtained from the upper eyelid of a 35-year-old man is shown in the figure below. Which of the following tissue types does it represent?

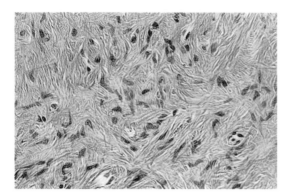

A. Areolar

B. White adipose

C. Embryonic

D. Dense connective, irregular

E. Dense connective, regular

10. A 16-year-old girl presents with acute-onset skin eruptions on her face. A punch biopsy obtained from her normal skin is shown in the figure below. Which of the following cells synthesize the structure labeled by the black arrow in the figure?

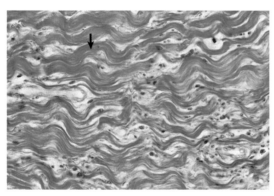

A. Fibroblasts

B. Mast cells

C. Plasma cells

D. Macrophages

E. White adipocytes

11. A 6-year-old boy presents with a prolapsed mitral valve and a dilated aorta. A general examination reveals abnormally elongated fingers (arachnodactyly) and severe pectus excavatum. Which of the following structures might be defective in the young boy?

A. Type I collagen fibers

B. Type II collagen fibers

C. Type IV collagen fibers

D. Reticular fibers

E. Elastic fibers

12. A 54-year-old man presents with acute-onset low-grade fever and swollen and tender axillary lymph nodes. A biopsy from an involved node reveals damage of a distinct tissue component that selectively stains with periodic acid Schiff (PAS) reagent. It also has high affinity for and stains black with silver stains. Which of the following is most likely defective in the individual?

A. Skeletal muscle fiber

B. Collagen type I fiber

C. Elastic fiber

D. Reticular fiber

E. Nerve fiber

13. While studying tissue architecture with the electron microscope, a pathology intern comes across the cell depicted in the figure. Which of the following is an important function for the cell?

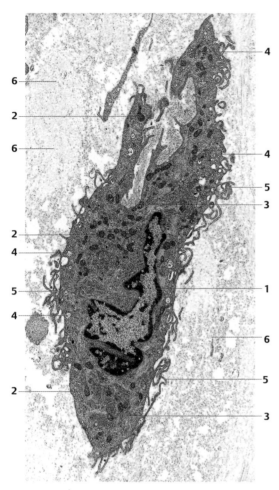

A. Synthesizes extracellular matrix

B. Synthesizes histamine

C. Synthesizes IgG

D. Engulfs bacteria

E. Stores metabolic energy

14. A first-year medical student is curious to find out the structure-function correlation of the cell depicted in the accompanying photomicrograph. She was advised to find out molecules that were contained within the structures indicated by yellow asterisks. Which of the following is such a molecule?

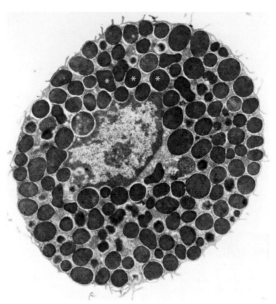

A. Hemoglobin

B. Mucinogen

C. Histamine

D. IgA

E. IgG

15. A 3-year-old girl presents with spontaneous fractures of her lower limbs while standing up. A physical examination reveals a bluish discoloration of the sclera. Her father, who had been diagnosed with osteoporosis, had suffered from more than a dozen fractures, including a hip fracture at age 34. A DNA analysis is most likely to reveal a defect in which of the following structures in the child?

A. Skeletal muscle fiber

B. Collagen type I fiber

C. Collagen type IV fiber

D. Elastic fiber

E. Reticular fiber

16. A 63-year-old man presents with a productive cough that is worse in the morning, and breathlessness. He has smoked 10 cigarettes per day for the past 40 years and has suffered from pneumonia in the previous month. Laboratory studies reveal moderate hypoxemia and mild hypercapnia (arterial blood gas), and a reduced serum α1-antitrypsin level. Which of the following structures is probably damaged in his lungs?

A. Skeletal muscle fiber

B. Collagen type I fiber

C. Collagen type IV fiber

D. Elastic fiber

E. Reticular fiber

17. A 16-year-old boy presents with short stature, stretchable skin, and moderate joint hypermobility. Cultured skin fibroblasts of the patient synthesized excessively soluble collagen and had low activity for a specific enzyme. Which of the following enzymes, with a major role in extracellular assembly of collagen fibrils, might have been deficient in him?

A. Prolyl 3-hydroxylase

B. Lysyl hydroxylase

C. Galactosyl transferase

D. Disulfide isomerase

E. Lysyl oxidase

18. A 52-year-old homeless alcoholic has lived eating out of trash cans for several years. She presents at the free clinic with bleeding and inflamed gums. She is irritable, clinically depressed, and fatigued with general muscle weakness. What might be the underlying mechanism for the symptoms in this patient?

A. Increased collagen secretion from fibroblasts

B. Stimulation of prolyl hydroxylase

C. Stimulation of lysyl hydroxylase

D. Formation of unstable collagen helices

E. Decreased collagen solubility

19. A 28-year-old previously healthy man presents with acute-onset pain in the right flank with radiation to the back. An emergency surgical exploration reveals ruptured dissection of the right common iliac artery. The surgical specimen shows deficiency of collagen type III. Which of the following is a true statement for him?

A. He is also suffering from arachnodactyly.

B. He is at high risk for intestinal rupture.

C. Joint hypermobility, affecting all joints, is extensive in him.

D. Synostosis, resulting in megalencephaly, should be an associated finding in him.

E. He is likely to have a bluish discoloration of sclera.

20. A 7-year-old child presents with chronic rhinitis, corneal clouding, and hepatomegaly. A deficiency of α-L-iduronidase was identified in his serum. Which of the following might be the underlying defect in him?

A. A decreased rate of synthesis of glycosaminoglycans

B. An increased rate of synthesis of glycosaminoglycans

C. A decreased rate of breakdown of glycosaminoglycans

D. An increased rate of breakdown of glycosaminoglycans

3.2 Answers and Explanations

Easy	Medium	Hard

1. Correct: Type IV collagen (D)

The patient is suffering from Alport's syndrome, which includes a group of inherited disorders affecting the kidneys, ears, and eyes. The most common and earliest manifestation of the syndrome is hematuria. Sensorineural deafness is a characteristic feature. Most patients have mutations in genes for the chains of type IV collagen, which is an important constituent of lamina densa.

Type I collagen (**A**) is found mainly in bones, tendons, etc. Type II collagen (**B**) is a major component of cartilage. Type III collagen (**C**) provides structural maintenance in expansible organs as reticular fibers. Fibrillin (**E**) forms the scaffold on which elastin is deposited during the synthesis and assembly of elastic fibers.

2. Correct: a (A)

The girl suffered from anaphylaxis (type I hypersensitivity reaction). This is caused by re-exposure to an allergen following prior sensitization, and is due to release of chemical mediators from mast cells (panel A, identified by nuclei obscured by granules) and basophils.

Macrophages (**B**, identified by giant size and eccentric nucleus), plasma cells (**C**, identified by basophilic cytoplasm, eccentric and cartwheel appearance of nucleus), adipocytes (**D**, identified by signet ring appearance), and fibroblasts (**E**, identified by flat nuclei, slender and branching cytoplasmic processes) are not responsible for the symptoms of anaphylaxis.

3. Correct: Synthesizes antibodies (D)

The cell in the figure is a plasma cell. It is identified by abundant rough endoplasmic reticulum within the cytoplasm, perinuclear stacks of Golgi apparatus (that produce the characteristic halo in light micrograph), eccentric nucleus, and distribution of heterochromatin giving the nucleus a cartwheel appearance. The patient might be suffering from multiple myeloma, which is characterized by proliferation of plasma cells.

Synthesis of collagen (**A**) and proteoglycans (**C**) involves fibroblasts. Histamine (**B**) is synthesized by mast cells and basophils, while lipoprotein lipase (**E**) is synthesized by adipocytes.

4. Correct: Achilles tendon (E)

The figure depicts collagen fiber bundles and fibroblasts arranged in a uniform parallel manner that impart maximum strength to the tissue. This is an example of dense regular connective tissue which is abundant in ligaments, tendons, and aponeuroses.

Lamina propria of the gastrointestinal tract (**A**) is rich in loose (areolar) connective tissue that is characterized by cellularity and vascularity, with sparse connective tissue fibers. Paranephric fat (**B**) is rich in adipose tissue (unilocular adipose cells: rim of cytoplasm and nucleus pushed to periphery by large lipid droplet, signet ring appearance). The neonatal umbilical cord (**C**) contains Wharton's jelly (embryonic mucoid tissue: large stellate-shaped mesenchymal cells with a jellylike matrix). Dermis (**D**) is mostly made up of dense irregular connective tissue (irregularly bundled collagen fibers, sparse cells).

5. Correct: Synthesizes matrix metalloproteinases (C)

The cell in the figure is a macrophage. It is identified by its irregular shape, cytoplasmic processes (pseudopodia), eccentric nucleus, and abundant lysosomes (primary, secondary, phagolysosomes or residual bodies). The patient might be suffering from multicentric reticulohistiocytosis, which is characterized by proliferation of histiocytes (macrophages). Macrophages, along with several other cells (fibroblasts, neutrophils, etc.), synthesize matrix metalloproteinases that play important role in matrix turnover.

Synthesis of type I collagen (**A**) involves fibroblasts. Histamine (**B**) is synthesized by mast cells and basophils. Immunoglobulins (**D**) are synthesized by plasma cells. Lipoprotein lipase (**E**) is synthesized by adipocytes.

6. Correct: Elastic fiber (D)

Desmosine and isodesmosine represent ideal biomarkers for monitoring elastin turnover, because these special cross-links are exclusively found in mature elastin. These amino acids are responsible for covalent bonding between elastin molecules, during synthesis and assembly of elastic fibers. The patient probably is suffering from pulmonary emphysema, which is characterized by destruction of elastic fibers in alveolar septa of the lung.

Degradation of skeletal muscle (**A**), nerve (**B**), collagen (**C**), or reticular (**E**) fibers will not result in increased serum or urinary desmosine levels.

7. Correct: Rough endoplasmic reticulum (B)

Synthesis of pro-α chains, hydroxylation of proline and lysine residues, glycosylation of hydroxylysyl residues, formation of the procollagen triple helices, and stabilization of the helices by formation of intracellular and intercellular bonds all occur within the rough endoplasmic reticulum.

Formation of mRNA occurs within the nucleus (**A**). Packaging of procollagen molecules into secretory vesicles for transport occurs within the Golgi apparatus (**D**). Cleavage of terminal peptides from procollagen to form collagen, and their subsequent assembly to form collagen fibrils (in case of type I collagen for example) occur in the extracellular environment (**E**). None of the events in collagen biosynthesis occurs within the mitochondria (**C**).

8. Correct: Activation of mast cells (E)

The woman suffered from anaphylaxis (type I hypersensitivity reaction). It is a potentially fatal multisystem reaction and is due to release of chemical mediators from mast cells and basophils. This is caused by re-exposure to an allergen following prior sensitization and involves IgE-mediated release of histamine and other mediators. The physiologic responses to the release of these mediators include smooth muscle spasm in the respiratory and gastrointestinal tracts, vasodilation, increased vascular permeability, and airway edema.

While choices **A–D** could arguably trigger non-IgE-mediated (anaphylactoid) reactions, degranulation of mast cells and basophils must be the terminal events responsible for the patient's symptoms.

9. Correct: Dense connective, irregular (D)

The figure depicts densely intertwined collagen fibers that run in various directions. Sparsity of cells and dominance of fibers classify the tissue as dense irregular. The arrangement is necessary to impart tensile strength necessary to withstand stress from different directions. This type of tissue is widely found in the dermis, organ capsules, dura mater, and sclera.

Areolar tissue (**A**) is characterized by cellularity and vascularity, with sparse fibers. White adipose tissue (**B**) predominantly comprises unilocular adipose cells (rim of cytoplasm and nucleus pushed to the periphery by a large lipid droplet with a signet ring appearance). Embryonic connective tissue (**C**) presents large stellate-shaped mesenchymal cells with branched cytoplasmic processes scattered in a gel-like matrix. Dense regular connective tissue (**E**) is characterized by regularly arranged collagen fiber bundles (with sparse cells) that impart maximum strength to the tissue.

10. Correct: Fibroblasts (A)

The arrow on the figure indicates collagen fiber, which is identified by its wavy, unbranched appearance. All fibers and matrix of connective tissue are synthesized by fibroblasts.

11. Correct: Elastic fibers (E)

The boy is suffering from Marfan's syndrome, which involves the musculoskeletal, cardiovascular, and ocular systems. Diagnosis is mainly clinical and comprises features described in the case. It is caused by a defect in the *FBN1* gene, which codes for fibrillin. During biosynthesis of elastic fibers, fibrillin microfibrils form the scaffold on which elastin is deposited. Any defect in its formation leads to abnormalities in tissue rich in elastic fibers (e.g., the aorta).

12. Correct: Reticular fiber (D)

Reticular fibers form delicate, branched, tight-meshed networks and grids. They form a supportive structure in walls of many organs, including lymph nodes. Argyrophilia (affinity for silver) is a standout property of reticular fibers that distinguishes them from other connective tissue fibers (e.g., collagen, elastic). Reticular fibers stain black with silver salt impregnation techniques (e.g., Gomori silver impregnation). Also, due to high carbohydrate content, these fibers can be readily stained with PAS.

13. Correct: Synthesizes extracellular matrix (A)

The cell in the figure is a fibroblast, which synthesizes extracellular matrix. Fibroblasts can be identified by the lobed nucleus (structure 1) with heterochromatin and euchromatin, prominent rough endoplasmic reticulum (structure 3), secretory vesicles (structure 4), and cell processes in the form of tentacles (structure 5). Collagen fibers (structure 6) can be identified in extracellular matrix.

Histamine (**B**) is synthesized by mast cells and basophils, immunoglobulins (**C**) are synthesized by plasma cells, macrophages engulf bacteria (**D**), and lipoprotein lipase (**E**) is synthesized by adipocytes.

14. Correct: Histamine (C)

The cell in the figure is a mast cell. It can be identified by the round- or oval-shaped electron-dense granules that occupy most of the cytoplasm. The granules contain histamine and heparin among several other mediators of anaphylaxis. Also, note the nucleus has characteristic peripheral heterochromatin. None of the other molecules (**A–B, D–E**) is contained in mast cell granules.

15. Correct: Collagen type I fiber (B)

The child is suffering from osteogenesis imperfecta (OI). It is a disorder of bone fragility chiefly caused by mutations in the *COL1A1* and *COL1A2* genes that encode type I procollagen, and he is usually diagnosed on the basis of clinical criteria. Type IA OI is the most prevalent and mildest form and is genetically transmitted in an autosomal-dominant or sporadic-mutation fashion. The presence of fractures together with blue sclerae, dentinogenesis imperfecta, or family history of the disease is usually sufficient to make the diagnosis. Blue sclera is probably caused by a thinness of the collagen layers of sclerae that allows the choroid layers to be seen.

16. Correct: Elastic fiber (D)

History, clinical features, and laboratory results indicate the diagnosis of pulmonary emphysema. It is defined as an abnormal permanent enlargement of air spaces distal to the terminal bronchioles, accompanied by the destruction of alveolar walls. α_1-antitrypsin neutralizes neutrophil elastase in the lung interstitium. Deficiency of α_1-antitrypsin is associated with the breakdown of the lung's elastic framework. Cigarette smoking is the most important risk factor for emphysema development.

17. Correct: Lysyl oxidase (E)

The patient is suffering from Ehlers-Danlos syndrome (type V), with a deficiency of lysyl oxidase. Lysyl oxidase is a copper-dependent amine oxidase that plays a critical role in the formation and repair of the extracellular matrix by oxidizing lysine residues in elastin and collagen, thereby initiating the formation of covalent cross-linkages that stabilize these proteins. These cross-links are essential for the tensile strength of collagens and the elastic properties of elastin.

Prolyl (**A**) and lysyl (**B**) hydroxylases catalyze the formation of hydroxyproline and hydroxylysine, respectively, in the rough endoplasmic reticulum during collagen biosynthesis. Galactosyl transferase (C) is involved in glycosylation (addition of sugar moieties) of hydroxylysyl residues, while disulfide isomerase (D) catalyzes the formation of disulfide bonds between procollagen triple helices in the rough endoplasmic reticulum during collagen biosynthesis.

18. Correct: Formation of unstable collagen helices (D)

The patient is suffering from scurvy, the disease of vitamin C deficiency. Humans are unable to synthesize vitamin C and therefore require it in their diet. Vitamin C is an antioxidant and essential cofactor for enzymes prolyl hydroxylase (B) and lysyl hydroxylase (C) in collagen biosynthesis. It is required for the hydroxylation of proline residues on procollagen, enabling the formation of hydrogen–hydrogen bonding in the triple helix of mature collagen. Without ascorbic acid, the polypeptides are unstable and unable to form stable triple helices. This results in decreased collagen secretion from fibroblasts (A), increased collagen solubility (E), and unstable collage fibrils. Defective collagen synthesis leads to defective dentine formation, hemorrhaging into the gums, and loss of teeth. Hemorrhaging is a hallmark feature of scurvy and can occur in any organ. Hair follicles are one of the common sites for cutaneous bleeding.

19. Correct: He is at high risk for intestinal rupture. (B)

The patient is suffering from the vascular type of Ehlers-Danlos syndrome (EDS). This is the most clinically significant EDS subtype due to the risk of arterial or major organ rupture. It is associated with mutations in the type III collagen gene (*COL3A1*), resulting in reduced amounts of type III collagen in the dermis, vessels, and viscera. The classic clinical features include a characteristic facial appearance: thin, translucent skin with a prominent venous pattern; extensive bruising or hematomas; and vascular or visceral rupture (or both). Arterial or intestinal rupture often presents as acute abdominal or flank pain; arterial rupture is the most common cause of death.

Joint hypermobility is usually minimal and limited to the digits (C). Arachnodactyly (A), synostosis (D), or blue sclera (E) is not associated with the syndrome.

20. Correct: A decreased rate of breakdown of glycosaminoglycans (C)

The patient is suffering from Hurler's syndrome (mucopolysaccharidosis type I, MPS I), which is an autosomal recessive disorder caused by deficiency of α-L-iduronidase. It often presents in infancy or early childhood as chronic rhinitis, clouding of corneas, and hepatosplenomegaly. The child also suffers from mental retardation and skeletal dysplasia. The diagnosis can also be established by increased urinary secretion of glycosaminoglycans (e.g., heparan sulfate and dermatan sulfate in MPS1). Mucopolysaccharidoses (MPS) are a group of lysosomal storage disorders that involve defective activity of the lysosomal enzymes, which blocks degradation of glycosaminoglycans (GAGs) and leads to their abnormal accumulation.

Rate of synthesis of GAGs is not altered (A–B), and increased rate of breakdown of GAGs (D) does not occur in MPS.

Chapter 4

Muscle Tissue Histology

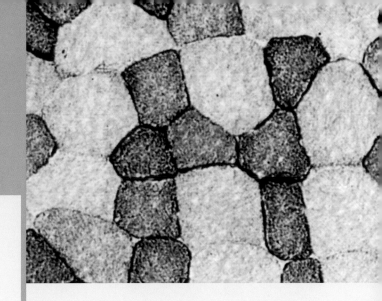

LEARNING OBJECTIVES

- ▶ Critique the microstructure of skeletal muscles in histologic sections. Analyze their distribution according to their functions.
- ▶ Describe the ultrastructure of a sarcomere.
- ▶ Describe the mechanism of skeletal muscle contraction.
- ▶ Describe the regulation of skeletal muscle contraction.
- ▶ Describe the etiopathogenesis of myasthenia gravis. Correlate this with its clinical features.
- ▶ Describe the etiopathogenesis of Guillain-Barré syndrome. Correlate this with its clinical features.
- ▶ Describe the etiopathogenesis of botulism. Correlate this with its clinical features.
- ▶ Critique the microstructure of cardiac muscle in histologic sections. Correlate its ultrastructure with its function.
- ▶ Describe the mechanism of cardiac muscle contraction.
- ▶ Describe the regulation of cardiac muscle contraction.

4.1 Questions

Easy	Medium	Hard

Consider the following case for questions 1 to 4:

Length of sarcomeres in human striated muscles influence the force that can be exerted by the muscle. A length-tension curve for gastrocnemius revealed resting length for the I-band to be 1.5 μm and for the A-band to be 2.0 μm. Contraction of the muscle fiber resulted in 10% shortening of the sarcomere length.

1. Which of the following is the resting length for the sarcomere?

A. 4.0 μm

B. 3.5 μm

C. 2.75 μm

D. 2.0 μm

E. 1.5 μm

2. Which of the following is the length of the A-band after the shortening produced during muscle contraction?

A. 2.0 μm

B. 1.8 μm

C. 1.7 μm

D. 1.6 μm

E. 1.5 μm

3. Which of the following is the length of the I-band after the shortening produced during muscle contraction?

A. 1.5 μm

B. 1.45 μm

C. 1.35 μm

D. 1.25 μm

E. 1.2 μm

4. Which of the following is the fate of the H-band after the shortening produced during muscle contraction?

A. Lengthens slightly

B. Doubles its length

C. Shortens slightly

D. Halves its length

E. Almost disappears

5. Which of the following helps spread depolarization of muscle cell membranes throughout the interior of muscle cells?

A. Actin

B. Myosin

C. Troponin

D. T tubules

E. Microtubules

Consider the following case for questions 6 to 11:

A first-year-medical student is leading her group for a muscle histology study session. She has chosen the accompanying image as a comprehensive guide for the subject and has prepared the following questions for the group.

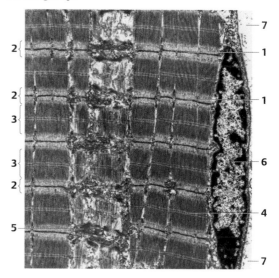

6. Which of the following might be the source for this tissue?

A. Esophagus

B. Stomach

C. Lungs

D. Heart

E. Kidneys

7. Which of the following proteins is directly attached to structure 1?

A. Actin

B. Myosin

C. Titin

D. A and B

E. A and C

F. B and C

8. Which of the following is true for structure 2?

A. Defines the contractile unit for the tissue

B. Is the seat for the enzyme creatine kinase

C. Comprises an overlap between actin and myosin filaments

D. Shortens during muscular contraction

E. Length is unaltered during muscular contraction

9. Which of the following is true for structure 3?

A. Defines the contractile unit for the tissue

B. Defined by the width of myosin filaments

C. Defined by the width of actin filaments

D. Is the seat for the enzyme α-actinin

E. Comprises the intermediate filament desmin

10. Which of the following is true for structure 4?

A. Defines the contractile unit for the tissue

B. Provides attachment for titin

C. Is the seat for the enzyme creatine kinase

D. Is the seat for the enzyme α-actinin

E. Comprises the intermediate filament desmin

11. A researcher develops antibodies against actin. Which of the following sites would most likely be spared from the action of such antibody?

A. Structure 1

B. Structure 2

C. Structure 3

D. Structure 4

Consider the following case for questions 12 to 13:

A 23-year-old girl was forced to pull her car over due to sudden blurring of vision. Soon after, she had trouble speaking when interrogated by a law enforcement officer. In the ER, she complained of nausea, had difficulty in swallowing fluids, and had trouble breathing. Her parents could not recall any recent health upsets for her, though they reported her spending the previous week on a farm with her grandparents. Her grandmother is famous in the neighborhood for home-canned vegetables and fruits that she grows on her farm. Physical examination revealed diplopia, dysarthria, dysphonia, bilateral ptosis and facial paralysis, and impaired gag reflex. Protein levels in her cerebrospinal fluid were normal.

12. Which of the following is the most probable diagnosis for her?

A. Guillain-Barré syndrome

B. Myasthenia gravis

C. Stroke affecting the genu of the left internal capsule

D. Botulism

E. Lambert-Eaton myasthenic syndrome

13. Which of the following is the most probable pathology in her case?

A. Deficient synthesis of acetylcholine

B. Deficient calcium ion entry into the axon terminal

C. Deficient release of acetylcholine in neuromuscular junction

D. Deficient transport of acetylcholine from cell body to axon terminal

E. Reduced number of available acetylcholine receptors in the postsynaptic membrane

14. Fascia adherens junctions are necessary for mechanically coupling and reinforcing cardiomyocytes. These always coincide with which of the following structures within the sarcomere?

A. A-band

B. H-band

C. I-band

D. Z disk

E. M line

15. Consider the following events: (1) Detachment of troponin I from actin; (2) Binding of myosin heads to actin filaments; (3) Binding of calcium to troponin C; (4) ADP on myosin head replaced by ATP; (5) Splitting of ATP into ADP and Pi.

Which of the following would be the correct order for these events to occur, following depolarization of the postsynaptic membranes, for skeletal muscles to contract?

A. 1, 2, 3, 4, 5
B. 1, 3, 2, 4, 5
C. 2, 1, 3, 5, 4
D. 3, 1, 2, 5, 4
E. 2, 1, 3, 5, 4

16. Cardiac troponin I is one of the most specific biomarkers for detection of acute myocardial infarction (AMI). Which of the following is true about the protein?

A. Binds the troponin complex to tropomyosin
B. Binds to calcium and initiates contraction
C. Binds to actin, inhibiting interaction of myosin and actin in the resting muscle cell
D. Binds to myosin, inhibiting interaction of myosin and actin in the resting muscle cell

Consider the following case for questions 17 to 18:

A 26-year-old woman complains that her "jaw gets tired" as she chews and that swallowing has become difficult. She also has blurring of vision that has worsened over the past month. Physical examination revealed diplopia, dysarthria, bilateral ptosis and facial paralysis, and impaired gag reflex. Her symptoms were reversed within 40 seconds of intravenous administration of edrophonium.

17. Which of the following is the most probable diagnosis for her?

A. Guillain-Barré syndrome
B. Myasthenia gravis
C. Stroke affecting the genu of the left internal capsule
D. Botulism
E. Lambert-Eaton myasthenic syndrome

18. Which of the following is the most probable pathology in her case?

A. Deficient synthesis of acetylcholine
B. Deficient calcium ion entry into the axon terminal
C. Deficient release of acetylcholine in the neuromuscular junction
D. Deficient transport of acetylcholine from cell body to axon terminal
E. Reduced number of available acetylcholine receptors in the postsynaptic membrane

Consider the following case for questions 19 to 20:

A male neonate was born with generalized hypotonia. Deep tendon reflexes were absent. Tongue fasciculation was observed. A skeletal muscle biopsy is seen in the figure.

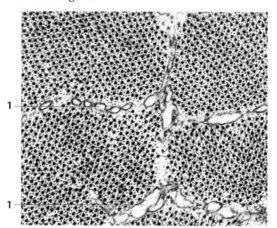

19. From where within the sarcomere is the section taken?

A. A-band
B. I-band
C. M line
D. Z disk
E. H-band

20. Which of the following is the function of structure 1?

A. Sequestration of enzyme that cross-links actin
B. Sequestration of enzymes that cross-links myosin
C. Sequestration of calcium during muscle relaxation
D. Sequestration of calcium during muscle contraction
E. Sequestration of sodium during muscle relaxation
F. Sequestration of sodium during muscle contraction

4.2 Answers and Explanations

Easy	Medium	Hard

Consider the following image for answers 1 to 4:

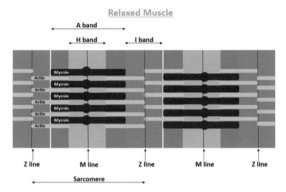

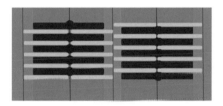

1. Correct: 3.5 µm (B)

Resting length of sarcomere is the total of the lengths of the resting A- and I-bands.

2. Correct: 2.0 µm (A)

Resting length of sarcomere is the total of the lengths of the resting A- and I-bands. Shortening of sarcomere during muscle contraction does not shorten the length of the A-band.

3. Correct: 1.35 µm (C)

Shortening of sarcomere during muscle contraction does not shorten the length of the A-band. It, therefore, occurs entirely due to shortening of the I-band. The process is illustrated in the figure.

4. Correct: Almost disappears (E)

The H-band completely disappears during the shortening. The process is illustrated in the figure.

5. Correct: T tubules (D)

To permit synchronous contraction of all sarcomeres in the muscle fiber, a system of T tubules extends transversely as tubular extensions of the muscle cell plasma membrane (sarcolemma) to surround each myofibril at the region of the junction of the A- and I-bands. Depolarization of the sarcolemma-derived T tubules is transmitted to the sarcoplasmic reticulum membrane (at the triad) with eventual release of sequestered calcium from the reticula. Actin (**A**), myosin (**B**), troponin (**C**), and microtubules (**E**) are not involved in this process.

Consider the following for answers 6 to 11:

The image key for the figure in the question is as follows:

1 - Z disk

2 - I-bands

3 - A-bands

4 - M line

5 - mitochondria

6 - nucleus

7 - ECM with collagen fibers

6. Correct: Esophagus (A)

The electron micrograph image has been obtained from skeletal muscle, given the striations, absence of intercalated disks, and peripheral nucleus.

The esophagus is the only organ from the list that contains skeletal muscle in its wall.

Consider the following image for answers 7 to 11:

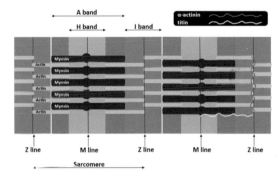

7. Correct: A and C (E)

Structure 1 is the Z disk. Actin (**A**) filaments of two successive sarcomeres are cross-linked by α-actinin at the Z disk. Also, titin (**C**) is the protein that anchors one end of myosin (**B**) to Z disk. Myosin (**B**), on the other hand, is not directly attached to the Z disk.

8. Correct: Shortens during muscular contraction (D)

Structure 2 is the I-band. It shortens and accounts entirely for sarcomere shortening during muscle contraction. The sarcomere defines the contractile unit for muscle tissue (**A**). The M line is the seat for creatine kinase (**B**). The A-band comprises an overlap between actin and myosin filaments (**C**) and does not shorten during contraction (**E**).

9.   Correct: Defined by the width of myosin filaments (B)

Structure 3 is the A-band. It is defined by the width of myosin (**B**) and not actin (**C**) filaments. The sarcomere defines the contractile unit for muscle tissue (**A**). The Z disk is the seat for intermediate protein desmin (**E**) and α-actinin (**D**).

10.   Correct: Is the seat for the enzyme creatine kinase (C)

Structure 4 is the M line. It bisects the H-band and is composed primarily of creatine kinase, which catalyzes formation of ATP. The sarcomere defines the contractile unit for muscle tissue (**A**). The Z disk provides attachment for the protein titin (**B**) and is the seat for intermediate protein desmin (**E**) and α-actinin (**D**).

11.   Correct: Structure 4 (D)

The M line does not provide attachment for actin. The Z disk provides attachment for actin, the I-band is composed of actin filaments only with no overlap of thick filaments, and the A-band is composed of actin filaments interdigitating with thick filaments. Therefore, all three would be affected by action of antibody against actin.

12.   Correct: Botulism (D)

She is most probably suffering from botulism, which is a neuroparalytic disease caused by botulinum toxin. The incubation period from ingestion of contaminated food (which in her case probably is canned vegetables and fruits given the highly suggestive history) to onset of symptoms is usually 8 to 36 hours. Symmetric cranial nerve palsies (diplopia, dysarthria, dysphonia, ptosis, ophthalmoplegia, facial paralysis, and impaired gag reflex) followed by bilateral descending flaccid paralysis that may progress to respiratory failure and death are hallmarks of the disease.

Guillain-Barré syndrome (**A**), an autoimmune demyelinating polyneuropathy that often follows an acute infection, presents most often as an ascending paralysis. Protein levels in cerebrospinal fluid are elevated. Myasthenia gravis (**B**) closely resembles the symmetrical descending paralysis that has occurred in this patient. However, the history (possible consumption of canned food) and the rapid evolution of symptoms tilt the diagnosis in favor of botulism. Stroke affecting the genu of the left internal capsule (**C**) should present with asymmetry of paralysis and upper motor neuron signs. Lambert-Eaton myasthenic syndrome (**E**) usually manifests as proximal limb weakness in a patient who is already, in most cases, debilitated by cancer (commonly small-cell lung carcinoma). Proximal muscles are more affected than distal muscles; lower extremity muscles are affected predominantly.

13.   Correct: Deficient release of acetylcholine (C)

Deficient release of acetylcholine in a neuromuscular junction occurs in botulism. Calcium-mediated fusion of synaptic vesicle membrane with the presynaptic membrane is impaired, resulting in decreased quantal content.

Defective acetylcholine synthesis (**A**) might be due to defective uptake of choline by the nerve terminal or defective enzymatic synthesis of acetylcholine from choline and acetyl-CoA; this might be encountered in congenital myasthenic syndrome. Muscle weakness typically begins in early childhood.

Deficient calcium ion entry into the axon terminal (**B**) results in a decreased probability of synaptic vesicle release and a low quantal content. The classic example is Lambert-Eaton myasthenic syndrome, in which antibodies are directed against voltage-gated calcium channels located in active zones of the presynaptic membrane.

Deficient transport of acetylcholine from cell body to axon terminal (**D**) can occur in microtubular (kinesin) defects but is not seen in botulism.

The underlying defect in myasthenia gravis is due to an antibody-mediated autoimmune attack directed against acetylcholine receptors (AChRs) at neuromuscular junctions, resulting in a decrease in the number of available AChRs (**E**).

14.   Correct: Z disk (D)

Fascia adherens, along with desmosomes and gap junctions, form intercalated disks that interconnect cardiomyocytes. Fascia adherens junctions anchor cells firmly by linking the cell membrane to the actin cytoskeleton. These are located in transverse sectors and coincide with the Z disk within the sarcomere of cardiac myocytes.

15. Correct: 3, 1, 2, 5, 4 (D)

The figure illustrates the excitation-contraction coupling within skeletal muscles.

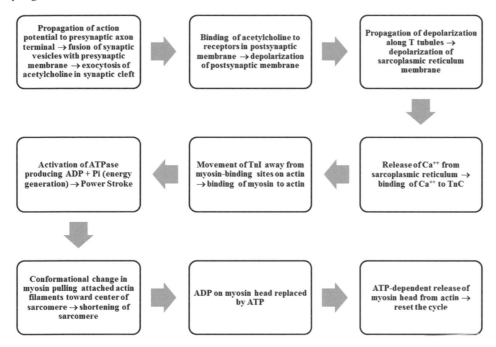

16. Correct: Binds to actin, inhibiting interaction of myosin and actin in the resting muscle cell (C)

Troponin I (TnI), in the resting muscle cell, binds to actin, thereby inhibiting the interaction of actin with myosin. Calcium binding by troponin C results in a conformational change that breaks the TnI-actin bond and exposes the myosin-binding sites of actin. Troponin T binds the troponin complex to tropomyosin (A). Troponin C binds calcium and initiates contraction (B). None of the troponin molecules binds to myosin (D).

17. Correct: Myasthenia gravis (B)

Myasthenia gravis (MG) is a neuromuscular disorder characterized by weakness and fatigability of skeletal muscles. The cranial muscles, particularly the lids and extraocular muscles, are typically involved early in the course of MG; diplopia and ptosis are common initial complaints. Facial weakness produces a "snarling" expression when the patient attempts to smile. Weakness in chewing is most noticeable after prolonged effort.

Edrophonium is an acetylcholinesterase inhibitor that prolongs presence of acetylcholine in the neuromuscular junction. It results in increased muscle strength in MG patients within a minute and lasts for ~ 5 minutes.

Guillain-Barré syndrome (A), an autoimmune demyelinating polyneuropathy that often follows an acute infection, presents most often as an ascending paralysis. An edrophonium test would be negative.

Stroke affecting the genu of the left internal capsule (C) should present with asymmetry of paralysis and upper motor neuron signs. Botulism (D) closely resembles the symmetrical descending paralysis that has occurred in this patient. However, an edrophonium test would be negative in botulism. Lambert-Eaton myasthenic syndrome (E) usually manifests as proximal limb weakness in a patient already debilitated by cancer (commonly small-cell lung carcinoma). Proximal muscles are more affected than distal muscles; lower extremity muscles are affected predominantly.

18. Correct: Reduced number of available acetylcholine receptors in the postsynaptic membrane (E)

The underlying defect in MG is due to an antibody-mediated autoimmune attack directed against acetylcholine receptors (AChRs) at neuromuscular junctions, resulting in decrease in the number of available AChRs.

Defective acetylcholine synthesis (A) might be due to defective uptake of choline by the nerve terminal or defective enzymatic synthesis of acetylcholine from choline and acetyl-CoA; this might be encountered in congenital myasthenic syndrome. Muscle weakness typically begins in early childhood.

Deficient calcium ion entry into the axon terminal (B) results in decreased probability of synaptic vesicle release and a low quantal content. The classic example is Lambert-Eaton myasthenic syndrome in which antibodies are directed against voltage-gated calcium channels located in active zones of the pre-synaptic membrane.

Deficient release of acetylcholine in a neuromuscular junction (**C**) occurs in botulism. Calcium-mediated fusion of the synaptic vesicle membrane with the presynaptic membrane is impaired, resulting in decreased quantal content. Calcium channels and flow of the ion through these into presynaptic terminal are normal.

Deficient transport of acetylcholine from the cell body to the axon terminal (**D**) can occur in microtubular (kinesin) defects but is not seen in MG.

19.   Correct: A-band (A)

This is a cross section through bundles of myofibrils of a skeletal muscle.

Hexagonal organization of cross-sectioned thick myosin filaments, and fine spotlike structures that correspond to cross-sectioned thin actin filaments indicate this to be sectioned from the zone that has overlap between actin and myosin, the A-band. Sections from the I-band (**B**) or the Z disk (**D**) would contain only actin, while that from the M line (**C**) or the H-band (**E**) will contain only myosin filaments. Note:

To complicate the issue, a section from the I-band might have thicker titin proteins scattered with thin actin, mimicking this section. Careful observation, however, can discriminate hexagonal organization of myosin from circular titin.

20.   Correct: Sequestration of calcium during muscle relaxation (C)

The structures labeled 1 are T tubules (network of sarcoplasmic reticulum). To permit synchronous contraction of all sarcomeres in the muscle fiber, a system of T tubules extends transversely as tubular continuations of the muscle cell plasma membrane (sarcolemma) to surround each myofibril at the region of the junction of the A- and I-bands. Depolarization of the sarcolemma-derived T tubules is transmitted to the sarcoplasmic reticulum membrane (at the triad) with eventual release of sequestered calcium from within the reticula. During repolarization (relaxation), calcium is resequestered within the lumen of the sarcoplasmic reticulum.

Sequestration of α-actinin (**A**, enzyme that cross-links actin) occurs at the Z disk. Sequestration of enzymes that cross-link myosin (**B**) occurs at the M line. Calcium is not sequestered but released from sarcoplasmic reticulum during contraction (**D**). Sodium is not sequestered within sarcoplasmic reticulum either during contraction (**F**) or relaxation (**E**).

Chapter 5

Cartilage and Bones Histology

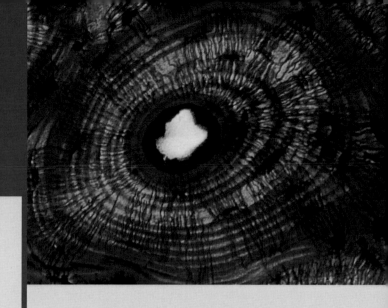

LEARNING OBJECTIVES

- ▶ Describe the etiopathogenesis of rickets. Correlate this with its clinical features.
- ▶ Describe the etiopathogenesis of osteomalacia. Correlate this with its clinical features.
- ▶ Describe the etiopathogenesis of Paget's disease. Correlate this with its clinical features.
- ▶ Describe the etiopathogenesis of osteoporosis. Correlate this with its clinical features.
- ▶ Describe the etiopathogenesis of osteogenesis imperfecta. Correlate this with its clinical features.
- ▶ Describe the etiopathogenesis of multiple myeloma. Correlate this with its clinical features.
- ▶ Describe the properties of hyaline cartilage. Analyze its distribution according to its functions.
- ▶ Describe the etiopathogenesis of osteoarthritis. Correlate this with its clinical features.
- ▶ Describe the properties of elastic cartilage. Analyze its distribution according to its functions.
- ▶ Describe the properties of fibrous cartilage. Analyze its distribution according to its functions.
- ▶ Describe the etiopathogenesis of rheumatoid arthritis. Correlate this with its clinical features.
- ▶ Describe the etiopathogenesis of renal osteodystrophy. Correlate this with its clinical features.

5.1 Questions

Easy	Medium	Hard

Consider the following case for questions 1 to 5:

A 5-year-old boy presents with outward bowing of both his legs. His family history is significant for a strict vegan diet that precludes intake of any animal protein and milk. A physical examination reveals mild tenderness of the legs and beaded swellings along the costochondral junctions.

1. Which of the following is the most probable diagnosis?

A. Paget's disease

B. Osteoporosis

C. Rickets

D. Multiple myeloma

E. Osteogenesis imperfecta

2. Which of the following is a likely associated finding in his serum?

A. Low calcium, low phosphate, low alkaline phosphatase

B. Low calcium, low phosphate, high alkaline phosphatase

C. High calcium, high phosphate, high alkaline phosphatase

D. High calcium, high phosphate, low alkaline phosphatase

E. Normal calcium and phosphate, low alkaline phosphatase

3. Which of the following is the most probable pathology for the child?

A. Decreased osteoblastic activity

B. Increased osteoclastic activity

C. Decreased osteoclastic activity

D. Defective synthesis of type I collagen

E. Defective mineralization of osteoid

4. Which of the following signs might be evident in a radiograph of his femur?

A. Alternate areas of sclerosis and lucencies

B. Homogeneously increased bone density with cortical thickening

C. Homogeneously decreased bone density

D. Widening of the metaphysis

E. Multiple pathological fractures

5. Which of the following layers within the growth plate should show an expansion in the child?

A. Reserve zone of chondrocytes

B. Proliferating zone of chondrocytes

C. Hypertrophic zone of chondrocytes

D. A and C

E. B and C

Consider the following case for questions 6 to 9:

A 75-year-old woman presents with a chronic painful hip. X-ray shows signs suggestive of osteoarthritis. She underwent total hip replacement. Histologic review of the surgical specimen revealed a significantly damaged articular surface with marked degeneration of articular cartilage.

6. Which of the following factors is primarily responsible for poor repair of her cartilage?

A. Being relatively avascular

B. Being relatively non-nervous

C. Presence of excessive interstitial water

D. Presence of excessive type II collagen fibers

E. Presence of excessive chondroitin sulfate

7. Which of the following is an expected finding for the synovial fluid from her hip joint?

A. Clear; increased neutrophils

B. Clear; increased mononuclear cells

C. Clear; no significant inflammatory cells

D. Purulent; increased neutrophils

E. Purulent; increased mononuclear cells

8. Which of the following did she increasingly excrete in urine prior to surgery?

A. Type I collagen

B. Type II collagen

C. Type III collagen

D. Type IV collagen

E. Type V collagen

9. Which of the following histological features, within an H & E stained section, is the most reliable indicator for the articular cartilage's ability to withstand compressive forces?

A. Thickness of the inner cellular layer of the periosteum

B. Thickness of the outer fibrous layer of the periosteum

C. Degree of basophilia

D. Concentration of chondrocytes

E. Concentration of adipose tissue

Consider the following case for questions 10 to 12:

A 65-year-old man presents with bone pain primarily affecting the right thigh. Physical examination reveals cutaneous erythema and warmth, and bony tenderness over the affected area. Laboratory findings are significant for increased serum alkaline phosphatase and increased urinary hydroxyproline. Radiograph reveals bowing of the right femur with cortical thickening, and a mixture of lytic and blastic lesions.

10. Which of the following is the possible diagnosis for the patient?

A. Osteoporosis

B. Osteomalacia

C. Multiple myeloma

D. Paget's disease

E. Osteitis fibrosa cystica

11. Which of the following cells is primarily responsible for the pathology?

A. Chondroblasts

B. Osteoblasts

C. Osteoprogenitor cells

D. Osteocytes

E. Osteoclasts

12. Which of the following is an expected additional finding in his serum?

A. Calcium ↓, phosphate ↓

B. Calcium ↑, phosphate ↑

C. Calcium ↓, phosphate ↑

D. Calcium ↑, phosphate ↓

E. Normal calcium and phosphate

Consider the following case for questions 13 to 15:

During a routine busy day in the laboratory, the technician forgets to label the image. The consultant pathologist asks her internist for interpretation of the image.

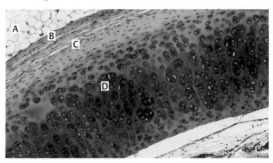

13. Which of the following might be a probable source for the tissue?

A. External ear

B. Meniscus of the knee

C. Symphysis pubis

D. Epiglottis

E. Trachea

14. Which of the following zones might be responsible for appositional growth of the tissue?

A. A

B. B

C. C

D. D

15. Which of the following zones might be responsible for interstitial growth of the tissue?

A. A

B. B

C. C

D. D

16. A 45-year-old woman presents with a four-week history of bilateral hand pain. Her hands are stiffer in the morning, and it gradually loosens up. Physical examination reveals a warm, erythematous wrist, metacarpophalangeal, and proximal interphalangeal joints bilaterally. Hand X-ray films show periarticular erosions, and blood test results are significant for a mild anemia and an elevated erythrocyte sedimentation rate. Which of the following is the most probable diagnosis for her?

A. Osteoarthritis

B. Rheumatoid arthritis

C. Paget's disease

D. Lupus erythematosus

E. Osteoporosis

Consider the following case for questions 17 to 18:

A 39-year-old woman presents with severe hip pain. A physical examination is significant for central obesity, tender bilateral hip joints, mild hypertension, and abdominal striae. Laboratory findings are significant for increased fasting glucose, increased urinary and plasma cortisol, and increased ACTH. A radiograph reveals generalized osteolysis with preservation of joint space and an intact articular cartilage.

17. Which of the following is the most likely diagnosis?

A. Rheumatoid arthritis

B. Osteoarthritis

C. Primary osteoporosis

D. Secondary osteoporosis

E. Paget's disease

18. Which of the following might be the most likely finding for her affected bones?

A. Decreased mineral-to-osteoid ratio

B. Scanty bony trabeculae

C. Increased thickness of cortical bone

D. Increased number of osteoclasts

E. Decreased number of osteoblasts

19. A 20-year-old man sustained a twisting injury to his right knee while playing football. He underwent partial medial meniscectomy. Which of the following is true for the resected tissue?

A. The cells are mostly present in isogenous groups.

B. The perichondrium is most pronounced.

C. Interstitial growth is more pronounced.

D. The collagen component is exclusively of type I.

E. The collagen component is exclusively of type II.

20. A 58-year-old female with a history of chronic renal failure presents with progressive bilateral ankle, foot, and hip pain of 4 weeks' duration. She has no history of trauma or of swelling or redness of the affected joints. The physical examination is unremarkable. The laboratory examination reveals low serum level of calcium and high serum levels of phosphorus, alkaline phosphatase, and parathyroid hormone (PTH). A radiograph of the hand reveals subperiosteal bone resorption. Which of the following is the probable diagnosis for her?

A. Renal osteodystrophy

B. Paget's disease

C. Osteomalacia

D. Rheumatoid arthritis

E. Multiple myeloma

5.2 Answers and Explanations

Easy	Medium	Hard

1. Correct: Rickets (C)

Nutritional rickets is a dietary deficiency of vitamin D that interferes with skeletal ossification. Abnormal mineralization in growing bone affects the transformation of cartilage into bone. As a result, disorganized, nonmineralized, degenerating cartilage appears, leading to widening of the epiphyseal plate (observed radiologically as a widened radiolucent zone) with flaring or cupping and irregularity of the epiphyseal-metaphyseal junctions. This latter problem gives rise to the clinically obvious beaded swellings along the costochondral junctions known as the rachitic rosary and the swelling at the ends of the long bones.

Paget's disease of the bone (**A**) is characterized by excessive abnormal bone remodeling. It usually presents in persons older than 55 years. Osteoporosis (**B**) is metabolic skeletal disease defined as a reduction of bone mass. Primary osteoporosis occurs in postmenopausal women or in older men and women due to age-related factors. Secondary osteoporosis results from specific clinical disorders, such as endocrinopathies, trauma, or inflammation. Multiple myeloma (**D**) is the most common primary malignant bone neoplasm in adults (> 70% of cases are diagnosed between 50 and 70 years of age) arising from red marrow due to monoclonal proliferation of the plasma cells. Destruction of bone manifests as osteolytic lesions, bone pain, and pathologic fractures. Osteogenesis imperfecta (**E**) is a disorder of collagen type I production, involving connective tissues and bones. Characteristic features of osteogenesis imperfecta are fragile bones that fracture easily, blue sclera, dental fragility, and hearing loss.

2. Correct: Low calcium, low phosphate, high alkaline phosphatase (B)

Vitamin D deficiency results in decreased intestinal absorption of calcium and phosphate. In conjunction with the resulting secondary hyperparathyroidism, it leads to an increase in bone resorption. The net result tends to be low to normal serum calcium, low serum phosphate, and elevated serum alkaline phosphatase.

3. Correct: Defective mineralization of osteoid (E)

Bone matrix comprises osteoid (secreted by osteoblasts) that requires mineralization (with calcium and phosphate) to form mature bone. Vitamin D deficiency results in decreased intestinal absorption of calcium and phosphate. Consequently, deficient mineralization of osteoid occurs. There is increased osteoblastic activity (A) in rickets laying down an increased amount of osteoid in an effort to compensate for weak bones. Osteoclast activity is normal (B, C). Defective synthesis of type I collagen (D) leads to osteogenesis imperfecta.

4. Correct: Widening of the metaphysis (D)

As mentioned earlier, disorganized, non-mineralized, and degenerating cartilage within the epiphyseal plate leads to widening of the plate, with flaring or cupping and irregularity of the epiphyseal-metaphyseal junctions. Alternate areas of sclerosis and lucencies (A) are common in Paget's disease. Homogeneously increased bone density with cortical thickening (B) is commonly seen in Paget's disease and osteopetrosis. Homogeneously decreased bone density (C) is a hallmark feature of osteoporosis. Multiple pathological fractures (E) can be commonly encountered in multiple myeloma and osteogenesis imperfecta.

5. Correct: Hypertrophic zone of chondrocytes (C)

Rickets associated with vitamin D deficiency is characterized by expansion of the hypertrophic layer. Cells in this layer are metabolically active that divide, produce matrix, and initiate vascular invasion. The expansion of the rachitic growth plate is a consequence of impaired apoptosis of the late hypertrophic chondrocytes, an event that precedes replacement of these cells by osteoblasts during endochondral bone formation. The reserve zone (A, D) normally exhibits no cellular proliferation or matrix production. The proliferating zone (B, E) contain cells that divide and form matrix (by collagen synthesis, etc.). However, these cells do not show any expansion in rickets.

6. Correct: Being relatively avascular (A)

Osteoarthritis is a noninflammatory degenerative joint disease that is characterized by joint space narrowing, sclerosis, and presence of osteophytes. Distal interphalangeal joints and large weight-bearing joints are most commonly involved.

Cartilage is vulnerable to damage primarily because cells of the immune system have limited access to it, mostly due to its avascular nature. None of the other listed factors contribute to poor repair of cartilage.

7. Correct: Clear; no significant inflammatory cells (C)

Osteoarthritis is not primarily an inflammatory process, and therefore the synovial fluid from her joint should resemble normal synovial fluid (clear and devoid of inflammatory cells).

Clear fluid with increased inflammatory cells (A, B) is commonly found in rheumatoid arthritis. Purulent fluid with increased inflammatory cells (D, E) is commonly seen in septic arthritis.

8. Correct: Type II collagen (B)

The pathologic hallmark of osteoarthritis is hyaline articular cartilage loss. Approximately 80% of collagen in hyaline cartilage is of type II. Therefore, an increased urinary excretion of this type of collagen is expected. Type I collagen (A) is found mainly in bones, tendons, etc. Type III collagen (C) provides structural maintenance in expansible organs as reticular fibers. Type IV collagen (D) is predominantly found in the basal lamina of epithelia. Type V collagen (E) normally localizes at the surface of type I collagen.

9. Correct: Degree of basophilia (C)

Chondroblasts synthesize the cartilage ground substance (cartilage matrix), which consists of water, glycosaminoglycans (GAGs—chondroitin sulfate, etc.), and collagen fibrils (type II collagen). Aggrecan, with side chains of chondroitin sulfate and keratan sulfate, is the most abundant proteoglycan of hyaline cartilage. Water bound to GAGs in the proteoglycans is responsible for the cartilage's ability to withstand compressive forces. Also, these proteoglycans are responsible for the basophilia of the cartilage matrix. Thickness of the periosteum (A, B), chondrocyte concentration (D), and adipose tissue (E) are not direct indicators of the amount of GAGs (and hence water) present in the tissue.

10. Correct: Paget's disease (D)

Paget's disease of the bone is characterized by excessive abnormal bone remodeling. It usually presents in persons older than 55 years. Cutaneous erythema and warmth and bone tenderness are found over affected areas of the skeleton, reflecting greatly increased blood flow through the bone. Initial lesions are typically osteolytic, with focal radiolucencies; process of accelerated bone remodeling leaves cortical thickening and coarse trabeculation, and alternating lytic and sclerotic lesions.

Osteoporosis (**A**) is a metabolic skeletal disease defined as a reduction of bone mass that presents as homogeneously osteolytic lesions. Primary osteoporosis occurs in postmenopausal women or in older men and women due to age-related factors. Secondary osteoporosis results from specific clinical disorders, such as endocrinopathies, trauma, and inflammation. Osteomalacia (**B**) is caused by vitamin D deficiency leading to abnormal mineralization of osseous tissue that occurs after the epiphyseal plates have closed. This results in wide osteoid seams, and a large fraction of bone is covered by non-mineralized osteoid. Multiple myeloma (**C**) is the most common primary malignant bone neoplasm in adults (> 70% of cases are diagnosed between 50 and 70 years of age) arising from red marrow due to monoclonal proliferation of the plasma cells. The destruction of bone manifests as osteolytic lesions, bone pain, and pathologic fractures. Osteitis fibrosa cystica (**E**) is a manifestation of hyperparathyroidism. Rise in the parathyroid hormone results in mobilization of skeletal calcium through rapid osteoclastic turnover of bone to maintain normal serum calcium levels. Radiographic features include well-defined, purely lytic lesions that provoke little reactive bone. The cortex is usually thinned and expanded.

11. Correct: Osteoclasts (E)

Paget's disease is characterized by increased osteoclast activity, causing lytic lesions in the bone; these cells initiate the bone remodeling cycle in a chaotic fashion, and the end result of remodeling is a mosaic pattern of lamellar bone.

12. Correct: Normal calcium and phosphate (E)

Even though local disparities in remodeling may result in areas with the radiographic appearance of osteolysis or dense new bone, a tight coupling between biochemical markers of bone resorption and formation is maintained in Paget's disease. Calcium and phosphate levels, therefore, are usually maintained despite enormously increased skeletal turnover rates.

13. Correct: Trachea (E)

The image represents hyaline cartilage, identified by isogenous groups of chondrocytes scattered in a glassy matrix.

Tracheobronchial cartilages are of hyaline type.

The external ear (**A**) and epiglottis (**D**) contain elastic cartilage. Meniscus (**B**) and symphysis pubis (**C**) contain fibrocartilage.

14. Correct: C (C)

Appositional growth forms new cartilage at the surface of existing cartilage and involves progenitor cells in the perichondrium (**C**) differentiating into chondroblasts.

Adipose tissue (**A**), dense connective tissue (**B**), and isogenous groups of chondrocytes in lacunae (**D**) are not involved.

15. Correct: D (D)

Interstitial growth forms new cartilage within existing cartilage and involves division of lacunar chondrocytes (**D**).

Adipose tissue (**A**), dense connective tissue (**B**), and perichondrium (**C**) are not involved.

16. Correct: Rheumatoid arthritis (B)

The history, physical, and laboratory findings in the patient are suggestive of an inflammatory process, and are very typical of rheumatoid arthritis (RA). RA is a chronic systemic inflammatory disorder characterized by the insidious onset of symmetric polyarthritis. In nearly all patients, the wrist, metacarpophalangeal joints, and proximal interphalangeal joints are affected, whereas the distal interphalangeal joints are spared. The typical X-ray finding in rheumatoid arthritis, periarticular bone erosion (loss of joint space), may not develop until later in the disease process.

Osteoarthritis (**A**) is a noninflammatory degenerative joint disease that is characterized by joint space narrowing, sclerosis, and presence of osteophytes. Distal interphalangeal joints and large weight-bearing joints are most commonly involved in osteoarthritis. Paget's disease of the bone (**C**) is characterized by excessive abnormal bone remodeling. It usually presents in persons older than 55 years. Initial lesions are typically osteolytic, with focal radiolucencies; process of accelerated bone remodeling leaves cortical thickening and coarse trabeculation, and alternating lytic and sclerotic lesions. Lupus (**D**), while it can have identical clinical features, often presents with asymmetric polyarthritis. Even if symmetric, it usually is characterized by the presence of other symptoms, such as malar rash, serositis (pleuritis and pericarditis), renal disease with proteinuria or hematuria, central nervous system (CNS) manifestations, as well as hematologic disorders, such as hemolytic anemia, leukopenia, lymphopenia, or thrombocytopenia. Osteoporosis (**E**) is a noninflammatory process that is characterized by uniform reduction in bone mass. While secondary osteoporosis can occur subsequent to inflammation, given the clinical features, this should not be the primary diagnosis in our patient.

17. Correct: Secondary osteoporosis (D)

The patient has osteoporosis (diagnosed by generalized osteolysis) secondary to Cushing's disease (diagnosed by central obesity, hypertension, abdominal stria, impaired glucose tolerance, elevated cortisol, and elevated ACTH).

Rheumatoid arthritis (**A**) is an autoimmune inflammatory disease that initially affects the hands and wrists in a characteristic symmetric, proximal distribution. The hip is not commonly affected, and concentric loss of joint space is a characteristic feature. Osteoarthritis (**B**) is a degenerative joint disease that is characterized by joint space narrowing, sclerosis, and the presence of osteophytes. Primary osteoporosis (**C**) occurs in postmenopausal women or in older men and women due to age-related factors. Paget's disease of the bone (**E**) is characterized by excessive abnormal bone remodeling. It usually presents in persons older than 55 years. A radiograph usually reveals alternate areas of sclerotic and lytic lesions.

18. Correct: Scanty bony trabeculae (B)

Decreased bone density in osteoporosis can be appreciated radiographically by decreased cortical thickness and loss of bony trabeculae.

Decreased mineral-to-osteoid ratio (**A**) is common in defective mineralization of bone (rickets, for example). Increased thickness of cortical bone (**C**) is common in Paget's disease and osteopetrosis. Numbers of both osteoblasts (**E**) and osteoclasts (**D**) are unaltered in osteoporosis.

19. Correct: Interstitial growth is more pronounced. (C)

The menisci of knees are made of fibrocartilage. Because this type of cartilage lacks definite perichondrium (**B**), interstitial but not appositional is the primary mode of cartilage growth. Cells in fibrocartilage mostly occur in isolation, rather than in isogenous groups (**A**). Matrix of fibrocartilage contains both type I (**D**) and type II (**E**) collagen.

20. Correct: Renal osteodystrophy (A)

In patients with renal osteodystrophy, the inability of the failing kidneys to convert 25-OH-vitamin D to the active form, 1, 25-OH-vitamin D causes impaired calcium absorption from the intestine, and bone resorption appears to become less sensitive to PTH. This leads to hypocalcemia. Also, phosphate excretion by the diseased kidney is decreased, resulting in hyperphosphatemia, which amplifies the fall in serum calcium and independently increases PTH secretion. Summing it up, these patients will have a low serum level of calcium and high serum levels of phosphorus, alkaline phosphatase, and PTH. Subperiosteal bone resorption is a classic radiographic finding for renal osteodystrophy.

Paget's disease (**B**) presents with normal calcium and phosphate levels. Osteomalacia (**C**) could have similar clinical features, but the patient will have hypocalcemia and hypophosphatemia (since without renal failure). Rheumatoid arthritis (**D**) is an inflammatory process. No strong suggestions about morning stiffness, absence of redness or swelling of the affected joints, and sparing of the hand practically precludes the diagnosis. Multiple myeloma (**E**) presents with anemia and hypercalcemia. In contrast to other types of osteolytic bone disease, serum alkaline phosphatase activity is decreased or within the normal range.

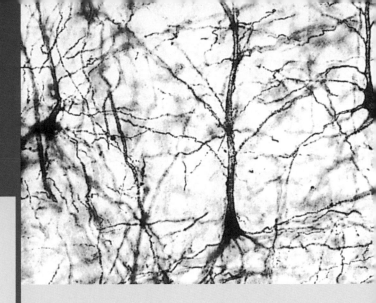

Chapter 6
Nerve Tissue Histology

LEARNING OBJECTIVES

- ▶ Describe axonal transport. Analyze the need for anterograde and retrograde transport.
- ▶ Describe the ultrastructure of a Schwann cell. Correlate this with its development, distribution, and functions.
- ▶ Describe the etiopathogenesis of Charcot-Marie-Tooth disease. Correlate this with its clinical features.
- ▶ Describe the microstructure of an astrocyte. Correlate this with its development, distribution, and functions.
- ▶ Describe the cells within the cerebellar cytoarchitecture. Analyze their roles in the cerebellar microscopic circuitry.
- ▶ Describe neural responses to injury within the central and peripheral nervous system. Analyze axonal and perikaryal changes in response to such injuries.
- ▶ Describe the microstructure of an oligodendrocyte. Correlate this with its development, distribution, and functions.
- ▶ Describe the organization of autonomic and spinal ganglia. Correlate this with their development, distribution, and functions.
- ▶ Describe the etiopathogenesis of alcoholic cerebellar degeneration. Correlate this with its clinical features.
- ▶ Describe the organization of connective tissue in a nerve. Correlate this with its functions.
- ▶ Describe the organization of neuron and neuropil within nerve tissue. Correlate this with their development, distribution, and functions.
- ▶ Describe the histological structure of neocortex. Correlate this with its distribution and functions.

6.1 Questions

Easy	Medium	Hard

1. A 26-year-old sexually active woman presents with vesicular lesions on the cervix and bilateral painful vesicles on the external genitalia. Following laboratory studies, she was diagnosed with genital herpes. She was treated with oral antivirals and was counselled carefully for prevention of recurrence. Virions travel from the initial site of infection on the mucosa to the dorsal root ganglion, where latency is established.Which of the following mechanisms is responsible for such movement of the virus?

A. Positive to negative terminal; molecular motor kinesin

B. Positive to negative terminal; molecular motor dynein

C. Negative to positive terminal; molecular motor kinesin

D. Negative to positive terminal; molecular motor dynein

E. Negative to positive terminal; molecular motor actin

Consider the following case for questions 2 to 3:

A 60-year-old man presents with a history of lower extremity weakness that began in his second decade. Weakness has progressed over time and is associated with significant muscle wasting of both lower extremities and hands. A review of the patient's family history reveals two similarly affected relatives in an autosomal dominant pattern of inheritance. Physical examination reveals a severely decreased vibration sense and proprioception. A nerve conduction velocity test performed on the median nerve confirms markedly reduced conduction velocity.

2. Which of the following cells is responsible for synthesizing the defective protein in this patient?

A. Fibroblasts

B. Schwann cells

C. Satellite cells

D. Skeletal muscle cells

E. Oligodendrocytes

3. Which of the following additional finding(s) might be expected in this patient?

A. Exaggerated deep tendon reflexes

B. Intact pain and temperature sensation

C. "Onion bulb" appearance in the nerve biopsy

D. A, B, and C

E. B and C

4. A biopsy obtained from the lower brainstem of a 26-year-old male is examined under the microscope. Which of the following is true about the cell labeled 1 in the figure?

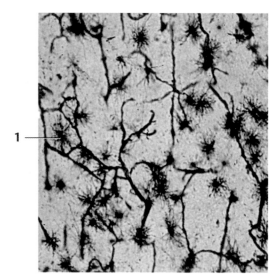

A. It is instrumental in synthesizing and secreting cerebrospinal fluid.

B. It is instrumental in forming glia limitans.

C. It is instrumental in laying down myelin sheath for neurons in the peripheral nervous system.

D. It is instrumental in laying down myelin sheath for neurons in the central nervous system.

E. It expresses neurofilament as the intermediate filament.

5. Medulloblastoma is a common malignant tumor in children that involves the cerebellar vermis. Precursors of an excitatory neuron and the molecular mechanisms involved in controlling their proliferation have been implicated in its pathogenesis. Predecessor of which of the following cells seems to be involved in the etiopathogenesis of the tumor?

A. Basket cell

B. Golgi cell

C. Granule cell

D. Purkinje cell

E. Stellate cell

6. A 39-year-old woman presents with weakness in right shoulder abduction 2 weeks following a right-sided axillary lymph node resection. A physical examination reveals decreased sensation over the upper and outer side of her right shoulder. Which of the following histological changes might be noted in a right anterior horn cell of her fourth cervical spinal segment?

A. Increased cytoplasmic basophilia

B. Increase in the number of cellular organelles

C. Decrease in volume (shrinkage)

D. Increase in Nissl granules

E. Peripheral movement of the nucleus

7. Mutations in genes coding for proteins responsible for transporting neurotransmitters synthesized in the cell body to the axon terminal have been identified as etiological factors for certain motor neuron diseases. Which of the following proteins might be a target for such mutation?

A. Kinesin

B. Dynein

C. Actin

D. Myosin

E. Tropomyosin

8. A 35-year-old man presents with a spastic-type of paralysis in the right lower extremity, visual impairment in his right eye, and fatigue. Magnetic resonance imaging (MRI) confirms areas of patchy demyelination in specific areas of the left cerebral hemisphere. Which of the following cells are specifically targeted in his condition?

A. Astrocytes

B. Oligodendrocytes

C. Ependymal cells

D. Schwann cells

E. Satellite cells

9. A 72-year-old man presents with severe peripheral vascular disease unsuitable for vascular reconstruction. Neurosurgery was advised and proved beneficial. The attached slide was obtained from a routine biopsy of the tissue procured is attached. Which of the following is/are true of the figure?

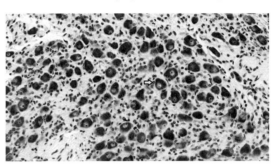

A. The chief source of the indicated cells is neuroectoderm.

B. The chief source of the indicated cells is neural crest.

C. The micrograph has probably been obtained from a dorsal root ganglion.

D. The micrograph has probably been obtained from a sympathetic ganglion.

E. A and C

F. A and D

G. B and C

H. B and D

10. A brain biopsy obtained from a 66-year-old man, who presented with an undifferentiated cerebral tumor, is attached (image). Which of the following is an important role for the cell in the center?

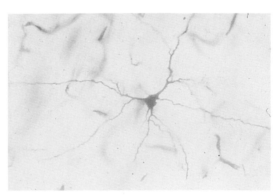

A. Producing myelin in the CNS

B. Lining ventricles in the CNS

C. Producing scar tissue in the CNS

D. Macrophage activity in the CNS

E. Producing CSF in the CNS

11. A chronic alcoholic presents with truncal instability and an uncoordinated gait. An MRI confirms alcoholic degeneration of the cerebellar vermis. Which of the following cells is most notably destroyed in this patient?

A. Basket cell

B. Golgi cell

C. Granule cell

D. Purkinje cell

E. Stellate cell

12. A 20-year-old male presents with progressive weakness of both legs that developed over several hours. A nerve biopsy confirmed immune-mediated damage to the blood-nerve barriers in his lower limbs. Which of the following is instrumental in establishing these barriers for the affected nerves?

A. Astrocytes

B. Endoneurium

C. Perineurium

D. Epineurium

E. Satellite cells

13. Unmyelinated axons are more vulnerable to degeneration than the myelinated ones in neuro-degenerative disorders. Which of the following cell types supports unmyelinated axons in the peripheral nervous system?

A. Ganglion cells

B. Satellite cells

C. Schwann cells

D. Astrocytes

E. Ependymal cells

14. A 2-month-old infant presents with poor muscle tone, muscle weakness, and feeding and breathing difficulty. A spinal cord biopsy (shown in the figure) was obtained to confirm a diagnosis. Which of the following is/are true of the structure indicated by the arrow?

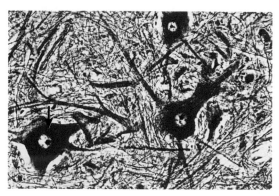

A. The chief source of the indicated structure is neuroectoderm.

B. The chief source of the indicated structure is neural crest.

C. It expresses neurofilament as the intermediate filament.

D. It expresses glial fibrillary acidic protein (GFAP) as the intermediate filament.

E. A and C

F. A and D

G. B and C

H. B and D

15. A 45-year-old female presents with recent onset dizziness and nausea. The symptoms are followed by vertigo, nystagmus, limb ataxia, and dysarthria. She has no history of hypertension, diabetes, stroke, or alcoholism. CSF sampling reveals autoantibodies against the chief output cells for cerebellum, and a diagnosis of paraneoplastic cerebellar degeneration was made. Which of the following cells is the target for the antibodies?

A. Basket cell

B. Golgi cell

C. Granule cell

D. Purkinje cell

E. Stellate cell

16. A biopsy (image) was obtained from the ventral horn of the spinal cord of a 16-year-old boy. Which of the following is/are true of the composition of the structure indicated by the arrow?

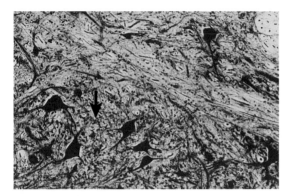

A. Cell bodies of glia
B. Processes of glial cells
C. Cell bodies of neurons
D. Processes of neurons
E. Capillaries
F. A, B, C, E
G. A, B, D, E
H. A, B, C, D, E

17. A section from the sciatic nerve is shown in the figure. Which of the following layers might have been subjected to a teratogenic insult during embryogenesis if the newborn suffered from a defect in synthesis of the coverings for structures labeled 1?

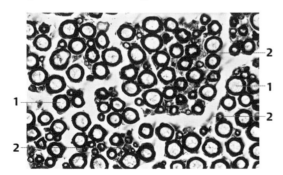

A. Surface ectoderm
B. Mesoderm
C. Endoderm
D. Neural crest cells
E. Neuroectoderm

Consider the following case for questions 18 to 20:

A 68-year-old man was admitted with sudden onset of severe neck pain. A CT scan of the brain revealed ventricular hematoma and acute hydrocephalus. Despite several attempts to resuscitate, he died on the 6th day from complications of the subarachnoid hemorrhage. The figure shows normal cortical (cerebral) tissue, which was obtained from him at autopsy.

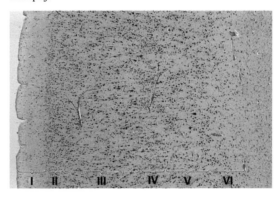

18. Which of the following cortical areas is most likely to be the source of the tissue?

A. Primary motor cortex
B. Primary sensory cortex
C. Primary visual cortex
D. Primary auditory cortex
E. Prefrontal association cortex

19. How would the image be different if it was obtained from the anterior paracentral lobule?

A. Disproportionately larger area II
B. Disproportionately larger area III
C. Disproportionately larger area IV
D. Disproportionately larger area V
E. Disproportionately larger area VI

20. How would the image be different if it was obtained from the posterior paracentral lobule?

A. Disproportionately larger area II
B. Disproportionately larger area III
C. Disproportionately larger area IV
D. Disproportionately larger area V
E. Disproportionately larger area VI

6.2 Answers and Explanations

Easy	Medium	Hard

1. Correct: Positive to negative terminal; molecular motor dynein (B)

The movements of the virus described can be identified as retrograde, occurring from the mucosa (peripheral axonal process, positive terminal) to the dorsal root ganglion (neuronal cell body, negative terminal). Dynein is the molecular motor for such transport.

Kinesin (**A, C**) is the molecular motor for anterograde axonal transport. This occurs from the cell body to the periphery. Actin (**E**) is not directly involved in axonal transport.

2. Correct: Schwann cells (B)

The patient is suffering from Charcot-Marie-Tooth disease (CMT), a member of the group of hereditary motor and sensory neuropathies (HMSN), a commonly inherited neurological disorder characterized by progressive motor weakness, decreased nerve conduction velocities, and nerve root enlargement. About 70 to 80% of these cases are caused by a mutation in the peripheral myelin protein-22 (PMP22) gene that results in abnormal myelin, which is unstable and spontaneously breaks down. Demyelination leads to uniform slowing of nerve conduction velocity, thereby causing weakness and numbness.

Schwann cells are responsible for synthesis of PMP22, a component protein of myelin for the peripheral nerves. Fibroblasts (**A**), satellite cells (**C**), and skeletal muscle cells (**D**) are not involved in the process, while oligodendrocytes (**E**) are responsible for myelin synthesis for the central nervous system.

3. Correct: B and C (E)

The patient is suffering from Charcot-Marie-Tooth disease (CMT), a member of the group of hereditary motor and sensory neuropathies (HMSN), a commonly inherited neurological disorder characterized by progressive motor weakness, decreased nerve conduction velocities, and nerve root enlargement. About 70 to 80% of these cases are caused by a mutation in the peripheral myelin protein-22 (PMP22) gene that results in abnormal myelin, which is unstable and spontaneously breaks down. Demyelination leads to uniform slowing of nerve conduction velocity, thereby causing weakness and numbness.

In response to demyelination, Schwann cells proliferate and form concentric arrays of myelin. Repeated cycles of demyelination and remyelination result in a thick layer of abnormal myelin around the peripheral axons. These changes cause the onion bulb appearance (**C**) evident in nerve biopsies. As expected with lower motor neuron lesions, deep tendon reflexes (DTRs) are markedly diminished or are absent (**A**). Pain and temperature sensations usually are not affected (**B**) because they are carried by unmyelinated (type C) nerve fibers.

4. Correct: It is instrumental in forming glia limitans. (B)

The cell labeled 1 is a protoplasmic astrocyte. It can be identified by a large number of processes radiating from the perikaryon, resembling spiders. The astrocyte foot processes form glia limitans (outermost layer of nervous tissue of the brain and spinal cord, lying directly under the pia mater) which serves as a functional barrier at the interface between non-neural tissue and CNS neural parenchyma. Ependymal cells secrete cerebrospinal fluid (**A**), Schwann cells are responsible for myelination of the peripheral nervous system (**C**), oligodendrocytes are responsible for myelination of the central nervous system (**D**), and neurons express neurofilament as intermediate filaments (**E**).

5. Correct: Granule cell (C)

From the list, the granule cell is the only excitatory neuron within the cerebellar cortex. The microscopic circuitry of the cerebellum is shown in the figure.

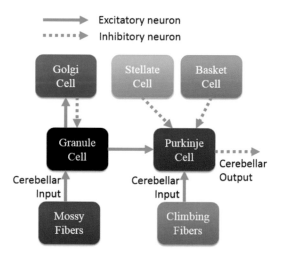

The excitatory inputs carried by mossy fibers (from the cerebral cortex, brainstem, and spinal cord) and climbing fibers (from the contralateral inferior olivary nuclear complex) synapse directly (climbing) or indirectly (mossy) onto Purkinje cells, which carry the outputs to the deep cerebellar and vestibular nuclei. Mossy fiber afferents project to the cerebellar glomerulus in the granular layer. In the cerebellar glomerulus, the mossy fiber afferents synapse with the granule cell. After this first processing stage, the granule cell conveys this afferent information to the Purkinje cell and the Golgi cell (through the excitatory parallel fibers). The Golgi (**B**) cell exerts an inhibitory (feedback) influence on the synapse between the mossy fiber and the granule cell, within the glomerulus. The Purkinje cell also receives direct afferent information (excitatory) through the climbing fiber. Further synapses with the Purkinje cell are from stellate (**E**) cells and basket (**A**) cells (both inhibitory). The Purkinje (**D**) cell then sends its efferent projection (inhibitory) to the deep cerebellar nuclei. The deep cerebellar nuclei serve as relay and processing stations for information coming from the cerebellar cortex to targets outside the cerebellum.

6. Correct: Peripheral movement of the nucleus (E)

The clinical features point toward an axillary nerve injury during the surgical procedure. Cell bodies of the motor axons (peripheral nerve) lie in the ventral horn cells of the 3rd, 4th, and 5th segments of the cervical cord. The histological changes that occur within a neuronal cell body following an axonal injury are referred to as chromatolysis. The features of chromatolysis are dissolution of the Nissl granules (rough endoplasmic reticulum), and hence decreased basophilia (**A, D**), cellular swelling (**C**), death of cell organelles (**B**), and peripheral displacement of the nucleus (**E**).

7. Correct: Kinesin (A)

The microtubule-associated protein families of kinesins and dyneins serve as the molecular motors that distribute intracellular cargo along microtubules, with kinesins working in the anterograde direction, from the cell body (-ve terminal) to the periphery (+ve terminal), and dyneins (**B**) working in the retrograde direction. Actin (**C**), myosin (**D**), and tropomyosin (**E**) are not directly involved in anterograde axonal transport.

8. Correct: Oligodendrocytes (B)

Oligodendrocytes are responsible for myelination in the central nervous system. Schwann cells (**D**) are responsible for myelination in the peripheral nervous system. Astrocytes (**A**), ependymal cells (**C**), and satellite cells (**E**) are not responsible for myelination.

9. Correct: B and D (H)

The micrograph has been obtained from a sympathetic ganglion. Autonomic ganglia can be distinguished from dorsal root ganglia (DRG) by presence of multipolar ganglion cells (as opposed to pseudounipolar neurons in DRG), eccentric nuclei of the ganglion cells (as opposed to central nuclei in DRG neurons), and loosely packed satellite cells. While the multipolarity of the neurons is not best demonstrated in the image (because of nonstaining of neuronal processes), the eccentricity of the nuclei and spreading out of satellite cells are the standout features. The arrows indicate satellite cells, which are peripheral glia that support ganglionic neurons. These cells (along with the ganglionic cells) are derived from the neural crest.

10. Correct: Producing scar tissue in the CNS (C)

The cell in the micrograph is a fibrous astrocyte. It can be identified by long and rarely branched processes of the perikaryon. Gliosis is the focal proliferation of glial cells in the CNS in response to insult. Astrocytes and the microglia are the glial cells predominantly responsible for tissue response to injury. Proliferation and hypertrophy of astrocytes play a huge role in formation of scar tissue within the CNS. Oligodendrocytes are responsible for myelination within the CNS (**A**). Ependymal cells line the ventricles (brain) and the central canal (spinal cord) and are functional in the production of cerebrospinal fluid (**B, E**). Microglia are the macrophages in the CNS (**D**).

11. Correct: Purkinje cell (D)

Alcohol is directly toxic to the cerebellum, causing degeneration primarily of the anterior superior vermis. This is due especially to either shrinkage or atrophy of Purkinje cells. Chronic alcoholism results in a risk of significant loss of Purkinje cells. This is worsened by associated vitamin B_1 deficiency, resulting from both a poor diet and a direct toxic effect on vitamin B_1 metabolism. Alcohol impairs thiamine uptake from the gastrointestinal tract, reduces thiamine-dependent enzyme activity, and depletes liver thiamine stores.

The Golgi (**B**) cell exerts an inhibitory influence on the synapse between the mossy fiber and the granule cell, within the cerebellar glomerulus. Basket (**A**) and stellate (**E**) cells provide direct inhibitory influences on the Purkinje cells. In the cerebellar glomerulus, the mossy fiber afferents synapse with the granule cell (**C**). After this first processing stage, the granule cell conveys this afferent information to the Purkinje cell and the Golgi cell (through excitatory parallel fibers).

12. Correct: Perineurium (C)

Perineurium is the specialized connective tissue surrounding a nerve fascicle that contributes to the formation of the blood-nerve barrier. Cells in this layer possess receptors, transporters, and enzymes that provide for the active transport of substances.

Astrocytes (**A**) help maintain a blood-brain barrier in the central nervous system. Endoneurium (**B**) comprises loose connective tissue wrapping around an individual nerve fiber. Macrophages in this layer phagocytose debris following nerve injury. Epineurium (**D**) comprises dense irregular connective tissue that binds nerve fascicles into a common bundle. It contains the larger blood vessels that supply the nerve. Satellite cells (**E**) provide support for ganglionic neurons and are not involved in forming the blood-nerve barrier.

13.   Correct: Schwann cells (C)

Schwann cells wrap around and support the unmyelinated axons in the peripheral nervous system. Ganglion cells (**A**) are neuronal cell bodies that are involved in the conduction of impulses. Satellite cells (**B**) are peripheral glial cells that surround and support the ganglion cells. Astrocytes (**D**) are glial cells found in the central nervous system that support neurons. Ependymal cells (**E**) line the ventricles (brain) and the central canal (spinal cord) and are functional in the production of cerebrospinal fluid.

14.   Correct: A and C (E)

The indicated structure is a multipolar neuron located in the ventral horn of the spinal cord. It is derived from neuroectoderm and not the neural crest (**B**). Also, neurons express neurofilaments. GFAP (**D**) is expressed by the glial cells.

15.   Correct: Purkinje cell (D)

The excitatory inputs carried by mossy fibers (from the cerebral cortex, brainstem, and spinal cord) and climbing fibers (from the contralateral inferior olivary nuclear complex) synapse directly (climbing) or indirectly (mossy) onto Purkinje cells, which carry the outputs to the deep cerebellar and vestibular nuclei (see figure for answer 5). The deep cerebellar nuclei serve as relay and processing stations for information coming from the cerebellar cortex to targets outside the cerebellum.

The Golgi (**B**) cell exerts an inhibitory influence on the synapse between the mossy fiber and the granule cell, within the cerebellar glomerulus. Basket (**A**) and stellate (**E**) cells provide direct inhibitory influences on the Purkinje cells. In the cerebellar glomerulus, the mossy fiber afferents synapse with a granule cell (**C**). After this first processing stage, the granule cell conveys this afferent information to the Purkinje cell and the Golgi cell (through the excitatory parallel fibers).

Paraneoplastic cerebellar degeneration is a complication of a malignancy (usually undetected), typically mediated by antibodies generated against tumor antigens. Similar proteins are also expressed on Purkinje cells, leading to their immunologic destruction. This is suspected in patients who present with acute or subacute cerebellar degeneration and no risk factors for cerebellar disorders (e.g., stroke, alcoholism, etc.).

16.   Correct: A, B, D, E (G)

The arrow indicates neuropil, the structure that fills the spaces between perikarya (**C**, neuronal cell bodies). Neuropils comprise glial cells (**A**) with their processes (**B**), processes of nerve cells (**D**), and capillaries (**E**).

17.   Correct: Neural crest cells (D)

The structures labeled 1 are myelinated nerve fibers. Since this is a peripheral nerve (sciatic), Schwann cells are responsible for the synthesis of myelin. Schwann cells are derived from neural crest cells.

Neuroectoderm (**E**) gives rise to oligodendrocytes, which are responsible for myelination in the CNS. Surface ectoderm (**A**), mesoderm (**B**), and endoderm (**C**) do not produce cells related to myelin synthesis.

18.   Correct: Prefrontal association cortex (E)

The histological organization of the neocortex can be summarized as:

Cell Layers of the Neocortex			
Layer	Name	Description	Major connections
I	Molecular layer	Cell sparse	Dendrites and axons from other layers
II	External granular layer	Scattered granular cells	Intra and inter cortical connections
III	External pyramidal layer	Scattered pyramidal cells	Intra and inter cortical connections
IV	Internal granular layer	Densely packed granular cells	Receives inputs from thalamus
V	Internal pyramidal layer	Densely packed pyramidal cells	Sends outputs to subcortical structures
VI	Multiform layer	Polymorphic layer	Sends output to thalamus

The larger size of area III compared with that of area IV and V, in the figure, indicates it to be from an association area rather than from a primary motor or a primary sensory area. The primary motor cortex (**A**) would have a disproportionately larger area V with minimal area IV representation (agranular cortex), while each of the primary sensory (**B**), primary visual (**C**), and primary auditory (**D**) areas would have a larger area IV (granular cortex).

19. Correct: Disproportionately larger area V (D)

The anterior area of the paracentral lobule is a primary motor area that controls movements of the contralateral lower limbs. This area would therefore represent the agranular cortex, with maximum thickness of area V, with pyramidal cells predominating (see figure for answer 18).

20. Correct: Disproportionately larger area III (C)

The posterior area of the paracentral lobule is primarily sensory and involves sensation from the contralateral lower limbs. This area would therefore represent the granular cortex, with maximum thickness of area IV (see figure for answer 18).

Chapter 7

Integumentary System Histology

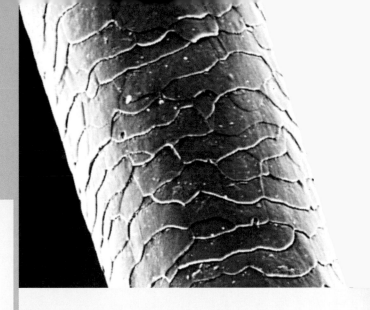

LEARNING OBJECTIVES

▶ Describe the microstructure of a sebaceous gland. Correlate this with its development, distribution, and functions.

▶ Describe the etiopathogenesis of acne vulgaris. Correlate this with its clinical features.

▶ Describe the microstructure of epidermis. Correlate this with its development and functions.

▶ Describe the etiopathogenesis of pemphigus vulgaris. Correlate this with its clinical features.

▶ Describe the mechanism of epidermal regeneration during wound healing.

▶ Differentiate between thick and thin skin.

▶ Describe the etiopathogenesis of psoriasis. Correlate this with its clinical features.

▶ Describe the etiopathogenesis of ichthyosis vulgaris. Correlate this with its clinical features.

▶ Describe the microstructure of an eccrine sweat gland. Correlate this with its development, distribution, and functions.

▶ Describe the microstructure of an apocrine sweat gland. Correlate this with its development, distribution, and functions.

▶ Describe the etiopathogenesis of hidradenitis suppurativa. Correlate this with its clinical features.

▶ Describe the ultrastructure of a Merkel cell. Correlate this with its development, distribution, and functions.

▶ Describe the etiopathogenesis of dermatitis herpetiformis. Correlate this with its clinical features.

7.1 Questions

Easy	Medium	Hard

1. A 16-year-old girl presents to the clinic complaining of pimples. Over the past 8 months, she has been using an over-the-counter face wash, but it has not helped. Physical examination reveals several erythematous papules and pustules on her face with scattered open and closed comedones. Hyperactivity of the structure in the figure was diagnosed to be partially responsible for her symptoms. Which of the following is a true statement for her?

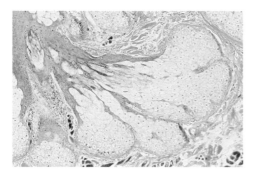

A. Her palm and sole will soon be severely affected.

B. Her condition has accelerated since she attained puberty.

C. Her condition should not alter during her menstrual cycle.

D. The indicated structure opens directly on the skin surface, so this will not involve any surrounding structures.

E. She should not expect to have similar lesions on her scalp.

Consider the following case for questions 2 to 4:

A 56-year-old man presents with painful oral ulceration that has appeared over the last 3 days. This has limited his ability to eat and drink. He also has developed some tender blisters in his neck, axilla, arm, and trunk, but his palms and soles are spared. Physical examination reveals fragile, flaccid blisters that easily rupture to produce extensive denudation of mucous membrane and skin.

2. Which of the following might be an associated finding in him?

A. Intraepidermal acantholysis

B. Subepidermal acantholysis

C. Dermoepidermal separation

D. Negative Nikolsky's sign

E. Blisters that heal without scarring if not traumatized

3. Which of the following epidermal layers predominantly contain structures that are targets in him?

A. Stratum corneum

B. Stratum lucidum

C. Stratum granulosum

D. Stratum spinosum

E. Stratum basalis

4. Which of the following proteins might be the targets in him?

A. Connexin

B. Desmoglein

C. BP 230

D. Type XVII collagen

E. Type IV collagen

Consider the following case for questions 5 to 6:

A 26-year-old woman presents with extensive abrasions over both of her forearms following a road traffic accident. On the left forearm, there is complete loss of epidermis, but the dermis seems to be intact. On the right, partial epidermal loss is seen.

5. Which of the following will be the chief source for regeneration of epithelium in her left forearm?

A. Endothelial cells lining capillaries within the dermis

B. Hair follicles within the dermis

C. Fibroblasts within the dermis

D. Macrophages within the dermis

E. Collagen fibers within the dermis

6. Which of the following will be the chief source for regeneration of epithelium in her right forearm?

A. Endothelial cells lining capillaries within the dermis

B. Hair follicles within the dermis

C. Fibroblasts within the dermis

D. Epidermal cells within the basal layer and wound edges

E. Collagen fibers within the dermis

Consider the following case for questions 7 to 9:

A 28-year-old woman presents with a progressing rash that has developed over the past 6 weeks. Physical examination reveals several erythematous plaques affecting the extensor surfaces of both the upper and lower extremities as well as similar lesions on her scalp. The plaques seem to be covered with tightly adherent silvery scales and are sharply demarcated. A biopsy obtained from her normal skin can be seen in the figure.

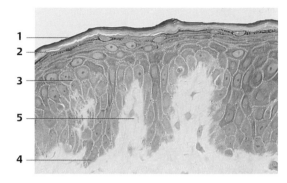

7. Which of the following is most likely responsible for her symptoms?

A. Intraepidermal acantholysis

B. Subepidermal acantholysis

C. Decrease in epidermal thickness with continual loss of cells

D. Increase in epidermal thickness with addition of immature cells

E. Restriction of inflammatory cells since epidermis is avascular

8. Increased epidermal turnover is a key pathogenic factor in the disease. Which of the following, as seen in the figure, are responsible for hyperproliferation of cells in her?

A. 1

B. 2

C. 3

D. 4

E. 5

F. 2 and 3

G. 3 and 4

H. 2, 3, and 4

9. Which of the following is true for the type of skin shown in the accompanying image?

A. Primarily present in the palm and sole

B. Absence of dermatoglyphics

C. Absence of hair follicles in the dermis

D. Abundance of Merkel's cells

E. Abundance of eccrine sweat glands

10. A 3-year-old boy presents with dry skin and fine scaling on the trunk and extensor surfaces of his extremities. Laboratory studies reveal null mutation in the gene encoding profilaggrin. A defect in which of the following layers, as seen in the figure, is most likely responsible for the symptoms in the child?

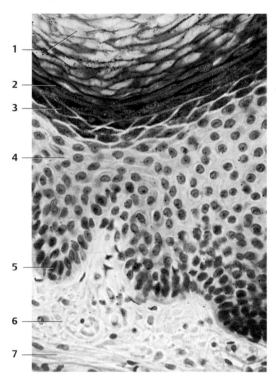

A. 1

B. 2

C. 3

D. 4

E. 5

F. 6

Consider the following case for questions 11 to 13:

A 16-year-old girl presents with tender nodular lesions in her axilla. She has a positive history for similar outbreaks (3 times in the past 6 months) in both axilla and groin. She states that it is painful to have them opened. Physical examination reveals several painful, firm, and erythematous nodules. A skin biopsy obtained from an unaffected area in her is seen in the figure.

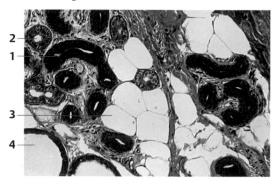

11. Involvement of which of the following structures is responsible for her symptoms?

A. 1
B. 2
C. 3
D. 4

12. Which of the following is a true statement for her?

A. Her palm and sole will soon be severely affected.
B. Her condition has accelerated since she attained puberty.
C. Smoking is not related to the disease process.
D. The affected structure opens directly onto the skin surface, so this will not involve any surrounding structures.
E. Her condition should not alter during her menstrual cycle.

13. Which of the following is true for structure 2?

A. This structure is most abundant in the vermillion zone of the lips.
B. This structure is most abundant in thin skin.
C. This structure opens directly onto the skin surface.
D. This structure is under parasympathetic cholinergic control.
E. Aldosterone has no effect on the final product from this structure.

Consider the following case for questions 14 to 18:

A pathology resident is analyzing the image, which was obtained from the normal skin of an elderly female.

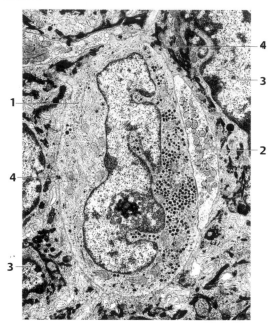

14. Which of the following is the possible area being examined within the biopsy?

A. Stratum granulosum
B. Stratum spinosum
C. Stratum basalis
D. Papillary layer, dermis
E. Reticular layer, dermis

15. Which of the following is true for structure 1?

A. These are abundant in thin skin.
B. These are abundant in the skin of the fingertips.
C. These are usually associated with blood capillaries.
D. These are usually associated with skeletal muscles.
E. These usually do not display keratin as intermediate filaments.

16. Which of the following is the primary function for structure 1?

A. Attachment between epidermal cells
B. Attachment of epidermis to the underlying dermis
C. Coloration of the skin
D. Processing of invading pathogens
E. Tactile two-point discrimination

17. Which of the following is the probable embryologic source for structure 1?

A. Surface ectoderm

B. Neuroectoderm

C. Visceral mesoderm

D. Parietal mesoderm

E. Endoderm

18. Which of the following is true for structures labeled 4?

A. These affect apical domain of cells.

B. These affect basal domain of cells.

C. These activities depend on extracellular Ca^{2+} concentration.

D. Their primary function is to synthesize pigments.

E. Their primary function is to generate energy for metabolic processes.

Consider the following case for questions 19 to 20:

A 24-year-old man presents with intensely pruritic, papulovesicular eruptions. These are symmetrically distributed over his elbows, knees, and buttocks. Characteristically, the mucous membranes are spared, as are the palms and soles. Each of the eruptions, according to him, appeared 8–12 hours following localized itching and burning.

19. Which of the following would you expect with an indirect immunofluorescence of the perilesional skin in him?

A. IgA bound to the cell surface of keratinocytes through the epidermis

B. IgG bound to the cell surface of keratinocytes through the epidermis

C. Linear pattern of IgG binding to the epidermal dermal junction

D. Granular pattern of IgA binding to the epidermal dermal junction

20. Which of the following might be an invariable associated finding in him?

A. Blunting of intestinal villi

B. Nonmotile respiratory cilia

C. Intraepidermal acantholysis

D. Nonmotile spermatozoa

7.2 Answers and Explanations

Easy	Medium	Hard

1. Correct: Her condition has accelerated since she attained puberty. (B)

The girl is suffering from acne vulgaris, and the indicated structure is a sebaceous gland. Acne vulgaris is a self-limited disorder of the pilosebaceous unit that is seen primarily in adolescents. Follicular epidermal proliferation and excess sebum production are key features in its pathogenesis. Both are stimulated by androgens and therefore accelerate on attaining puberty.

Sebaceous glands are exocrine glands that occur in all thin skin, most often in association with the hair follicles into which their ducts empty (**D**), but are most numerous in the skin of the face, forehead, and scalp (**E**). Thick skin (**A**) has fewer sebaceous glands, and acne is not a common association. Flareup of the disease in the luteal phase of the menstrual cycle (**C**) occurs after a boost in ovarian androgens, establishing the role of androgens in the pathogenic process. As indicated previously, epidermal proliferation and inflammation of hair follicles are keys to pathogenesis of acne (**D**).

2. Correct: Intraepidermal acantholysis (A)

The patient seems to suffer from pemphigus vulgaris (PV), which is a mucocutaneous blistering disease that predominantly occurs in patients over 40 years of age. PV typically begins on mucosal surfaces and often progresses to involve the skin. This disease is characterized by fragile, flaccid blisters that rupture to produce extensive denudation of mucous membranes and skin. The mouth, scalp, face, neck, axilla, groin, and trunk are typically involved, not the palms and soles.

PV presents with intraepidermal blistering characterized by loss of cohesion between epidermal cells (acantholysis). Nikolsky's sign is considered positive if application of pressure on either the blister, the perilesional skin, or the adjacent normal skin results in both peripheral extension of a blister and separation of the epidermis. This sign is positive in pemphigus vulgaris.

Choices **B, C, D**, and **E** are true for bullous pemphigoid (BP). It typically occurs in patients over 60 years of age and rarely involves oral mucosa. Also, subepidermal blisters in BP are tense and do not rupture easily. When ruptured, these usually do not cause denudation of mucosa or skin.

3.   Correct: Stratum spinosum (D)

Desmosomal proteins are targets for autoantibodies in PV. Desmosomes are most abundant within cells of stratum spinosum and anchor large bundles of keratin filaments between adjacent keratinocytes to provide the mechanical strength essential for resistance to physical trauma.

4.   Correct: Desmoglein (B)

Patients with PV have IgG autoantibodies to desmogleins, transmembrane desmosomal glycoproteins that belong to the cadherin family of calcium-dependent adhesion molecules.

Connexin (**A**, proteins forming gap junctions), BP 230 (**C**, hemidesmosomal protein), collagen type XVII (**D**, BP 180, hemidesmosomal protein), and type IV collagen (**E**, lamina densa, basal lamina) are not involved in PV.

5.   Correct: Hair follicles within the dermis (B)

In general, there are four recognized phases that characterize the cutaneous repair process: (1) coagulation (dominated by platelets), (2) inflammatory phase (dominated by leukocytes), (3) proliferative and migratory phase (tissue formation dominated by keratinocytes, endothelial cells, and fibroblasts), and (4) remodeling phase (dominated by myofibroblasts). Regeneration of epithelium (epidermis) belongs to the third phase.

In wounds that remove the entire epidermis, keratinocytes in the external root sheath of the hair follicles divide and migrate to cover the granulation tissue.

6.   Correct: Epidermal cells within the basal layer and wound edges (D)

Wounds with incomplete epidermal loss are typically recovered by dividing keratinocytes arising from the stratum basale and wound edges.

7.   Correct: Increase in epidermal thickness with addition of immature cells (D)

The patient is suffering from psoriasis, which is diagnosed by the classical appearance and distribution of the lesions. It is an immune-mediated disease clinically characterized by erythematous, sharply demarcated plaques covered by silvery scale with symmetrical involvement of extensor surfaces of the extremities and scalp.

In psoriasis, there is shortening of the usual duration of the keratinocyte cell cycle and excessive epidermal proliferation. This results in skin thickening (**C**) and plaque formation. Truncation of the cell cycle leads to an accumulation of immature cells within the cornified layer with retained nuclei. This pattern is known as parakeratosis and results in neutrophil migration (**E**) into the cornified layer. Together these form the silvery scale characteristic of psoriasis. Finally, psoriasis induces endothelial cell proliferation, resulting in pronounced dilation, tortuosity, and increased permeability of the capillaries in the superficial dermis (**E**) and causing erythema. Acantholysis (**A, B**) is not a usual finding in psoriasis.

8.   Correct: 3 and 4 (G)

The image key for the figure for questions 7 to 9 is as follows:

1 - stratum corneum

2 - stratum granulosum

3 - stratum spinosum

4 - stratum basale

5 - dermal papilla

Cell proliferation by mitosis occurs only in the Malpighian layer, which includes the stratum basale and stratum spinosum.

9.   Correct: Absence of dermatoglyphics (B)

Absence of stratum lucidum indicates that this section has been obtained from thin skin. Dermatoglyphics are the unique patterns of ridges and grooves formed in an individual that are characteristically found in thick skin. Also, choices **A, C, D**, and **E** are characteristics of thick skin.

10.   Correct: 3 (C)

The image key for the figure is as follows:

1 - stratum corneum

2 - stratum lucidum

3 - stratum granulosum

4 - stratum spinosum

5 - stratum basale

6 - papillary layer, dermis

7 - reticular layer, dermis

The child is suffering from ichthyosis vulgaris (IV). In IV, loss-of-function mutations in the profilaggrin gene causes impaired keratinization. Filaggrin is synthesized as a high-molecular weight precursor, profilaggrin, which contains multiple filaggrin molecules and is localized to keratohyalin granules. The granular layer cells are recognized by characteristic basophilic keratohyalin granules in the cytoplasm composed primarily of keratin filaments, filaggrin, and loricrin. Through their association with mature filaggrin, keratin filaments aggregate and form disulfide bonds, and a cornified cell envelope is assembled.

11. Correct: 4 (D)

The image key for the figure is as follows:

1 - duct of eccrine sweat gland (identified by compound epithelium—outer basal and inner luminal cells)

2 - acinus of eccrine sweat gland (identified by pseudostratified epithelium, narrow lumen)

3 - adipocyte

4 - acinus of apocrine sweat gland (identified by simple cuboidal epithelium enclosing a wide lumen)

She is suffering from hidradenitis suppurativa (HS), which is a recurrent inflammatory skin disease of the hair follicle (with consequent occlusion of surrounding apocrine glands). It usually presents after puberty with painful, deep-seated, inflammatory lesions in the apocrine gland-bearing areas of the body.

As indicated, secondary occlusion of apocrine sweat glands plays a key role in pathogenesis of HS.

12. Correct: Her condition has accelerated since she attained puberty. (B)

Apocrine glands are most common in axillary, inguinal, and anogenital regions. These are not found in the palm or sole (A). Poor hygiene, smoking (C), alcohol consumption, and bacterial involvement are thought to exacerbate the disease process. In contrast to eccrine glands, whose ducts open in the skin surface, apocrine glands empty their content into the follicular canal (D), just above the sebaceous gland duct. The primary histopathologic event is follicular hyperkeratosis with plugging and dilatation of the hair follicle, with secondary apocrine involvement. Flareup of the disease in the luteal phase of the menstrual cycle (E) occurs after a boost in ovarian androgens, establishing the role of androgens in the pathogenic process.

13. Correct: This structure opens directly onto the skin surface. (C)

Structure 2 indicates the acinus of an eccrine sweat gland, which is lined by a pseudostratified epithelium; its duct opens directly onto the skin surface. These glands are most abundant in thick skin (B) and absent in tympanic membrane, glans penis, glans clitoridis, and the vermilion border of the lips (A). Sweat is secreted in response to thermal, emotional, and taste stimuli, mediated by sympathetic cholinergic fibers (D). Sweat is modified as it passes along the duct by the action mainly of the basal cells, which resorb sodium, chloride, and water. Aldosterone enhances this activity (E).

14. Correct: Stratum basalis (C)

The image key for the figure is as follows:

1 - merkel cell (identified by large and lobed nucleus, and osmiophilic granules localized to cytoplasmic area that contacts the expanded nerve ending)

2 - unmyelinated nerve terminal with mitochondria

3 - keratinocyte

4. Macula adherens (desmosome)

Merkel cells are mostly scattered in the stratum basalis but are also found in bases of some hair follicles.

15. Correct: These are abundant in the skin of the fingertips (B)

Merkel cells are sensitive mechanoreceptors essential for light touch sensation. They are abundant in highly sensitive skin like that of fingertips.

They are more numerous in thick skin (A), associated with free nerve endings (C, D), and display keratin intermediate filaments (E).

16. Correct: Tactile two-point discrimination (E)

Merkel cells function as mechanoreceptors and are important in fine touch sensation for two-point discrimination.

Attachment between epidermal cells (A) is primarily achieved with desmosomes of keratinocytes within stratum spinosum, while attachment between epidermis and dermis (B) is primarily achieved by hemidesmosomes of keratinocytes within stratum basale. Keratinocytes will not present with such osmiophilic granules. Synthesized by melanocytes, melanin contributes to skin, eye, and hair color (C). Melanocytes might contain several melanin granules but will not be associated with a free nerve ending. Langerhans cells function as antigen-presenting cells within the epidermis (D). Ultrastructurally, these cells can be identified by Birbeck granules, which are flattened, discoid, membrane-bound granules showing a layer of latticed matrix material sandwiched by the granule membrane. In a cross section they appear as characteristic rod-like profiles with a dotted line of matrix down the midline.

17. Correct: Surface ectoderm (A)

Merkel cells originate from the same stem cells as keratinocytes (surface ectoderm), although their origin from neural crest cells has been debated for a long time.

18.   Correct: Its activity depends on extracellular Ca²⁺ concentration. (C)

Desmosomes utilize calcium-dependent transmembrane proteins, cadherins (desmoglein and desmocollin), to bind intermediate filaments of adjacent cells. These affect the lateral domain of cells (**A, B**) and primarily function to resist shearing forces (**D, E**).

19.   Correct: Granular pattern of IgA binding to the epidermal dermal junction (D)

The patient is suffering from dermatitis herpetiformis (DH), which is an intensely pruritic, papulovesicular skin disease characterized by lesions symmetrically distributed over extensor surfaces (i.e., elbows, knees, buttocks, back, scalp, and posterior neck). Mucous membrane lesions are uncommon, as are lesions on the palms and soles. Patients sometimes report that their pruritus has a distinctive burning or stinging component; the onset of such local symptoms reliably heralds the development of distinct clinical lesions 12 to 24 hours later.

Patients with DH have granular deposits of IgA in their epidermal basement membrane zone.

IgG (**B**), but not IgA (**A**), bound to the cell surface of keratinocytes through the epidermis is a feature of desmosomal affection in pemphigus vulgaris. A linear pattern of IgG binding to the epidermal dermal junction (**C**) occurs in bullous pemphigoid (autoantibodies against hemidesmosomal proteins).

20.   Correct: Blunting of intestinal villi (A).

Almost all DH patients have associated, usually subclinical, gluten-sensitive enteropathy. Biopsies of the small bowel usually reveal blunting of intestinal villi and a lymphocytic infiltrate in the lamina propria. Nonmotile cilia (**B**) or spermatozoa (**D**) could be encountered in ciliary dyskinesia. Subepidermal, but not intraepidermal (**C**), acantholysis occurs in DH.

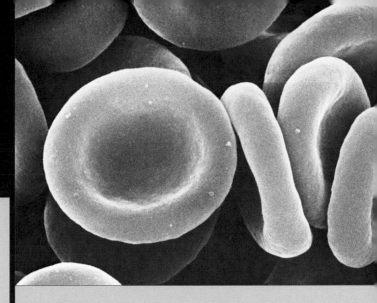

LEARNING OBJECTIVES

- ▶ Describe the microstructure of the spleen. Correlate this with its functions.
- ▶ Describe the microstructure of bone marrow. Correlate this with its functions.
- ▶ Describe the microstructure of a tonsil. Correlate this with its functions.
- ▶ Describe the formed elements found in peripheral blood. Correlate their structure with their functions.
- ▶ Describe the etiopathogenesis of anaphylaxis (type I hypersensitivity reaction). Correlate this with its clinical features.
- ▶ Describe the microstructure of a lymph node. Correlate this with its functions.
- ▶ Describe the etiopathogenesis of pernicious anemia. Correlate this with its clinical features.
- ▶ Describe the microstructure of the thymus. Correlate this with its functions.

8.1 Questions

Easy	Medium	Hard

Consider the following case for questions 1 to 2:

A 16-year-old boy, following an educational tour of Brazil, presents with fever accompanied by chills and rigor. Thin blood smears obtained from him were positive for *Plasmodium vivax*. The biopsy of an organ obtained from him can be seen in the figure.

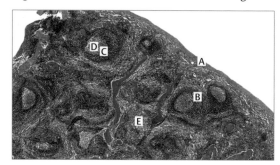

1. Which of the following areas would, most likely, sequester plasmodium-containing erythrocytes?

A. A

B. B

C. C

D. D

E. E

2. Which of the following zones will atrophy in case of a developmental disorder involving the third pharyngeal pouch?

A. A

B. B

C. C

D. D

E. E

3. A 66-year-old man presents with pallor, low-grade fever, and moderate hepatosplenomegaly. Bone marrow aspirate obtained from his right iliac crest can be seen in the figure. Which of the following is true for the space indicated by Y?

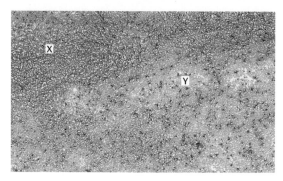

A. Primarily contains cells secreting factors responsible for hemopoiesis

B. Primarily contains mature cells to be released into the peripheral bloodstream

C. Primarily contains hematopoietic cell population

D. Primarily contains leukocytes and their precursors

E. Primarily contains erythrocytes and their precursors

4. In an attempt to review formed elements in a peripheral blood smear before your block final, you obtain the figure. For reviewing, which of the following cells would you require additional slides from your collection?

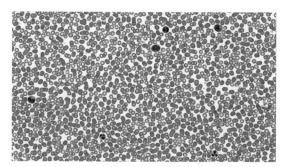

A. Erythrocytes

B. Thrombocytes

C. Lymphocytes

D. Basophils

E. Eosinophils

F. Neutrophils

G. Monocytes

Consider the following case for questions 5 to 7:

A 6-year-old boy presents with acute malaise and shivering. For the past 12 hours, he had complained of a dry, sore throat and had vomited twice. Physical examination revealed fever (104°F), tachycardia, and tender, bilateral, cervical lymphadenopathy. A surgical specimen obtained from the child was biopsied (image).

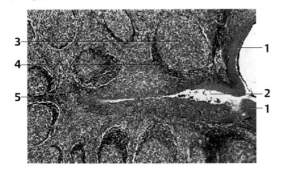

5. Which of the following is the likely source of the biopsy?

A. Spleen

B. Nasopharyngeal tonsil

C. Palatine tonsil

D. Deep cervical lymph node

E. Thymus

6. Which of the following is a primary function of the organ?

A. Positive selection of lymphocytes for MHC recognition

B. Negative selection of lymphocytes for autoantigen recognition

C. Filtration of foreign antigen transported across epithelium

D. Filtration of foreign antigen from lymph

E. Filtration of foreign antigen from blood

7. Which of the following is correct about the histological structure of the organ?

A. It is surrounded by a complete well-formed capsule.

B. Lymphocytes are present only in diffuse lymphatic tissue.

C. Lymphoid nodules are exclusively secondary.

D. Afferent and efferent lymphatics pierce the capsule.

E. Overlying epithelium is infiltrated with lymphocytes.

8. A 56-year-old man presents with a complicated anemia. Preliminary investigations reveal defective hematopoiesis. To help further in diagnosis, you order a biopsy from his chief hematopoietic organ. Which of the following would be a potential source of biopsy for the individual?

A. Spleen

B. Inguinal lymph nodes

C. Iliac crest

D. Liver

E. Tibia

Consider the following case for questions 9 to 11:

A 12-year-old boy presents to the ER with wheezing. He was well until he was stung by a bee while playing in the yard. He initially complained of localized pain and swelling. Twenty minutes later, he could not breathe. He also complained of dizziness. Physical examination reveals edema and erythema of the bee-stung area, and severe wheezing with reduced air entry to bilateral lungs.

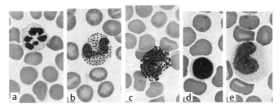

9. Which of the following panels contain cells that are responsible for his symptoms?

A. A

B. B

C. C

D. D

E. E

10. Which of the following is true for the cell responsible for his symptoms?

A. The specific granules stain intensely with eosin.

B. The cell expresses high-affinity IgG receptors on the surface.

C. The cell produces and secretes IgG in response to antigen.

D. The cell expresses high-affinity IgE receptors on the surface.

E. The cell produces and secretes IgE in response to antigen.

11. Which of the following should be unaltered in the boy, such that the attending physician does not need to worry about it immediately?

A. Mean corpuscular hemoglobin

B. Smooth muscle contraction

C. Gastric secretion

D. Vascular permeability

E. Blood pressure

Consider the following case for questions 12 to 14:

A 46-year-old female presents with advanced-stage breast carcinoma. Biopsies were obtained from the primary growth and secondarily involved organs. One such specimen can be seen in the figure.

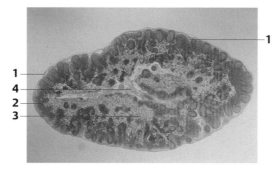

12. Which of the following is a primary function for the organ?

A. Positive selection of lymphocytes for MHC recognition

B. Negative selection of lymphocytes for autoantigen recognition

C. Filtration of foreign antigens transported across epithelium

D. Filtration of foreign antigen from lymph

E. Filtration of foreign antigen from blood

13. Which of the following zones is a primary source for IgG in response to antigens?

A. 1

B. 2

C. 3

D. 4

14. Which of the following zones serves as the entry point for circulating (blood) lymphocytes?

A. 1

B. 2

C. 3

D. 4

Consider the following case for questions 15 to 18:

A 42-year-old woman presents with complaints of progressive fatigue and weakness for the past 3 months. She is short of breath after walking several blocks. Physical examination reveals tachycardia, pale conjunctivae, and a beefy red tongue with loss of papillae. A peripheral blood smear obtained from her is seen in the figure.

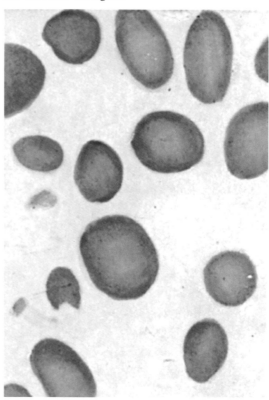

15. Which of the following is the most likely diagnosis for her?

A. Iron deficiency anemia

B. Hereditary spherocytosis

C. Pernicious anemia

D. Hemolytic anemia

E. Aplastic anemia

16. Which of the following might be a probable cause for her symptoms?

A. Menorrhagia

B. Autoimmune destruction of gastric parietal cells

C. Alteration of gene encoding for spectrin

D. Bone marrow failure

E. Bleeding peptic ulcer

17. Which of the following might be an additional finding in her blood smear?

A. Basophilic stippling

B. Spherocytes

C. Target cells

D. Howell-Jolly bodies

E. Hypersegmentation of neutrophils

18. Which of the following might be an associated clinical feature in her?

A. Hyperacidity

B. Hematochezia

C. Peripheral neuropathy

D. Splenomegaly

E. Moderate jaundice

Consider the following case for questions 19 to 20:

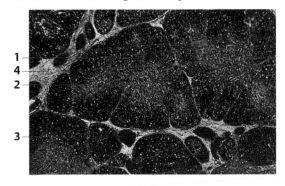

19. Which of the following is absent in patients with congenital agenesis of the organ?

A. T lymphocytes

B. CD4+ cells

C. Plasma cells

D. Monocytes

E. Mast cells

20. Which of the following is a function for structure 1?

A. Major site for generation of immune responses

B. Positive selection for MHC recognition

C. Negative selection for autoantigen recognition

D. Filtration of foreign antigen from lymph

E. Filtration of foreign antigen from blood

8.2 Answers and Explanations

Easy	Medium	Hard

1. Correct: E (E)

The boy is suffering from malaria. The organ in the figure can be identified as spleen by presence of red pulp and white pulp.

The image key for the figure is as follows: A, capsule; B, periarteriolar lymphatic sheath (PALS); C, germinal center; D, mantle zone; E, red pulp.

Red pulp is a unique mechanical filter that clears particulate matter from the blood. Blood cells containing large, rigid inclusions, such as plasmodium-containing erythrocytes, are sequestered in the red pulp.

The connective tissue capsule (**A**) dives into the substance of the spleen as trabeculae that convey splenic vessels and nerves. The PALS (**B**) is the zone rich in immunocompetent T lymphocytes; hence it plays an important role in cell-mediated immunity. The germinal center (**C**, active B lymphocytes) and mantle zone (**D**, resting B lymphocytes) form secondary lymphoid follicles within the white pulp of the spleen.

2. Correct: B (B)

The periarteriolar lymphatic sheath (PALS, identified by the adjacent "eccentric" arteriole) is the zone within the spleen that primarily contains immunocompetent T lymphocytes. In disorders of the third pharyngeal pouch (as in DiGeorge's syndrome), thymic aplasia will deplete the supply of such cells, resulting in thinning out of the PALS.

3. Correct: Primarily contains mature cells to be released into the peripheral blood stream (B)

X indicates hematopoietic cords and Y indicates sinusoids of bone marrow. Bone marrow contains specialized blood capillaries (sinusoids) into which newly developed mature blood cells and platelets are released, subsequently to be delivered into the peripheral circulation.

Adventitial (reticular) cells partially line the sinusoids and produce reticular fibers that support the hematopoietic cords. These cells secrete hematopoietic factors (**A**). Hematopoietic cells (i.e., the precursors of formed elements) constitute the marrow cords. These cells are not found in the marrow sinuses in normal health (**C–E**).

4. Correct: Basophils (D)

The micrograph, as shown in the figure, contains each of the listed cells in the question except the basophils. Basophils are identified by metachromatic cytoplasmic granules obscuring the nucleus. Therefore, you would require additional slides for reviewing those.

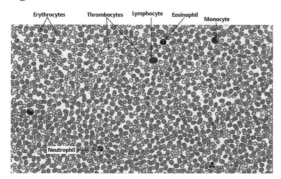

Erythrocytes (**A**) can be identified as uniformly staining eosinophilic circles without nuclei. Thrombocytes (**B**) can be identified as small basophilic fragments, often in clusters. Lymphocytes (**C**) can be identified by their round, dense nuclei almost filling up the agranular cytoplasm. Eosinophils (**E**) can be identified by their bilobed nuclei with eosinophilic specific granules. Neutrophils (**F**) can be identified by their multilobed nuclei held together by thin strands. Monocytes (**G**) can be identified by their large size, eccentric kidney-shaped nuclei, and finely granular cytoplasm (azurophilic granules).

5. Correct: Palatine tonsil (C)

The child had acute tonsillitis and underwent a tonsillectomy.

The organ can be identified as palatine tonsil by characteristic epithelial invagination into the underlying connective tissue, forming crypts (structure 2), nonkeratinized stratified squamous oral epithelium (structure 1), and plenty of secondary lymphatic follicles (nodules) containing germinal centers (structure 3).

The spleen (**A**) is identified by white and red pulp. The nasopharyngeal tonsil (**B**) is identified by respiratory (pseudostratified ciliated columnar with goblet cells) epithelium; tonsillar crypts are not prominent, and the capsule is thinner. A lymph node (**D**) is identified by lymphoid tissue comprising outer dark cortex and inner pale medulla. The thymus (**E**) is identified by the presence of lobules, each of which is seen to comprise outer dark cortex and inner pale medulla.

6. Correct: Filtration of foreign antigen transported across epithelium (C)

Tonsils function in filtration of inhaled or ingested foreign antigen across oral epithelium.

Positive selection of T lymphocytes for MHC recognition (**A**) occurs in the cortex of the thymus.

Negative selection of T lymphocytes for autoantigen recognition (**B**) occurs in medulla of the thymus. Filtration of foreign antigen from lymph (**D**) and blood (**E**) are primary functions of lymph nodes and spleen, respectively.

7. Correct: Overlying epithelium is infiltrated with lymphocytes. (E)

Epithelial lining of the crypts is densely infiltrated with lymphocytes.

Tonsils are partially encapsulated (**A**, formed by connective tissue) lymphoid aggregates that might form nodules (**B**) or stay diffused. Primary and secondary lymphoid follicles are both seen (**C**) depending on the immunologic status at any given time. Unlike lymph nodes, palatine tonsils do not possess afferent lymphatics (**D**). Efferent lymphatics pass through the capsule and drain primarily into jugulodigastric (deep cervical) lymph nodes.

8. Correct: Iliac crest (C)

Bone marrow is the chief hematopoietic organ after birth. While long bones (**E**) are dependable sources of red marrow before the age of 20, flat bones (iliac crest [most common], ribs, sternum, vertebrae, etc.) are frequently used for aspiration in adults. The liver (**D**) and spleen (**A**) serve as hematopoietic organs in the fetus and during some disease processes in adults. Lymph nodes (**B**) are not hematopoietic organs.

9. Correct: C (C)

The boy is suffering from anaphylaxis, a type I hypersensitivity reaction. These reactions are initiated by interaction of antigen with specific IgE antibodies bound to mast cells and basophils (via high-affinity FcεRI receptors) with subsequent release of inflammatory mediators. Interaction of mediators with specific target organs and cells frequently induces a biphasic response: an early effect on blood vessels, smooth muscle, and secretory glands marked by vascular leakiness, smooth-muscle constriction, and mucus hypersecretion, and a late response characterized by mucosal edema and the influx of inflammatory cells.

Panel C contains a basophil, identified by the presence of coarse basophilic granules obscuring the nucleus. Panel A contains a neutrophil, identified by the hypersegmented nucleus. Panel B contains an eosinophil, identified by coarse eosinophilic granules and bilobed nucleus. Panel D contains a lymphocyte, identified by a rim of agranular cytoplasm and the large spherical nucleus. Panel E contains a monocyte, identified by the large size, kidney-shaped nucleus, and fine granules (azurophilic) within the cytoplasm.

10. Correct: The cell expresses high-affinity IgE receptors on the surface. (D)

As mentioned above, anaphylaxis is initiated by interaction of antigen with specific IgE antibodies bound to mast cells and basophils (via high affinity FcεRI receptors) with subsequent release of inflammatory mediators.

Specific granules of basophils are not acidophilic, and therefore do not stain with eosin (**A**). Basophils do not express high affinity IgG receptors on the surface (**B**), nor do they produce antibodies (**C, E**) in response to antigen. Production of antibodies is a function of plasma cells.

11. Correct: Mean corpuscular hemoglobin (A)

Mean corpuscular hemoglobin is defined as the amount of hemoglobin in the average red cell. It is increased in macrocytosis (e.g., megaloblastic anemia), decreased in microcytosis (e.g., iron deficiency), and not affected by anaphylaxis.

Mediators of anaphylaxis (histamine, slow-reacting substance of anaphylaxis, eosinophil chemotactic factor of anaphylaxis, serotonin, prostaglandin, thromboxane, platelet-activating factor, etc.) cause vasodilation, increased vascular permeability (**D**), smooth muscle contraction (**B**), bronchospasm, and hypotension (**E**). Histamine is also a potent stimulator of gastric secretion (**C**).

12. Correct: Filtration of foreign antigen from lymph (D)

The organ can be identified as a lymph node by the characteristic division of lymphoid tissue into outer darker cortex, containing secondary lymphoid follicles with germinal centers, and inner pale medulla. Lymph nodes generate antigen-primed B and T lymphocytes and filter lymph-borne antigens.

Positive selection of T lymphocytes for MHC recognition (**A**) occurs in the cortex of the thymus. Negative selection of T lymphocytes for autoantigen recognition (**B**) occurs in the medulla of the thymus. Tonsils function in filtration of inhaled or ingested foreign antigen across oral epithelium (**C**). Filtration of foreign antigen from blood (**E**) occurs in the spleen.

13. Correct: 2 (B)

Immunoglobulins are produced by activated B lymphocytes, which reside in the germinal centers of the secondary lymphoid follicles. These are concentrated in the cortex of the lymph node.

The capsule (**A**) is pierced by afferent lymphatics that empty next into subcapsular sinuses. The deep cortex or paracortex (**C**) is primarily populated by T cells. The medulla (**D**) contains lymphocytes and plasma cells, but these are less densely packed than in the cortex. Macrophages are the predominant cell population here.

14. Correct: 3 (C)

Postcapillary high-endothelial venules (HEV) are abundant in the paracortex. These contain homing receptors for circulating (blood) lymphocytes and serve as their point of entry into the organ.

15. Correct: Pernicious anemia (C)

The patient presents with typical features of anemia, and in this case megaloblastic anemia. This can be diagnosed from the peripheral blood smear that shows numerous macro-ovalocytes with anisocytosis and poikilocytosis. Pernicious anemia is a megaloblastic anemia in which there is abnormal erythrocyte nuclear maturation due to severe lack of IF consequent to gastric atrophy.

Iron deficiency (**A**) will present as a microcytic hypochromic anemia. Hereditary spherocytosis (**B**), hemolysis (**D**), and aplastic anemia (**E**) present as normocytic anemias.

16. Correct: Autoimmune destruction of gastric parietal cells (B)

The gastric parietal cells (secrete HCl and intrinsic factor) are initially affected by an autoimmune phenomenon that leads to achlorhydria and loss of intrinsic factor. Pernicious anemia interferes with both the initial availability and the absorption of vitamin B_{12}. HCl is required for the release of cobalamin from foodstuff, and intrinsic factor binds cobalamin and is required for the effective absorption of cobalamin in the terminal ileum.

Menorrhagia (**A**) or bleeding peptic ulcer (**E**) will present as iron deficiency (microcytic hypochromic) anemia; alteration of gene encoding for spectrin (**C**) will present with spherocytosis; and bone marrow failure (**D**) will present as aplastic anemia.

17. Correct: Hypersegmentation of neutrophils (E)

The classic picture in pernicious anemia reveals significant anisocytosis and poikilocytosis of the red cell line, and hypersegmented neutrophils, revealing the nuclear dysgenesis from abnormal DNA synthesis.

Basophilic stippling (**A**) is diffuse fine or coarse blue dots in the red cell usually representing RNA residue. This is especially common in lead poisoning. Spherocytes (**B**) are red cells without the central pallor. They can be seen in hereditary spherocytosis and other hemolytic anemias. Target cells (**C**) have an area of central pallor that contains a dense center, or bull's eye. These cells are classically seen in thalassemia, but they are also present in iron deficiency, cholestatic liver disease, and some hemoglobinopathies. Howell-Jolly bodies (**D**) are dense blue circular inclusions that represent nuclear remnants. Their presence commonly implies defective splenic function.

18.   Correct: Peripheral neuropathy (C)

Peripheral neuropathy is an important finding in vitamin B_{12} deficiency states. Subacute combined degeneration of the spinal cord presents with paresthesias in the hands and feet, loss of vibration and position sensation, and a progressive spastic and ataxic weakness. Loss of reflexes due to an associated peripheral neuropathy (LMN sign) in a patient who also has Babinski signs (UMN sign) is an important diagnostic clue.

Gastric atrophy and achlorhydria (therefore, not hyperacidity [**A**]) are chief features of pernicious anemia. Hematochezia (**B**) will present as iron deficiency due to blood loss. Splenomegaly (**D**) and jaundice (**E**) are both prominent features of hemolytic anemia.

19.   Correct: CD4+ cells (B)

The organ can be identified as the thymus by the characteristic lobulated appearance, and each lobule presenting a darker staining cortex and a pale medulla.

T lymphocytes become immunocompetent and acquire surface receptors in the thymus. Thus, in its absence, CD4+ cells will be absent in circulation.

In the absence of the thymus, circulating T lymphocytes will stay naïve, but will still be present in circulation (**A**). Plasma cells (**C**, activated B lymphocytes, derived in bone marrow and activated in secondary lymphoid organs), monocytes (**D**, derived in bone marrow), or mast cells (**E**, derived in bone marrow, activated in peripheral tissue) will not be affected in thymic agenesis.

20.   Correct: Positive selection for MHC recognition (B)

The image key for the figure is as follows: 1, cortex; 2, medulla; 3, blood vessels; 4, trabecular connective tissue.

The thymic cortex is the site for positive selection of T lymphocytes for MHC recognition, while the thymic medulla is the site for negative selection of T lymphocytes for recognition of autoantigens (**C**). Secondary lymphoid organs (like lymph nodes) are sites where immune responses are generated (**A**). Filtration of foreign antigen from lymph (**D**, lymph node) or blood (**E**, spleen) does not occur in the thymus.

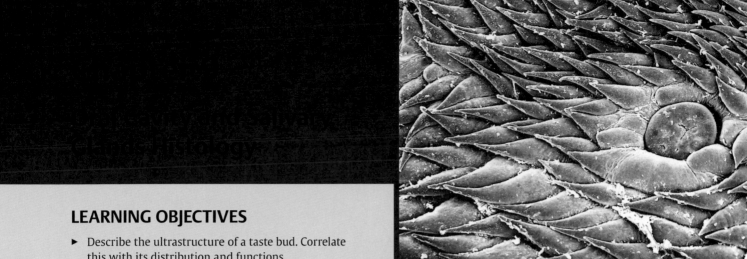

LEARNING OBJECTIVES

▶ Describe the ultrastructure of a taste bud. Correlate this with its distribution and functions.

▶ Correlate innervation of the tongue with its development.

▶ Describe the blood supply of the tongue.

▶ Describe microstructure of major salivary glands. Correlate their structural difference with their functions.

▶ Analyze the microstructure of serous, mucous, myoepithelial, and ductal cells within salivary glands. Correlate these with their functions.

▶ Describe the secretomotor supply to major salivary glands.

▶ Describe the microstructure of the lip. Correlate its innervation to its function.

▶ Illustrate the mucocutaneous transition at the vermilion zone.

9.1 Questions

Easy | Medium | Hard

Consider the following case for questions 1 to 2:

When attempting to pierce the tip of her tongue, a 15-year-old damages the indicated structures in the figure.

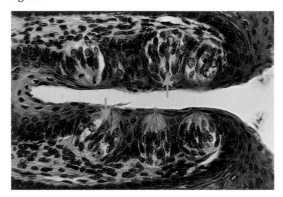

1. Primary afferents from the indicated structures travel through which of the following cranial nerves?

A. V, trigeminal

B. VII, facial

C. IX, glossopharyngeal

D. X, vagus

E. XII, hypoglossal

2. If the sensory loss involves damage of neuronal perikaryon, which of the following structures might be affected?

A. Trigeminal ganglion

B. Pterygopalatine ganglion

C. Geniculate ganglion

D. Inferior glossopharyngeal (petrosal) ganglion

E. Inferior vagal (nodose) ganglion

3. A 36-year-old male patient presents with sialorrhea that apparently has developed as a side effect from antipsychotics. A physical examination reveals enlargement of multiple salivary glands. Biopsies obtained from several of these are being observed under the microscope. Which of the following statements is true for the gland in the figure?

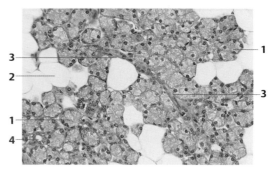

A. It is predominantly a mucus-secreting gland.

B. It is traversed by the facial nerve.

C. Its ducts open in the floor of the oral cavity at a papilla, one on each side of the frenulum linguae.

D. Its secretomotor fibers are carried in the facial nerve.

E. It lacks intercalated ducts in its structure.

4. A 39-year-old man comes to his physician because of a painful ulcer located in the tip of the organ depicted in the figure. The cranial nerve that transmits this patient's pain is also involved in which of the following functions?

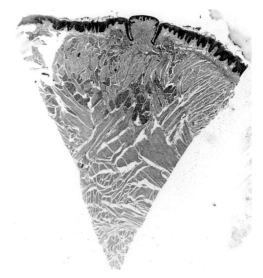

A. Lacrimation

B. Salivation

C. Mastication

D. Speech articulation

E. Tongue protrusion

5. A 45-year-old woman presents with painful swelling on the left side of her face. The swelling has enlarged over the past three days, and the pain radiates to the left ear and aggravates when she is chewing. A physical examination reveals enlargement of several major salivary glands. Excision biopsies obtained from one of these are examined under the microscope. Which of the following is true of the gland in the figure?

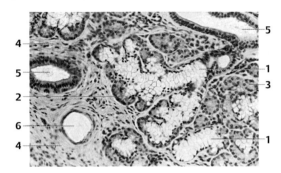

A. It is a predominantly serous-secreting gland.

B. It is an exclusively serous-secreting gland.

C. Its secretomotor fibers are carried in the facial nerve.

D. Its secretomotor fibers are carried in the glossopharyngeal nerve.

E. Its duct opens at a small elevation on the mucosal surface of the cheek opposite the second upper molar tooth.

Consider the following case for questions 6 to 7:

A 24-year-old woman presents to the outpatient department with complaints of foreign body sensation of the throat for the last 1 year. A physical examination and contrast enhanced CT scan of the neck revealed a pleomorphic adenoma affecting the base of the tongue, and a midline glossotomy was performed. The image is obtained from her biopsy specimen.

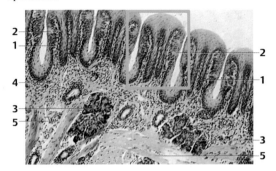

6. Which of the following is true for the structure contained within the blue rectangle in the figure?

A. It is devoid of taste buds.

B. It is heavily keratinized.

C. It lies parallel and anterior to sulcus terminalis.

D. It is not frequently found in the adult human.

E. The connective tissue underneath is devoid of lingual glands.

7. Which of the following cranial nerves innervates the structures labeled 5 in the figure?

A. V, trigeminal

B. VII, facial

C. IX, glossopharyngeal

D. X, vagus

E. XII, hypoglossal

8. During facial reconstruction surgery following a trauma in a 68-year-old man, normal glandular tissue from several of his major salivary glands was removed. A histological slide obtained from one such tissue specimen is seen in the figure. Which of the following is true for the cell outlined in blue?

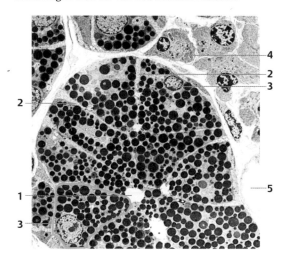

A. It is the primary cell found in the sublingual gland.

B. It is the primary cell found in the parotid gland.

C. It is the only cell found in the submandibular gland.

D. It produces a thick, viscid secretion.

E. The basal portion of the cell stains strongly acidophilic in H&E preparations.

9. A 36-year-old man presented with a tumor encroaching the middle ear cavity and compressing the chorda tympani nerve. Which of the following structures might be functionally impaired?

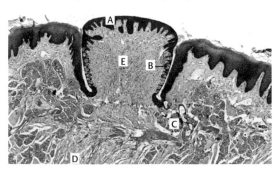

A. A

B. B

C. C

D. D

E. E

Consider the following case for questions 10 to 11:

A 44-year-old woman presents with a 6-month history of a painless swelling in the region of the right parotid gland. Fine needle aspiration shows presence of hyperplastic glandular cells. Surgical excision of the mass included a portion of the normal parotid gland. A Masson-Goldner stained paraffin section is being examined under the microscope (image).

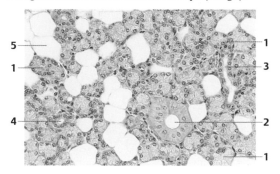

10. Which of the following is true for the structure labeled 2?

A. The cells actively secrete Cl^- in saliva.

B. The cells actively absorb K^+ from saliva.

C. The cells actively secrete HCO_3^- in saliva.

D. It has no major role in modifying the composition of saliva.

E. Its length is shortest in the sublingual gland among the major salivary glands.

11. Which of the following is correct for the structure labeled 4 in the figure?

A. The cells actively secrete Cl^- in saliva.

B. The cells actively secrete K^+ from saliva.

C. The cells actively secrete HCO_3^- in saliva.

D. It has no major role in modifying the composition of saliva.

E. It is lined by tall columnar cells.

12. A 65-year-old woman presents with a five-month history of a painful ulcer on the tongue. It did not improve with topical therapy, and an incisional biopsy was performed. A histopathological slide obtained from the specimen is being examined. Which of the following is true for structure 1 in the figure?

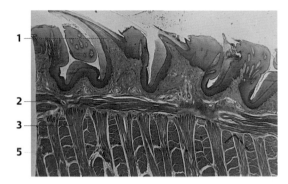

A. It is rarely found in the human tongue.

B. It is devoid of taste buds.

C. It is associated with a thick smooth muscle layer.

D. It is distributed predominantly parallel and anterior to the sulcus terminalis.

E. It is distributed predominantly parallel and posterior to the sulcus terminalis.

Consider the following case for questions 13 to 15:

A 13-year-old child reports to the clinic with a small swelling on the right lower lip for the past two months. The swelling was diagnosed as a mucocele and was surgically resected along with a surrounding rim of normal lip tissue (image).

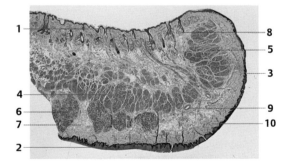

13. Which of the following is true for structure 1?

A. Lined by simple columnar epithelial cells

B. Characterized by absence of keratin

C. Associated with numerous sebaceous glands

D. Associated with pronounced smooth muscles

E. Associated with sensory nerve endings of the facial nerve

14. Which of the following is true for structure 2?

A. Characterized by a thick keratin layer

B. Associated with numerous sebaceous glands

C. Associated with pronounced smooth muscles

D. Characterized by a deep stratum granulosum layer

E. Characterized by stratified squamous epithelial lining thicker than skin

15. Which of the following is true for structure 4?

A. This would be paralyzed in a lesion involving the nucleus ambiguus.

B. This would be paralyzed in a midline tumor affecting the floor of the 4th ventricle.

C. This would be paralyzed in a patient with absent jaw jerk reflex.

D. This would be paralyzed in a lesion involving the pterygopalatine ganglion.

E. This would be paralyzed in a stroke affecting the posterior limb of the internal capsule.

Consider the following case for questions 16 to 17:

While reviewing histological structures pertinent to gastrointestinal (GI) organs before the block final, you come across the figure.

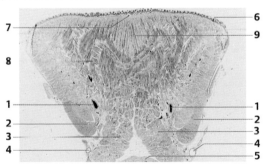

16. Which of the following structures will you be able to review from the image?

A. Simple columnar epithelium

B. Villi

C. Goblet cells

D. Striated muscles

E. Smooth muscles

17. Which of the following is the source of an infarct, if structure 1 was affected?

A. Vertebral artery

B. Basilar artery

C. Internal carotid artery

D. External carotid artery

E. Superior mesenteric artery

18. A 48-year-old female patient was admitted with a pleomorphic adenoma of the hard palate. Surgical removal of the mass accompanied excision of minimal normal glandular tissue from the sublingual salivary gland (image). Which of the following is true for structure 3?

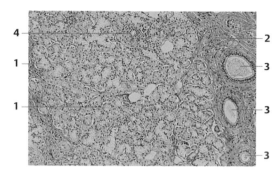

A. It is lined by simple cuboidal epithelium.

B. Basal cytoplasm of its cells presents infoldings lodging numerous mitochondria.

C. The cells actively secrete K^+ in saliva.

D. The cells actively secrete HCO_3^- in saliva.

E. It has no major role in modifying the composition of saliva.

19. A 69-year-old man presented with a tumor of the right submandibular gland. A histological slide prepared from the biopsy specimen has been attached. Which of the following is true for the structure indicated by 2 in the figure?

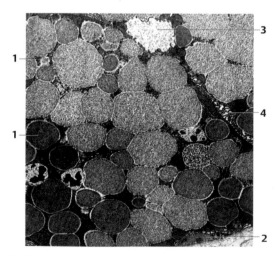

A. It secretes watery fluid rich in enzymes.

B. It secretes viscid fluid rich in mucus.

C. Contraction helps to expel secretory product from acinar lumen into the ducts.

D. It is the primary cell type in any salivary gland.

E. It possesses desmin as intermediate filaments.

20. An 81-year-old woman presented with a 2-year history of a nonpainful mass in the right cheek that recently increased in size. The patient underwent a wide local tumor resection via a transoral approach, which included normal glandular tissue from a major salivary gland (image). Which of the following is true of the gland in the figure?

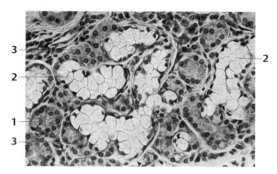

A. It is predominantly a mucous gland.

B. It is exclusively a serous gland.

C. It is traversed by the facial nerve.

D. Its secretomotor fibers are carried in the facial nerve.

E. Its secretomotor fibers are carried in the glossopharyngeal nerve.

9.2 Answers and Explanations

Easy	Medium	Hard

1. Correct: VII, facial (B)

The arrows indicate taste buds (identified by shape and component cells [sensory, supporting, and basal]).

Taste sensation from the tip of the tongue is carried by the chorda tympani, a branch of the facial nerve. The glossopharyngeal (**C**) nerve conveys taste fibers from the posterior third of the tongue (including vallate papillae), and the vagus (**D**) nerve carries such fibers from the epiglottis, vallecula, and soft palate. Trigeminal (**A**) or hypoglossal (**E**) nerves are not involved with taste sensation.

The chorda tympani nerve hitchhikes with the lingual nerve (branch of mandibular division, V_3, of trigeminal) to reach the tongue. This does not mean that the taste fibers are carried by the trigeminal—a common confusion among students.

2. Correct: Geniculate ganglion (C)

Cell bodies for first-order neurons of the chorda tympani nerve involved in taste sensation are located in the geniculate ganglion of the facial nerve. The second-order neurons lie in the rostral nucleus solitarius (gustatory nucleus), and the third-order neurons in the ventral posteromedial (VPM) nucleus of the thalamus. The third-order neurons project to the gustatory area (43) of the cerebral cortex.

The trigeminal ganglion (**A**) contains cell bodies of sensory fibers (discriminative touch, pain, temperature, etc.) carried by the trigeminal nerve from the face. The pterygopalatine ganglion (**B**), functionally related to the facial nerve, contains cell bodies of postganglionic parasympathetic (secretomotor) fibers for lacrimal, nasal, and palatine glands. The inferior glossopharyngeal ganglion (**D**) contains cell bodies for first order neurons of the glossopharyngeal nerve, involved in taste sensation from the posterior third of the tongue. The inferior vagal ganglion (**E**) contains cell bodies for first-order neurons of the vagus nerve, involved in taste sensation from the epiglottis and vallecula.

3. Correct: It is traversed by the facial nerve. (B)

The image, as identified by exclusively serous acini (structure 1), is the parotid salivary gland. The identity of the gland is further established by abundance of adipose tissue (structure 2) seen in the slide (a distinguishing histological feature). The facial nerve traverses this gland and, within the substance of the gland, gives off branches that supply facial muscles. Structures 3 and 4 are intercalated ducts in longitudinal and transverse sections, respectively.

The sublingual is predominantly a mucous gland (**A**), while the parotid is exclusively serous. The submandibular duct (Wharton's) opens in the floor of the oral cavity at a sublingual papilla, one on each side of the frenulum linguae (**C**). The parotid duct (Stenson's) opens at the parotid papilla, a small elevation on the mucosal surface of the cheek opposite the second upper molar tooth. Secretomotor fibers for the parotid gland are carried in the glossopharyngeal nerve, while those for the submandibular and sublingual glands are carried in the facial (chorda tympani) nerve (**D**). None of the major salivary glands lack intercalated duct (**E**), and parotid actually has the largest representation of it amongst the three.

4. Correct: Mastication (C)

The image can be identified as the tongue from the lining stratified squamous epithelium, papillae, and skeletal muscle fibers that run in three different planes (each arranged at right angles to the other two). Pain sensation from the tip of the tongue is carried by mandibular division of the trigeminal nerve, which also supplies motor fibers to the muscles of mastication.

Lacrimation (**A**, facial nerve), salivation (**B**, facial and glossopharyngeal nerve), articulation (**D**, vagus nerve), and protrusion of the tongue (**E**, hypoglossal nerve) are not functions of the trigeminal nerve.

5. Correct: Its secretomotor fibers are carried in the facial nerve. (C)

The image can be identified as the sublingual salivary gland by predominant mucous tubules (structure 1), a few serous acini (structure 3), and serous demilunes (structure 2). Secretomotor fibers for the gland are carried in the chorda tympani branch of the facial nerve. Structures 4 to 7 denote connective tissue, interlobular duct, vein, and striated duct, respectively.

The sublingual is a predominantly mucous gland, while the submandibular is predominantly serous (**A**), and the parotid is exclusively serous (**B**). Secretomotor fibers for the parotid gland are carried in the glossopharyngeal nerve (**D**), and its duct (Stensen's) opens at the parotid papilla, a small elevation on the mucosal surface of the cheek opposite the second upper molar tooth (**E**).

6. Correct: It is not frequently found in the adult human. (D)

The structure contained within the blue rectangle is a foliate papilla (identified by its leaf-like shape, and appearance of similar papillae in rows separated by deep clefts). In human beings, these are well developed only in children.

Foliate papillae are covered by stratified squamous nonkeratinized epithelium (**B**) containing numerous taste buds (**A**) on their lateral surfaces. Filiform papillae do not possess taste buds and are composed of keratinized epithelium. Vallate papillae are found parallel and anterior to sulcus terminalis (**C**). The connective tissue within and underneath the foliate papillae contain serous glands (von Ebner's) that open via ducts into the cleft between neighboring papillae (**E**).

7. Correct: XII, hypoglossal (E)

Image key:

1 – connective tissue cords
2 – taste buds
3 – serous glands
4 – lamina propria
5 – skeletal muscle

The hypoglossal nerve is the motor supply to all extrinsic and intrinsic tongue muscles (with the exception of the palatoglossus).

The trigeminal nerve (**A**) is responsible for general sensation from the anterior two-thirds of the tongue. The facial nerve (**B**) is responsible for taste sensation from the anterior two-thirds of the tongue and for supplying secretomotor fibers to serous glands (von Ebner's). The glossopharyngeal nerve (**C**) is responsible for general and taste sensation from the posterior third of the tongue. The vagus nerve (**D**) is responsible for taste sensation from the epiglottis and the vallecula.

8. Correct: It is the primary cell found in the parotid gland. (B)

Image key:

1 – acinar lumen

2 – intercellular secretory canaliculi

3 – cell nuclei

4 – plasma cell

5 – capillary; blue outlined cell—serous cell

The cell outlined in blue can be identified as a serous (protein-secreting) cell by conspicuous, secretory granules spread through the cell. These granules are homogeneously osmiophilic under the electron microscope, as opposed to the variably dense granules of mucus-secreting cells. The acinar cells of the parotid gland are exclusively serous.

Mucus-secreting cells are the major cells of the sublingual gland (**A**). While serous cells predominate, mucous cells are also found in the submandibular acini (**C**). Serous cells produce a thin, watery secretion rich in enzymes (**D**).

In H&E sections, the basal cytoplasm of the serous cell stains with hematoxylin (basophilic) because of the abundant rough endoplasmic reticulum and the free ribosomes (**E**).

9. Correct: C (C)

Image key:

A – stratified squamous epithelium

B – taste bud

C – serous (von Ebner's) glands

D – striated muscles

E – connective tissue

Identify the vallate papilla in the center of the slide. This is covered by stratified squamous epithelium that may be slightly keratinized. Each papilla is surrounded by a deep trench or cleft. Numerous taste buds are on the lateral walls of the papillae. The connective tissue near the papillae also contains several minor salivary serous (von Ebner's) glands that open via ducts into the bottom of the trench. Secretomotor supply to these glands is by the facial nerve (through its chorda tympani branch).

The lining epithelium (**A**) is nonnervous, and the connective tissue (**E**) will contain nerve endings responsible for general sensation (trigeminal nerve). Striated muscles (**D**) for the tongue are supplied by the hypoglossal nerve (with the exception of the palatoglossus). Taste buds (**B**) from vallate papillae are supplied by the glossopharyngeal nerve (this is an exception where taste buds anterior to sulcus terminalis are not supplied by the chorda tympani nerve).

10. Correct: Its length is shortest in the sublingual gland among the major salivary glands. (E)

Image key:

1 – serous acini

2 – striated duct

3 – intercalated duct, longitudinal section

4 – intercalated duct, cross section

5 – adipocytes

Striated duct has the smallest in the sublingual gland among major salivary glands. These ductal cells are tall columnar and have numerous infoldings of the basal plasma membrane. These are ion-transporting cells that absorb Na^+ and Cl^- ions (**A**) from luminal fluid, and actively pump K^+ ions (**B**) into it, thereby significantly modifying salivary composition (**D**). Intercalated ducts actively secrete HCO_3^- in saliva (**C**).

11. Correct: The cells actively secrete HCO_3^- in saliva. (C)

The cells of intercalated ducts possess carbonic anhydrase activity. In serous-secreting glands, they secrete HCO_3^- and absorb Cl^- (**A**) from the acinar product, thereby altering the composition of saliva (**D**). Mucous glands have very poorly developed intercalated ducts since their secretion is not modified significantly.

Striated duct cells remove Na^+ and Cl^- ions from luminal fluid and actively pump K^+ ions (**B**) into it. These are tall columnar cells (**E**), as opposed to the simple cuboidal cells that line intercalated ducts.

12. Correct: It is devoid of taste buds. (B)

Image Key:

1 – filiform papilla

2 – lingual aponeurosis

3 – vertical striated muscles

4 – horizontal striated muscles

Filiform papillae are conical projections of the epithelium. They are most numerous (**A**) and widely spread in humans, do not possess taste buds, and are composed of keratinized epithelium. These, like other papillae, are associated with skeletal muscles (**C**). Vallate papillae are distributed predominantly parallel and anterior to the sulcus terminalis (**D**), and papillae, in general, are not found posterior to the sulcus terminalis (**E**).

Image Key:

1 – epidermis (skin)

2 – oral mucosa

3 – vermilion zone

4 – orbicularis oris muscle (striated)

5 – labial glands

Epidermis is lined by keratinized stratified squamous epithelium (**A, B**). It is associated with numerous sweat and sebaceous glands. Oral mucosa of the lip is associated with striated muscle, orbicularis oris (**D**). Sensory nerve endings associated with oral mucosa should be of the trigeminal nerve (**E**).

The oral mucosa is lined by a nonkeratinized (parakeratinized in some areas) stratified squamous epithelium much thicker than the keratinized epithelium of the skin of the lip.

Epidermis of skin is lined by keratinized stratified squamous epithelium (**A**) and contains a deep stratum granulosum layer (**D**). The stratum granulosum layer ceases to exist beyond the vermilion zone (mucocutaneous junction). Epidermis, but not the oral mucosa, is associated with numerous sweat and sebaceous glands (**B**). Oral mucosa of the lip is associated with striated muscle, orbicularis oris (**C**).

The orbicularis oris muscle is supplied by the facial nerve. The motor root of the facial nerve winds around the abducens nucleus at the level of the pons to produce the facial colliculi—a pair of bumps one on each side adjacent to the midline in the floor of the 4th ventricle. A tumor affecting the colliculus will produce paralysis of (lower motor neuron type) muscles supplied by the facial nerve, including orbicularis oris.

Nucleus ambiguus (**A**) supplies striated muscles that derive from pharyngeal arches 3, 4, and 6 (innervated by the glossopharyngeal and vagus nerves). An intact jaw jerk (**C**) indicates a functioning trigeminal nerve (and its mesencephalic nucleus, etc.) and is not related to supply of orbicularis oris. The pterygopalatine ganglion (**D**), functionally related to the facial nerve, contains cell bodies of postganglionic parasympathetic (secretomotor) fibers for lacrimal, nasal, and palatine glands. The motor fibers of the facial nerve do not pass through this ganglion. The posterior limb of the internal capsule (**E**) conveys corticopontine, thalamocortical, and corticospinal fibers. The orbicularis oris will not be affected in a stroke involving the posterior limb. It will be paralyzed (upper motor neuron type of palsy) in a stroke involving the contralateral genu of the internal capsule, which conveys corticobulbar fibers.

The image can be identified as the tongue from the lining stratified squamous epithelium, papillae, and striated muscle fibers that run in three different planes (each arranged at right angles to the other two).

Image Key:

1 – lingual artery

2, 3, 5 – striated muscle

4 – submandibular duct

6 – lining epithelia and papillae

7 – lingual aponeurosis

Simple columnar epithelium (**A**) lines various parts of the GI tract (stomach, intestines, etc.), but not the tongue. Villi (**B**) are unique to the small intestine. Goblet cells (**C**) are found distal to the stomach. Smooth muscles (**E**) are found onward and include the middle third of the esophagus.

The lingual artery is a branch from the external carotid artery and would therefore be affected if the parent artery lodged an infarct. Vertebral (**A**), basilar (**B**), internal carotid (**C**), and superior mesenteric (**E**) arteries are not the sources for lingual arteries.

Image Key:

1 – mucus glands

2 – connective tissue

3 – interlobular duct

4 – intercalated duct

The structures labeled 3 can be identified as interlobular ducts by their stratified epithelial lining, interlobular position, and larger size. These stratified ducts are lined initially by cuboidal, then columnar, and terminally by squamous cells. Their major function is to carry saliva without significantly modifying its content.

Striated ducts are lined with simple columnar epithelial cells (**A**) that have numerous infoldings of the basal plasma membrane (**B**). These are ion-transporting cells that remove Na⁺ and Cl⁻ ions from luminal fluid, and actively pump K⁺ ions (**C**) into it. Intercalated ducts actively secrete HCO_3^- in saliva (**D**).

19. Correct: Contraction helps to expel secretory product from acinar lumen into the ducts. (C)

Image Key:

1 – mucus secretory granules

2 – myoepithelial cell

3 – lumen

4 – intercellular space

Structure 2 can be identified as a myoepithelial cell from its flattened shape and its location between the basal plasma membrane of the acinar cell and the basement membrane. The function of the cell is to contract and expel secretory product from acinar lumen to the duct system. It is not related to secretion of enzymes (**A**) or mucus (**B**), nor is it the primary cell type in any salivary gland (**D**). It shows characteristics of epithelial differentiation and possesses keratin as the intermediate filament (**E**).

20. Correct: Its secretomotor fibers are carried in the facial nerve. (D)

The image can be identified as the submandibular salivary gland by predominant serous acini (structure 1), scattered mucous tubules (structure 2), and serous demilunes (structure 3). Secretomotor fibers for the gland are carried in the chorda tympani branch of the facial nerve.

The sublingual is a predominantly mucous gland (**A**), and the parotid is exclusively serous (**B**). The parotid gland is traversed by the facial nerve (**C**), and its secretomotor fibers are carried in the glossopharyngeal nerve (**E**).

Chapter 10

Gastrointestinal Tract Histology

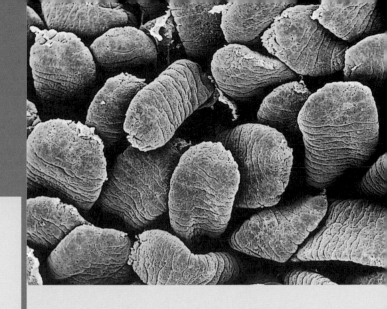

LEARNING OBJECTIVES

- ▶ Describe the microstructure of the small intestine. Correlate this with its development and functions. Describe its blood supply.

- ▶ Differentiate regions of the gastrointestinal tract based on variations in the mucosa, submucosa, muscularis, and serosa/adventitia.

- ▶ Describe the microstructure of the esophagus. Correlate this with its development and functions. Describe its blood supply.

- ▶ Analyze structural changes to the lower esophagus due to chronic acid reflux as occurs in Barrett's esophagus.

- ▶ Describe the microstructure of the colon. Correlate this with its development and functions. Describe its blood supply.

- ▶ Describe the microstructure of the anal canal. Correlate this with its development and functions. Describe its blood supply.

- ▶ Describe the microstructure of the stomach. Correlate this with its development and functions. Describe its blood supply.

- ▶ Describe the etiopathogenesis of infantile hypertrophic pyloric stenosis. Correlate this with its clinical features.

- ▶ Describe the microstructure of the appendix. Correlate this with its development and functions. Describe its blood supply.

10.1 Questions

Easy	Medium	Hard

1. A 30-year-old woman presents with chronic diarrhea of 3 months' duration. A biopsy obtained from her can be seen in the figure. Which of the following is true for the organ?

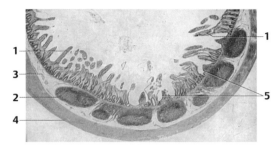

A. Develops from the foregut

B. Develops from the midgut

C. Develops from the hindgut

D. Is characterized by sacculations and haustrations

E. Is identified by prominent tenia coli

2. A 68-year-old man presents with indigestion, vomiting, postprandial fullness, loss of appetite, and weight loss. The symptoms have worsened over several months. An endoscopy-guided biopsy obtained from a suspicious area was examined under the microscope. While no histological abnormality was detected, the pathologist noted simple columnar cells lining the organ, deep pits consisting almost exclusively of mucus-secreting cells, and well-defined layers of smooth muscles. Interestingly, a smaller portion of the slide also revealed goblet cells, villi, and pronounced submucosal glands. Which is the most likely segment of the gastrointestinal tract that is being examined?

A. Gastroesophageal junction

B. Pectinate line

C. Gastroduodenal junction

D. Pharyngo-esophageal junction

E. Vermilion zone of lips

3. A 36-year-old man presents with dysphagia of acute onset. A biopsy obtained from a suspicious area during routine endoscopy was found to be normal histologically. Presence of submucosal glands, skeletal muscles, and a prominent muscularis mucosal layer was noted in the section. Which of the following additional features might be found in the specimen?

A. Teniae coli

B. Mucosa lined by stratified squamous epithelium

C. Mucosa lined by simple columnar epithelium

D. Prominent villi

E. Abundant goblet cells

4. A 68-year-old man presents with intestinal obstruction. An emergency exploration was done and a section of the intestine was removed. A biopsy obtained from the surgical specimen is attached. Which of the following is true regarding the organ?

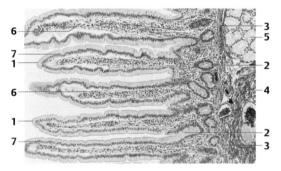

A. Its wall is characterized by the presence of skeletal muscles.

B. It develops exclusively from the cranial limb of the primary intestinal loop.

C. It develops exclusively from the caudal limb of the primary intestinal loop.

D. It is supplied by branches of the superior mesenteric artery.

E. It is supplied by branches of the inferior mesenteric artery.

5. A first-year medical student seeks help to identify lymphoid follicles. She pulls out a slide that, in addition to abundant aggregation of lymphoid follicles, demonstrates prominent villi. Which of the following structures might she also be able to identify using the same slide?

A. Submucosal glands

B. Plicae circulares

C. Epiploic appendages

D. Tenia coli

E. Parietal (oxyntic) cells

6. A tissue sample reveals simple columnar epithelium, straight and unbranched tubular glands extending through the full thickness of the mucosa, and extensive goblet cells. A thorough search failed to demonstrate villi. Which of the following areas is probably the source for the sample?

A. Esophagus

B. Fundic stomach

C. Duodenum

D. Ileum

E. Transverse colon

7. A histological section of the digestive tract revealed presence of skeletal muscles in the muscularis externa and small compound tubuloalveolar mucous glands in submucosa. Which of the following is true for the organ being examined?

A. The lower third of the organ is lined by simple columnar epithelium.

B. The lower third of the organ will reveal both striated and smooth muscles in its wall.

C. The lower third of the organ is susceptible to squamous cell carcinoma consequent to intestinal metaplasia in patients suffering from chronic acid reflux.

D. The lower third of the organ is often supplied by branches from the celiac artery.

E. The lower third of the organ is supplied by veins that mostly terminate in the inferior vena cava.

8. Which of the following statements concerning the histological structure of the organ in the figure is correct?

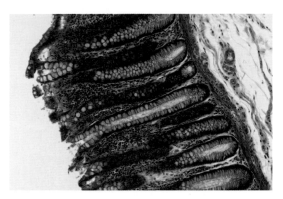

A. The mucosal lining is composed of simple squamous cells.

B. Goblet cells form a large proportion of the mucosal cells.

C. Villi significantly increase the mucosal surface area.

D. Glands traverse less than half the thickness of the mucosa.

E. Longitudinal muscle fibers are absent in the wall.

Consider the following case for questions 9 to 10:

A 48-year-old man comes to your clinic presenting with epigastric pain that appears a short time after eating. While over-the-counter antacids worked well initially, the response is gradually fading. He admits that he is stressed at work. An endoscopic biopsy was obtained from his gastric mucosa and counter-stained with periodic acid–Schiff (PAS) reagent (image).

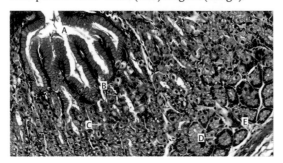

9. Hypersecretion from which of the following cells is most likely responsible for his symptoms?

A. A

B. B

C. C

D. D

E. E

10. Which of the following might occur if the cell marked B was absent in an individual?

A. Anemia

B. Jaundice

C. Peptic ulcer

D. Barrett's esophagus

■■■ A pathology resident is reviewing normal anatomy and histology for the gastrointestinal tract. Which of the following blood vessels is/are the source of supply to the region in the figure?

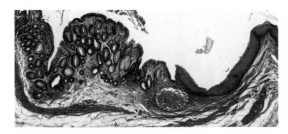

A. Celiac trunk

B. Thoracic aorta and celiac trunk

C. Inferior mesenteric artery

D. Inferior mesenteric and internal pudendal arteries

E. Superior mesenteric artery

Consider the following case for questions 12 to 13:

A 60-year-old man underwent laparoscopically assisted subtotal colectomy. A biopsy obtained from the surgical specimen is seen in the figure.

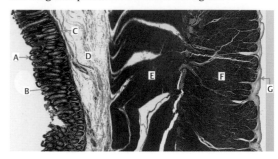

12. Tenia coli, sacculations, and epiploic appendages are unique to the large intestine. In which of the following layers are teniae coli represented?

A. C

B. B and C

C. E

D. F

E. E and F

13. Which of the following is/are component(s) of the mucous membrane of the colon?

A. A

B. A and B

C. A, B, and C

D. A, B, C, and D

E. G

14. A transition from simple columnar epithelium with simple tubular glands (predominant cells are goblet) to nonkeratinized stratified squamous epithelium is revealed in a histological slide. Based on the tissue types, which part of the GI tract is under examination?

A. Junction of the esophagus and cardia of the stomach

B. Junction of the pylorus of stomach and duodenum

C. Junction of the excretory duct of the salivary glands and oral cavity

D. Junction of the sigmoid colon and rectum

E. Pectinate line of the anal canal

15. A 24-day-old infant presents with abdominal pain. His mother reports that he was suddenly unable to hold down any milk after 3 weeks of normal breastfeeding. She states that the infant forcefully vomits at ~ 20 minutes following every feeding. The vomitus, she is confident, is not bluish-green or red. Which of the following layers is most likely pathologic in the infant?

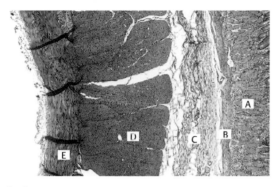

A. A
B. B
C. C
D. D
E. E

16. A 42-year-old woman presents with a 2-day history of central colicky abdominal pain, abdominal distension, and vomiting. A plain X-ray abdominal film showed distended small bowel loops and multiple gas fluid levels. An emergency exploration was done, and a section of the intestine was removed. A biopsy obtained from the surgical specimen is being examined. Which of the following is true for the structures labeled 1 in the figure?

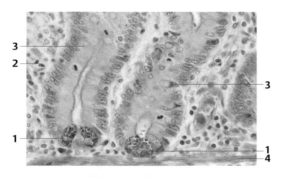

A. Secretory vesicles contain HCl.
B. Secretory vesicles contain zinc.
C. Secretory vesicles contain digestive enzymes.
D. Secretory vesicles contain mucinogen.

17. A 16-year-old girl presents with chronic heartburn that does not respond to over-the-counter antacids. An endoscopy was performed to obtain biopsies from different areas of her upper gastrointestinal tract. Which of the following is true for the indicated zone in the figure?

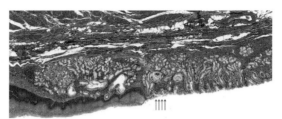

A. It is identified by glands in the submucosa.
B. It is the primary contributor to gastric juice.
C. It primarily contains mucus-secreting glands.
D. It lodges a sphincter that prevents regurgitation of bile into the organ.
E. It possesses the maximum proportion of goblet cells in the alimentary tract.

18. A 20-year-old man presents with severe pain in his abdomen. A biopsy obtained from the surgically removed inflamed organ is found in the figure. Which of the following is true for the organ?

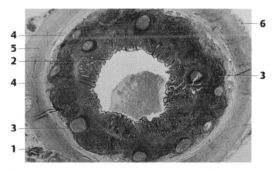

A. It might have both skeletal and smooth muscles in its wall.
B. It might have both mucosal and submucosal glands in its wall.
C. Inflammation of the organ might initially manifest as periumbilical pain.
D. It is the terminal part of the small gut.
E. It is the terminal part of the large gut.

19. A 66-year-old man attends the clinic for an excision biopsy from a definite segment of the alimentary tract. The biopsy, obtained from apparently normal mucosa, shows both smooth and striated muscles in the same section. The lining epithelium could be identified as stratified squamous for the most part. However, a small section of the slide also exhibits simple columnar epithelium with goblet cells. Which of the following is the probable source of the biopsy?

A. Tongue

B. Esophagus

C. Pyloric part of the stomach

D. Anal canal

E. Gastroesophageal junction

20. Bile, produced by hepatocytes, is carried to the alimentary tract by intrahepatic and extrahepatic biliary channels. Which of the following is true for the segment of the GI tract where bile first enters?

A. It has a stratified surface epithelium.

B. It is identified by aggregated lymphoid follicles that surround the entire lumen.

C. It is identified by aggregated lymphoid follicles that are restricted to a side of the lumen.

D. It is identified by expansion of its circular smooth muscle layer.

E. It is identified by the submucosal glands.

10.2 Answers and Explanations

Easy	Medium	Hard

1. Correct: Develops from the midgut (B)

The image can be identified as ileum, by the presence of extensively branched villi (structure 1) and aggregated lymphoid follicles or Peyer's patches (structure 2) confined to a side of the tube (antimesenteric border). The segment of the gastrointestinal tract (GIT) from the major duodenal papilla through proximal two-thirds of the transverse colon develops from midgut.

The segment of GIT from the esophagus through the major duodenal papilla develops from foregut (**A**), while that from the distal third of the transverse colon through the pectinate line of the anal canal develops from hindgut (**C**). Sacculations and haustrations (**D**) and tenia coli (**E**) are characteristics of the large gut.

2. Correct: Gastroduodenal junction (C)

Presence of simple columnar cells, deep pits comprising almost exclusively mucus-secreting cells, and well-defined layers of smooth muscles hint toward the pyloric end of the stomach. Villi, goblet cells, and pronounced submucosal glands confirm a portion of the slide to be duodenum. Hence, the gastroduodenal junction is the most likely region that is being examined.

The gastroesophageal junction (**A**) is characterized by stratified squamous nonkeratinized epithelium and submucosal glands for the esophageal part, and simple columnar epithelium with pits traversing half of the mucosa, branched, tubular, mucus-secreting gastric glands for the stomach. The pectinate line (**B**) is characterized by epithelial transition from proximal simple columnar to distal nonkeratinized stratified squamous. Presence of villi in the concerned slide precludes any part of the large gut from being present. The pharyngoesophageal junction (**D**) would be characterized by nonkeratinized stratified squamous epithelium lining both organs. In the pharyngeal part, muscularis mucosae (pronounced in the esophagus) would be replaced by a prominent layer of elastic fibers. The vermilion zone (**E**) of the lips presents a mucocutaneous junction: thin keratinized stratified squamous epithelium of skin of the lip transitions into thick nonkeratinized (para-keratinized in some areas) stratified squamous epithelium of the oral mucosa.

3. Correct: Mucosa lined by stratified squamous epithelium (B)

Presence of submucosal glands, skeletal muscles, and a prominent muscularis mucosal layer confirm the specimen as the upper or middle third of the esophagus. It is lined by nonkeratinized stratified squamous epithelium. Teniae coli (**A**) are present in the large gut; simple columnar epithelium (**C**) lines the gastrointestinal tract starting at and distal to the stomach; villi (**D**) are characteristics of the small gut; and goblet cells (**E**) are found in the gastrointestinal tract distal to the stomach.

4. Correct: It is supplied by branches of the superior mesenteric artery. (D)

Presence of simple columnar epithelium, branching villi (structure 1), and submucosal or Brunner's glands (structure 5) confirm the specimen as duodenum. Duodenum is supplied from branches of both the celiac (gastroduodenal) and superior mesenteric (inferior pancreaticoduodenal) arteries.

Skeletal muscles (**A**) in the gastrointestinal tract are seen only proximal to the middle third of the esophagus. While distal duodenum develops from the cranial limb (**B**) of the primary intestinal loop, proximal duodenum develops from the foregut. Structures that develop from the caudal limb (**C**) of the primary intestinal loop are lower ileum, cecum, appendix, ascending colon, and proximal two-thirds of the transverse colon. The inferior mesenteric artery (**E**) supplies the segment of the gastrointestinal tract that develops from the hindgut.

5. Correct: Plicae circulares (B)

Presence of abundant aggregated lymphoid follicles (Payer patches) and villi confirm the slide to be from the ileum. Plicae circulares are permanent folds (containing the mucosa and submucosa) that characterize the small gut (most developed in jejunum).

Submucosal glands (**A**) are characteristic of duodenum and esophagus; epiploic appendages (**C**) and tenia coli (**D**) characterize the large gut; parietal cells (**E**) secrete hydrochloric acid from the fundic stomach.

6. Correct: Transverse colon (E)

Presence of simple columnar epithelium, straight and unbranched tubular glands extending through the full thickness of the mucosa, and extensive goblet cells are highly indicative of the large gut. The esophagus (**A**) is lined by nonkeratinized stratified squamous epithelium; goblet cells are not present in the stomach (**B**); absence of villi precludes the slide from being either duodenum (**C**) or ileum (**D**).

7. Correct: The lower third of the organ is often supplied by branches from the celiac artery. (D)

Presence of skeletal muscles in muscularis externa and small compound tubuloalveolar mucous glands in submucosa confirm the organ as the esophagus. The lower third of the esophagus is commonly supplied by esophageal branches of the left gastric artery (off the celiac trunk).

The esophagus is lined by nonkeratinized stratified squamous epithelium (**A**); the upper third presents striated muscles, the middle third presents both striated and smooth muscles, and the lower third presents smooth muscles (**B**). The lower esophagus might undergo intestinal metaplasia (Barrett's esophagus) in patients with chronic gastroesophageal reflux disease, This precancerous condition has a 10% risk of progression to adenocarcinoma (**C**) and not squamous cell carcinoma (which is otherwise the more common cancer of the esophagus). Veins (**E**) draining the lower third of the esophagus belong to both systemic (esophageal tributaries of azygos that drain into the superior vena cava) and portal (esophageal tributaries of the left gastric) veins. This is an important region for portosystemic anastomosis.

8. Correct: Goblet cells form a large proportion of the mucosal cells. (B)

The micrograph can be identified as a section from the colon, given the simple columnar epithelium (**A**), straight and unbranched tubular glands extending through the full thickness of the mucosa (**D**), and extensive goblet cells. Villi (**C**) are features of the small gut; longitudinal smooth muscle fibers in large gut (**E**) condense to form bands (teniae coli).

9. Correct: B (B)

Image key:

A – surface mucous cell

B – parietal cell

C – mucous neck cell

D – chief cell

E – smooth muscle cell

Given the clinical scenario, excess secretion of hydrochloric acid (HCl) by the parietal (oxyntic) cells of the fundic stomach seems to be the pathology. These large eosinophilic (fried-egg appearance) cells are scattered largely near the neck of the glands and often are binucleate.

Surface mucous cells (**A**) line the inner surface of the gastric pits, and each possesses a large apical mucus cup that stains intensely with PAS. The insoluble alkaline mucus secreted by these cells forms a thick coat that adheres to the epithelial surface and protects it from abrasion or acid damage. Mucous neck cells (**C**), localized near the neck of the glands, secrete soluble mucus on vagal stimulation. While they might appear similar to surface mucous cells, mucinogen content of these cells is considerably lower. Chief (zymogenic) cells (**D**), localized predominantly near the base of the glands and secreting pepsinogen, are typical protein-secreting cells with basal cytoplasm staining basophilic (rough endoplasmic reticulum ++) and apical cytoplasm staining eosinophilic (secretory vesicles ++). Smooth muscle cells (**E**) are not involved in gastric HCl secretion.

10. Correct: Anemia (A)

The parietal cell secretes hydrochloric acid and intrinsic factor. The acid activates enzymes for protein digestion, and intrinsic factor is necessary for absorption of vitamin B_{12} from the small gut. Defective absorption of the vitamin can cause megaloblastic anemia.

Jaundice (**B**) results from disorders of bilirubin metabolism or defective bile transport and is not related to parietal cell function. Both peptic ulcer (**C**) and Barrett's esophagus (**D**) are commonly caused by mucosal damage by hydrochloric acid.

11. Correct: Inferior mesenteric and internal pudendal arteries (D)

The photograph has been obtained from the squamocolumnar junction at the pectinate line of the anal canal. This can be identified by normal colorectal mucosa (simple columnar epithelium, tubular glands extending through the full thickness of mucosa, and extensive goblet cells) at the left and nonkeratinized stratified squamous epithelium at the right of the micrograph. Part of the anal canal proximal to the pectinate line is supplied by the superior rectal (off the inferior mesenteric) artery, and that distal to the line is supplied by the inferior rectal (off the internal pudendal) artery.

The celiac trunk (**A, B**) supplies the segment of the alimentary tract derived from the foregut (lower esophagus, stomach, proximal duodenum, etc.), while the thoracic aorta (**B**) supplies the thoracic esophagus. For the attached image, squamocolumnar transition at the gastroesophageal junction can be ruled out by presence of goblet cells. The inferior mesenteric artery (**C**), continuing as the superior rectal artery, does not supply the area below the pectinate line. The superior mesenteric artery (**E**) supplies the segment of the alimentary tract derived from the midgut (distal duodenum, jejunum, ileum, cecum, appendix, ascending colon, and proximal two-thirds of the transverse colon).

12.   Correct: F (D)

Image Key:

A – epithelium (simple columnar) with goblet cells

B – lamina propria

C – muscularis mucosae

D – submucosa

E – inner circular layer of smooth muscle

F – outer longitudinal layer of smooth muscle

G – serosa (simple squamous epithelium)

Teniae coli are prominent longitudinal bands of smooth muscle formed by the condensed outer layer of muscularis externa.

13.   Correct: A, B, and C (C)

The mucous membrane comprises (starting from the luminal side) the epithelium, lamina propria, and the muscularis mucosae.

14.   Correct: Pectinate line of the anal canal (E)

The pectinate line, in the lower anal canal, is characterized by the epithelial transition from proximal colorectal mucosa (simple columnar epithelium, plenty of goblet cells, simple tubular glands, etc.) to distal nonkeratinized stratified squamous.

The gastroesophageal junction (**A**) is characterized by stratified squamous nonkeratinized epithelium and submucosal glands for the esophageal part, and simple columnar epithelium, with pits traversing half of the mucosa, and branched, tubular, mucus-secreting gastric glands for the stomach. Presence of goblet cells in the specimen precludes it from being the gastroesophageal junction. The pyloroduodenal junction (**B**) is lined by simple columnar epithelium, with villi and submucosal (Brunner's) glands for the duodenum. The junction of excre-

tory salivary duct and oral cavity (**C**) might present an epithelial transition from stratified columnar to nonkeratinized stratified squamous. Again, the presence of goblet cells in the specimen precludes it from being such junction. The junction of the sigmoid colon and rectum (**D**) would not present any notable epithelial transition.

15.   Correct: D (D)

Image Key:

A – epithelium

B – muscularis mucosae

C – submucosa

D – inner circular smooth muscle layer

E – outer longitudinal smooth muscle layer

Nonbilious and projectile vomiting following feeding in a 3- to 4-week-old infant is highly suggestive of hypertrophic pyloric stenosis. It occurs secondary to a hypertrophic pyloric sphincter, which is an expanded circular layer of smooth muscle in the muscularis externa of the gastric wall.

16.   Correct: Secretory vesicles contain zinc. (B)

The structures labeled 1 are Paneth cells. These cells, occupying the base of the crypts, are identified by intensely eosinophilic apical secretory vesicles that contain lysozyme, α-defensin, and zinc. These play a role in regulation of normal bacterial flora of the small intestine.

HCl-containing vesicles (**A**) would be seen in parietal cells, which are large eosinophilic cells that are often binucleate. Enzyme-containing vesicles (**C**) would be seen in chief cells (adjacent to Paneth cells in the image), which are otherwise similar to Paneth cells histologically, less the intense apical eosinophilia. Secretory vesicles containing mucinogen (**D**) would be seen in goblet cells (the structures labeled 3) with large demonstrable apical mucus cups.

17.   Correct: It primarily contains mucus-secreting glands. (C)

The image can be identified as the gastroesophageal junction and the indicated zone as the cardiac end of the stomach. To the left bottom is nonkeratinized stratified squamous epithelium of the esophagus, and toward the right bottom is the simple columnar epithelium of the stomach with characteristic branched tubular mucus-secreting glands of cardia that extend about half the length of mucosa.

Submucosal glands (**A**) are characteristic of the duodenum and esophagus. Fundic glands are chief contributors of the gastric juice (**B**). The pyloric stomach lodges the sphincter that prevents bile regurgitation to the stomach (**D**), while goblet cells are absent in the stomach (**E**).

18. Correct: Inflammation of the organ might initially manifest as periumbilical pain. (C)

The image can be identified as the appendix (simple columnar epithelium, less regular crypts (structure 2), large lymphoid follicles with germinal centers (structure 3) occurring all around the lumen—most important). Pain afferents from the appendix are carried by sympathetics to the T_{10} segment of the spinal cord. Therefore, pain is referred to the periumbilical area (T_{10} dermatome) initially. Pain is localized later to the right iliac fossa with involvement of the parietal peritoneum.

Skeletal muscles (**A**) or submucosal glands (**B**) are not found in the wall of the appendix. It is not the terminal part of either the small (**D**) or the large (**E**) gut.

19. Correct: Anal canal (D)

The histological findings in the slide are strongly indicative of the region surrounding the pectinate line of the anal canal. The normal colorectal mucosa (simple columnar epithelium with goblet cells) proximal to the pectinate line transitions into non-keratinized stratified squamous epithelium distally.

Presence of both skeletal and smooth muscle fibers are indicative of the external and internal anal sphincters, respectively, being present in the slide.

The tongue (**A**) would not have smooth muscle fibers or goblet cells in its wall. The esophagus (**B**) and pyloric stomach (**C**) would not have goblet cells in their walls. The findings in the slide are also typical for the gastroesophageal junction (**E**), except for the presence of goblet cells.

20. Correct: It is identified by the submucosal glands. (E)

The common bile duct enters the second part of the duodenum at the major duodenal papilla. The duodenum is characterized by the submucosal (Brunner's) glands.

The epithelial lining of duodenum is simple columnar (**A**); the appendix is identified by aggregated lymphoid follicles that surround the entire lumen (**B**); the ileum is identified by aggregated lymphoid follicles that are restricted to a side of the lumen (**C**); sphincters are formed by expansion of the circular smooth muscle layer—the pyloric stomach is an example (**D**).

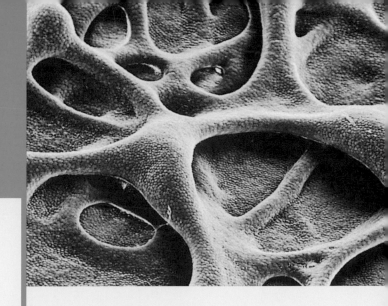

Chapter 11

Hepatobiliary System and Pancreas Histology

LEARNING OBJECTIVES

► Describe the types of liver lobules. Analyze their functional relationships to the direction of bile and blood flow.

► Describe the microstructure of the gallbladder. Correlate this with its development and functions.

► Describe the blood supply for the gallbladder.

► Describe the etiopathogenesis of acute cholecystitis. Correlate this with its clinical features.

► Describe the biliary apparatus. Correlate the structures of its components with their functions.

► Describe the microstructure of the liver. Correlate this with its development and functions.

► Describe the blood supply of the liver.

► Describe the microstructure of the pancreas. Correlate this with its development and functions.

► Describe the blood supply of the pancreas.

11.1 Questions

Easy	Medium	Hard

1. A 66-year-old female patient was admitted to the hospital with complaints of pruritus and jaundice. She has no history of liver disease, and a liver biopsy shows changes consistent with intrahepatic cholestasis. Hepatocytes from which of the following zones, as seen in the image, might initially be affected in the patient?

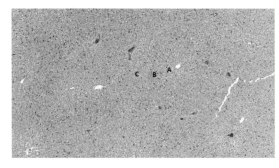

A. A

B. B

C. C

D. A and B would be affected simultaneously

E. A, B, and C would be affected simultaneously

Consider the following case for questions 2 to 3:

A 56-year-old woman presents with nausea and abdominal pain that worsen after meals. Physical examination and imaging indicates chronic inflammation of the organ in the image.

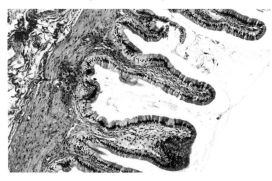

2. Which of the following organs is at the greatest risk to develop a communicating fistula, in case of inflammation of the organ in the image, breaking through its wall?

A. Appendix

B. Ileum

C. Spleen

D. Pancreas

E. Transverse colon

3. Which of the following arteries should be clamped for surgical removal of the organ?

A. Splenic

B. Common hepatic

C. Left gastric

D. Left hepatic

E. Superior mesenteric

Consider the following case for questions 4 to 7:

While reviewing histology slides before the block final, you pull out the slide (image) from a box labeled "gastrointestinal organs."

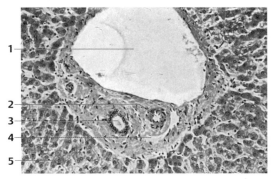

4. Which of the following structures is a component of the intrahepatic biliary apparatus?

A. 1

B. 2

C. 3

D. 4

E. 5

5. Which of the following structures synthesizes bile?

A. 1

B. 2

C. 3

D. 4

E. 5

6. Which of the following structures might be affected in an embolism consequent to splenic vein thrombosis?

A. 1

B. 2

C. 3

D. 4

E. 5

7. Which of the following structures will supply a drug, administered by a central venous (internal jugular) catheter, to the liver?

A. 1
B. 2
C. 3
D. 4
E. 5

Consider the following case for questions 8 to 9:

A 48-year-old woman presents with severe epigastric pain. She has a history of similar pain that had typically resulted in hospital admission. Physical examination, laboratory workup, and imaging reveal chronic inflammation affecting the anterior wall of the body of the organ in the image. She was admitted and treated extensively with intravenous fluids and antibiotics.

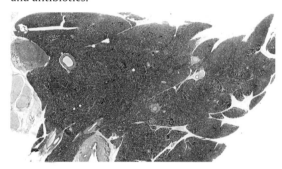

8. Which of the following statements is true regarding the organ?

A. It produces bile.
B. It produces HCl.
C. It is primarily supplied by branches from the splenic artery.
D. It is primarily supplied by branches from the external carotid artery.
E. It is primarily supplied by branches from the right hepatic artery.

9. Which of the following spaces would initially be affected if the inflammation resulted in an organ rupture?

A. Lesser sac
B. Greater sac
C. Right hepatorenal pouch (of Morrison)
D. Right paracolic gutter
E. Left paracolic gutter

Consider the following case for questions 10 to 11:

A 50-year-old woman presents with acute abdominal pain, nausea, and vomiting. Physical exam, laboratory workup, and imaging revealed an inflammation of the organ indicated by the black asterisks in the figure.

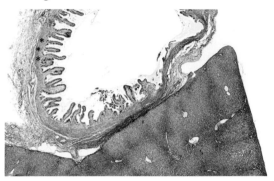

10. Which of the following is a true statement regarding the inflamed organ?

A. The organ has a primary role in absorption of nutrients from the alimentary tract.
B. The organ has a primary role in storing and concentrating bile.
C. The organ has a primary role in acid (HCl) secretion.
D. The organ has a primary role in synthesis of bile.
E. It is a retroperitoneal organ.

11. Which of the following might be an additional finding in the patient?

A. Pain shooting from right loin to groin
B. Pain at the tip of her right shoulder
C. Pain localized at the right iliac fossa
D. Pain localized at the lateral third of the right spinoumbilical line
E. Pain localized at the periumbilical area

12. A 45-year-old woman presents with a mass affecting the head of the pancreas. She was treated with a partial pancreaticoduodenectomy. The biopsy obtained from the surgical specimen is being examined. Which of the following is true regarding structure 1 in the image?

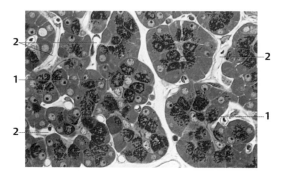

A. Produces bile

B. Removes Na^+ from pancreatic exocrine secretion

C. Secretes insulin

D. Secretes enzymes for protein digestion

E. Adds HCO_3^- to pancreatic exocrine secretion

13. A 64-year-old man presents with shortness of breath, progressive over the past 5 days. Physical examination reveals engorged neck veins, tender hepatomegaly, and bilateral pitting edema of lower extremities. Which of the following zones in the image might initially be affected in the patient?

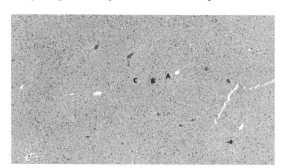

A. A

B. B

C. C

D. A and B would be affected simultaneously

E. A, B, and C would be affected simultaneously

14. A 54-year-old man presents with a history of constant right upper-quadrant abdominal pain and persistent fever and chills. An abdominal ultrasound demonstrates a mass in the right liver lobe. Segmental resection of the right lobe was performed. A biopsy obtained from the specimen is being examined. Which of the following, as labeled in the image, is the site for exchange of material between the hepatocyte and the hepatic sinusoid?

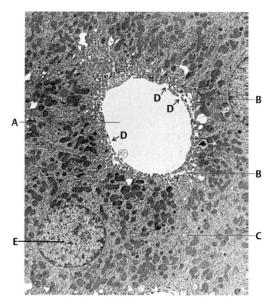

A. A

B. B

C. C

D. D

E. E

15. On a routine busy day in the laboratory, the technician forgets to label a biopsy specimen obtained from a 25-year-old woman. To make a diagnosis, the pathologist points to a prominent structure at the center of the field in the image. Which of the following is true for the indicated structure?

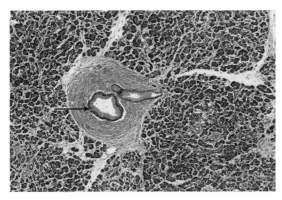

A. This will ultimately drain into the floor of the mouth.

B. This will ultimately drain in the mucosal surface of the cheek opposite the second upper molar tooth.

C. This will ultimately drain into the second part of the duodenum.

D. This will ultimately drain into the inferior vena cava.

E. This will ultimately drain into the hepatic portal vein.

Consider the following case for questions 16 to 18:

A 66-year-old man presents with acute abdominal pain, poorly localized to the right hypochondrium. A thorough physical examination followed by laboratory workup and imaging reveals an abscess affecting the organ in the image. Panel B represents a magnified view of the area within the black rectangle in panel A.

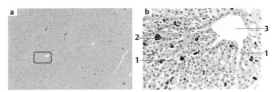

16. Which of the following is true for structure 1?

A. Blood flows through it toward the center of a classic hepatic lobule.

B. Blood flows through it toward the periphery of a classic hepatic lobule.

C. The gap between its lining endothelial cells is bridged by a diaphragm.

D. The gap between its lining endothelial cells lacks a diaphragm.

E. A and C

F. A and D

G. B and C

H. B and D

17. Which of the following is true for structure 2?

A. It has an important role in bilirubin synthesis.

B. It has an important role in vitamin A storage.

C. It has an important role in synthesis of albumin.

D. It has an important role in synthesizing extracellular matrix in hepatic fibrosis.

E. It has an important role in detoxifying drugs.

18. Which of the following is true for structure 3?

A. It is a direct branch of the hepatic artery.

B. It drains into the interlobular bile duct.

C. It drains into the thoracic duct.

D. It drains into the portal vein.

E. It drains into the inferior vena cava.

19. A 56-year-old man presents with a growth affecting the organ in the image. A histologic section obtained from the surgical biopsy specimen is being examined. Which of the following is true for the indicated structure?

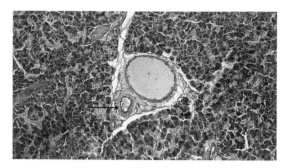

A. It drains into the superior mesenteric vein.

B. It is derived from a vessel that supplies foregut.

C. It is derived from a vessel that supplies midgut.

D. It could be derived from a vessel that supplies either foregut or midgut.

E. It carries exocrine secretion of the organ.

20. A 58-year-old man presents with severe epigastric pain unrelated to food ingestion. A CT angiogram revealed a critical celiac artery stenosis at its origin. Which of the following zones in the image might initially be affected by such a lesion?

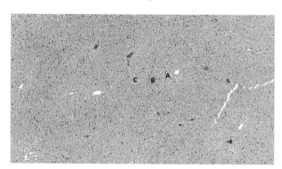

A. A

B. B

C. C

D. A and B would be affected simultaneously.

E. A, B, and C would be affected simultaneously.

11.2 Answers and Explanations

Easy	Medium	Hard

1.   Correct: C (C)

The liver acinus of Rappaport comprises 3 zones of liver cells, zone 1 (**C**) being the nearest and zone 3 (**A**) being the farthest from terminal branches of the portal triad that lie along the border between two classic hepatic lobules (image). Hepatocytes in zone 1 will initially show morphologic changes due to intrahepatic biliary stasis, given its proximity to branches of the interlobular bile ductules.

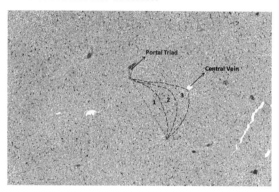

2.   Correct: Transverse colon (E)

The organ in the image is a gallbladder. This can be identified by the folded mucosa lined by simple columnar cells. The wall lacks muscularis mucosae and submucosa. Immediately deep to the lamina propria is the muscularis externa.

Chronic cholecystitis consequent to cholelithiasis may break down the wall between the gallbladder and the duodenum or the transverse colon due to their proximity, resulting in a cholecystoenteric fistula.

The appendix (**A**), ileum (**B**), spleen (**C**), and pancreas (**D**) are not at risk, given their location in the abdominal cavity, to develop such fistulas.

3.   Correct: Common hepatic (B)

The gallbladder is supplied by the cystic artery, which is a branch off the right hepatic artery, which itself is a terminal branch off the common hepatic artery. The splenic (**A**, mostly supplying the spleen and pancreas), left gastric (**C**, mostly supplying the lesser curvature of the stomach), left hepatic (**D**, mostly supplying the left physiologic hepatic lobe), and superior mesenteric (**E**, supplying structures derived from midgut) arteries do not supply the gallbladder.

4. Correct: 3 (C)

Image Key:

1 – portal vein (interlobular branch)

2 – hepatic artery (interlobular branch)

3 – bile ductule (interlobular)

4 – lymphatic vessel

5 – hepatocytes (cords)

Bile ductules can be identified by their darker-stained lining with simple cuboidal epithelial cells. These ductules, along with biliary canaliculi, canals of Hering, and intrahepatic bile ducts, form the intrahepatic biliary apparatus.

5. Correct: 5 (E)

Bile is synthesized by hepatocytes. In the image, cords of hepatocytes (structure 5) are seen to surround the portal triad.

6. Correct: 1 (A)

Structure 1 can be identified as an interlobular branch of the portal vein by the lining endothelium, thinner tunica media compared with tunica adventitia, and a large lumen. The portal vein is formed, behind the neck of the pancreas, by the union of the superior mesenteric and splenic veins. An embolus consequent to splenic venous thrombosis might affect the portal vein during its upstream course.

7. Correct: 2 (B)

Any drug administered via the central venous route will make its way to an organ via the arterial system. Structure 2 can be identified as an interlobular branch of the hepatic artery by the lining endothelium, tunica media of comparable thickness to tunica adventitia, and a smaller lumen compared with the vein (A).

8. Correct: It is primarily supplied by branches from the splenic artery. (C)

The image can be identified as the pancreas by presence of exclusive serous acini interrupted by the islets of Langerhans.

Being derived from the foregut, the pancreas is primarily supplied by branches from the celiac trunk (pancreatic branches from the splenic artery).

Bile (A) is produced in the liver, and HCl (B) is produced in the stomach. The parotid gland is supplied by branches from the external carotid artery (D); the presence of the islets of Langerhans, and the case history, preclude the organ from being the parotid gland. The pancreas is not supplied by branches off the right hepatic artery (E).

9. Correct: Lesser sac (A)

Because the inflammation has affected the anterior surface of the body of the pancreas, rupture of the part would initially spill the contents to the lesser sac, which lies immediately in front of the pancreatic body (and behind the stomach). The right hepatorenal pouch (C), right paracolic gutter (D), and left paracolic gutter (E) are all part of the greater sac (B). These are not directly related to the anterior wall of the body of the pancreas and will not be initially affected by its rupture.

10. Correct: The organ has a primary role in storing and concentrating bile. (B)

The organ indicated in the image is the gallbladder. This can be identified by folded mucosa lined by simple columnar cells. The wall lacks muscularis mucosae and submucosa. Immediately deep to the lamina propria is the muscularis externa. The photomicrograph also shows part of the liver tissue surrounding the gallbladder in the lower right corner.

The gallbladder has a primary role in storing and concentrating bile. Absorption of nutrients from the alimentary tract (A) is the primary function of the small intestine, and absence of goblet cells in the epithelial lining precludes it from being the small intestine. Acid (HCl) secretion is a primary function of the stomach, and bile synthesis (D) is a primary function of the liver. The fundus of the gallbladder is completely (and the inferior and lateral surfaces of the body and neck are usually) covered with serosa. The gallbladder, therefore, is not retroperitoneal (E).

11. Correct: Pain at the tip of her right shoulder (B)

Inflammation of the gallbladder may irritate the right hemidiaphragm and consequently the right phrenic nerve ($C_{3,4,5}$). Involvement of the right phrenic nerve results in pain referred to the tip of the right shoulder. Patterns of pain listed in the other choices are not typical of cholecystitis.

12. Correct: Adds HCO_3^- to pancreatic exocrine secretion (E)

Structure 1 is a centroacinar cell within the exocrine acinus of pancreas. These pale-staining squamous cells are initial components of the duct system that secrete HCO_3^--rich fluid. Hepatocytes produce bile (A), centroacinar or pancreatic duct cells do not absorb Na^+ (B), β cells of the pancreatic islets secrete insulin (C), and acinar cells secrete enzymes for protein digestion (D).

13. Correct: A (A)

The patient is suffering from congestive cardiac failure (right heart failure), where pressure eventually builds up in the veins and causes symptoms and signs related to systemic venous congestion. The liver acinus of Rappaport comprises 3 zones of liver cells, zone 1 (**C**) being the nearest and 3 (**A**) being the farthest from terminal branches of the portal triad that lie along the border between two classic hepatic lobules (short axis of the acinus). Hepatocytes in zone 3 will be the first to show morphologic changes consequent to congestive cardiac failure, given its proximity to the central vein.

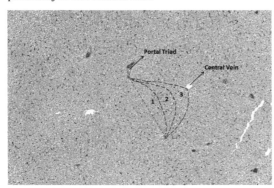

14. Correct: B (B)

Image Key:

A – hepatic sinusoid

B – space of Disse

C – bile canaliculi

D – fenestrated endothelium

E – hepatocyte nucleus

Between the basal surfaces of hepatocytes and endothelial cells is the perisinusoidal space of Disse. Occupied by hepatocyte microvilli, this is the site of exchange of material between blood and liver cells. This is also the location of hematopoietic cells in the fetus and the anemic adult.

15. Correct: This will ultimately drain into the second part of the duodenum. (C)

The image can be identified as the pancreas by the presence of exclusive serous acini, interrupted by a few islets of Langerhans. The indicated structure is an interlobular duct, given its location and the moderate amount of surrounding connective tissue. The presence of simple tall columnar epithelial cells confirms this as an interlobular pancreatic duct (as opposed to multilayered epithelial lining of similar salivary gland ducts). The pancreatic duct joins the common bile duct at the major duodenal papilla and empties into the second part of the duodenum.

Ducts from the submandibular and sublingual glands open into the floor of the mouth (**A**) The parotid (Stensen's) duct opens at the parotid papilla, a small elevation on the mucosal surface of the cheek opposite the second upper molar tooth (**B**). Pancreatic veins eventually drain into the hepatic portal vein (**E**), but not into the inferior vena cava (**D**). However, the tall columnar epithelium precludes the indicated structure from being a vein.

16. Correct: A and D (F)

Image key:

1 – hepatic sinusoid

2 – Kupffer cells

3 – central vein

Oxygen- and nutrient-rich blood from the portal vein and the hepatic artery flows through the hepatic sinusoids from the periphery (portal triad and its branches) to the center (central vein) of the classic hepatic lobules. Hepatic sinusoids are lined by fenestrated endothelium, but unlike renal glomeruli, these fenestrations are not bridged by diaphragms.

17.   Correct: It has an important role in bilirubin synthesis. (A)

The structures labeled 2 are Kupffer cells. These are hepatic macrophages that exhibit endocytic activity against blood-borne materials entering the liver. Heme oxygenase, expressed in Kupffer cells, is essential in the production of bilirubin. Hepatocytes are primarily related to albumin synthesis (**C**) and drug detoxification (**E**). Ito cells are the main place of vitamin A storage (**B**) in characteristic lipid droplets. Moreover, they demonstrate the synthetic activity of collagens and other extracellular matrix proteins involved in hepatic fibrosis (**D**).

18.   Correct: It drains into the inferior vena cava. (E)

Structure 3 indicates the central vein. These veins from adjacent lobules form interlobular veins that unite as hepatic veins and drain into the inferior vena cava. Central veins are not branches off an artery (**A**), or biliary (**B**) or lymphatic structures (**C**), and they do not drain into the portal vein (**D**).

19.   Correct: It could be derived from a vessel that supplies either foregut or midgut. (D)

The micrograph can be identified as the pancreas by the presence of exclusive serous acini, interrupted by a few islets of Langerhans. The indicated structure is a small artery, given the presence of an internal elastic lamina, a tunica media comparable in thickness to the tunica adventitia, and a smaller lumen (compared with the adjacent vein). The pancreas is supplied both by the celiac trunk (**B**, supply to the foregut) through its superior pancreaticoduodenal and splenic branches, and by the superior mesenteric artery (**C**, supply to the midgut) through its inferior pancreaticoduodenal branch. The indicated structure is not a vein (given the thick wall and small lumen) and therefore does not drain into the superior mesenteric vein (**A**). Absence of tall columnar epithelial cells precludes it from being an interlobular pancreatic duct, and hence it does not carry exocrine pancreatic secretion (**E**).

20. Correct: A (A)

The liver acinus of Rappaport comprises 3 zones of liver cells, zone 1 (**C**) being the nearest and 3 (**A**) being the farthest from terminal branches of the portal triad that lie along the border between two classic hepatic lobules (short axis of the acinus). Hepatocytes in zone 3, situated at the greatest distance from the branches of the interlobular arteries, will be the first to show morphologic changes consequent to arterial stenosis.

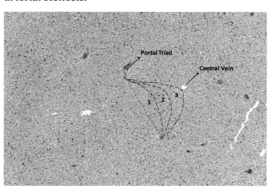

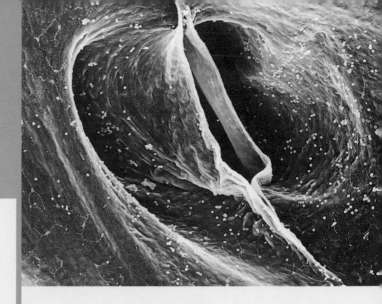

Chapter 12

Cardiovascular System Histology

LEARNING OBJECTIVES

- ▶ Describe the organization of elastic arteries. Critique their microstructure in histologic sections. Correlate their distribution with their functions.

- ▶ Describe the organization of muscular arteries. Critique their microstructure in histologic sections. Correlate their distribution with their functions.

- ▶ Describe the organization of arterioles. Critique their microstructure in histologic sections. Correlate their distribution with their functions.

- ▶ Describe the organization of capillaries. Critique their microstructure in histologic sections.

- ▶ Classify types of capillaries based on structure. Correlate their distribution with their functions.

- ▶ Describe the organization of lymphatic vessels. Critique their microstructure in histologic sections. Correlate their distribution with their functions.

- ▶ Describe the general organization of a blood vessel; correlate the structure with functions of individual layers.

- ▶ Describe the organization of microcirculation. Critique the microstructure of arteriovenous shunts in histologic sections. Correlate their structure with functions.

- ▶ Describe the etiopathogenesis of von Willebrand's disease. Correlate this with its clinical features.

- ▶ Describe the origin and distribution of the ventral branches of the abdominal aorta.

- ▶ Describe the organization and distribution of the large and medium veins, and venules; correlate their structures with their functions.

- ▶ Describe the formation and distribution of the hepatic portal vein.

12.1 Questions

Easy	Medium	Hard

1. A 35-year-old man presents with an anterior mediastinal mass. A CT-guided biopsy was obtained for tissue diagnosis. The image indicates a blood vessel found within the tissue mass. Which of the following is an important function for the vessel?

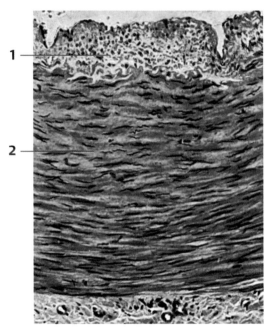

A. Primary contributor to regulate peripheral vascular resistance

B. Adjust the rate of blood flowing in an organ by vasoconstriction or vasodilation

C. Regulate amount of blood flowing into the capillary bed

D. Minimize blood pressure difference during ventricular systole and diastole

E. Bring in deoxygenated blood from the periphery to the heart

Consider the following case for questions 2 to 4:

A 72-year-old woman presented to the ER with hypertension, headache, and palpitation. She was diagnosed with multiple endocrine neoplasia type 2A and died on the second day from admission due to a sudden cardiac arrest. Several organs from her were being examined for pathology at autopsy. Panels A and B in the image indicate tissue obtained from two such organs.

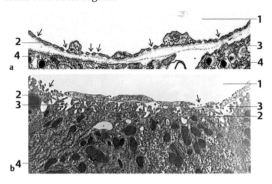

2. Which of the following are the likely sources of tissues for the image?

A. A – CNS; B – Liver

B. A – CNS; B – Pancreas

C. A – CNS; B – Lungs

D. A – Pancreas; B – Liver

E. A – Liver; B – Pancreas

3. Which of the following is true for the type of blood vessel depicted in panel A?

A. There is no gap between endothelial cells.

B. Diameter is larger than the blood vessel in panel B.

C. Characteristic feature of the endothelial cells is numerous pinocytic vesicles.

D. An intact basal lamina surrounds the endothelium.

E. It is widely found in connective tissue.

4. Which of the following is true for the type of blood vessel depicted in panel B?

A. There is no gap between endothelial cells.

B. Gap between endothelial cells is bridged by the diaphragm.

C. Diameter is larger than the blood vessel in panel A.

D. An intact basal lamina surrounds the endothelium.

E. It is widely found in connective tissue.

5. A 40-year-old man presents with a painless abdominal mass gradually increasing in size over the last 3 months. An ultrasound demonstrated a large mass of heterogeneous echogenicity arising from the left lateral rectus abdominis muscle. Radical resection of full thickness of the affected abdominal wall was performed that included a moderate peripheral margin of healthy tissue. The tissue was sent for histopathologic examination (image). Which of the following is the function for the vessel seen within the tissue mass?

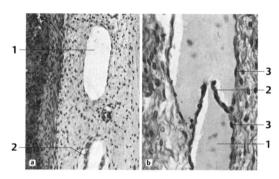

A. Adjusts the rate of blood flowing in an organ by vasoconstriction or vasodilation

B. Regulates the amount of blood flowing into the capillary bed

C. Minimizes the blood pressure difference during ventricular systole and diastole

D. Major contributor to regulating peripheral vascular resistance

E. Collects fluid from interstitial space and returns it to the bloodstream

Consider the following case for questions 6 to 9:

A 60-year-old man presents with generalized vasculitis affecting several different-sized vessels following long-standing untreated rheumatoid arthritis. Biopsies were obtained from different-sized vessels from several locations, and one such specimen is seen in the image.

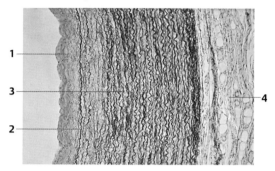

6. Which of the following is true for the blood vessel?

A. It could be directly involved in a humeral neck fracture.

B. It could be directly involved in a supracondylar humeral fracture.

C. It could be directly involved in compartment syndrome of the posterior leg.

D. It could be directly involved with aneurysms in Marfan's syndrome.

E. It could be directly involved in ischemia of the vermiform appendix.

7. Which of the following is an important function for the structure labeled 3?

A. Major contributor to regulate peripheral vascular resistance

B. Adjusts the rate of blood flowing in an organ by vasoconstriction or vasodilation

C. Regulates the amount of blood flowing into the capillary bed

D. Minimizes the blood pressure difference during ventricular systole and diastole

E. Brings in deoxygenated blood from the periphery to the heart

8. Which of the following is the primary function for the structure labeled 2?

A. Enables diffusion of O_2 and nutrients to deeper layers

B. Produces contraction and relaxation that affect the diameter of the vessel

C. Produces vasoactive agents that regulate the diameter of the vessel

D. Oxidizes cholesterol-rich circulating LDLs (low-density lipoproteins)

E. Forms a nonthrombogenic platform that prevents blood clotting

9. Which of the following is true for the structure labeled 4?

A. Forms the thinnest layer in the large veins

B. Produces contraction and relaxation that affect the diameter of the vessel

C. Produces vasoactive agents that regulate the diameter of the vessel

D. Mostly contains smooth muscle cells

E. May contain smaller blood vessels and nerve fibers

10. A 32-year-old construction worker presents with an ulcerated mass affecting his right palm. A biopsy from the tumor and a peripheral rim of normal tissue was obtained (image). Which of the following is the primary function for the structure (denoted by labels 1 and 2), apparently seen within normal tissue?

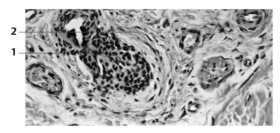

A. Adjusts the rate of blood flowing into the palm

B. Reroutes the bloodstream directly from arterial to venous circulation

C. Brings in deoxygenated blood from the palm to the heart

D. Collects fluid from interstitial space and returns it to the bloodstream

Consider the following case for questions 11 to 15:

A first-year medical student is reviewing structures of the cardiovascular system prior to her board finals. She creates a panel (image) that depicts components of vessel walls for different blood vessels from the human body.

■ Endothelium   ■ Smooth Muscle
■ Elastic Fibers   ■ Collagen Fibers

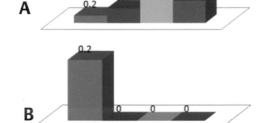

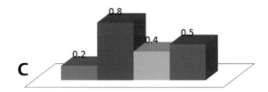

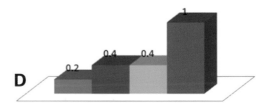

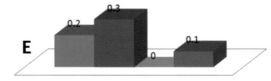

11. Which of the following is a section from the pulmonary artery?

A. A

B. B

C. C

D. D

E. E

12. Which of the following is a section from the popliteal artery?

A. A
B. B
C. C
D. D
E. E

13. Which of the following is a section from an arteriole?

A. A
B. B
C. C
D. D
E. E

14. Which of the following is a section from a capillary?

A. A
B. B
C. C
D. D
E. E

15. Which of the following is a section from the femoral vein?

A. A
B. B
C. C
D. D
E. E

Consider the following case for questions 16 to 17:

A 65-year-old woman was diagnosed with advanced breast cancer with palpable supraclavicular and axillary lymph nodes. Extensive axillary and mediastinal lymph node resection was performed with an accompanying peripheral rim of normal tissue (image).

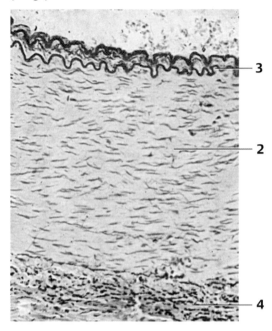

16. Which of the following is true for the blood vessel depicted within the normal tissue?

A. It could be a branch off the axillary artery.
B. It could be arising directly out of the left ventricle.
C. It could be arising directly out of the right ventricle.
D. It could be draining into the right atrium.
E. It could be a tributary of the inferior vena cava.

17. Which of the following is the primary function for structure 2?

A. Affects permeability of the structure
B. Produces contraction and relaxation that affect the diameter of the structure
C. Produces vasoactive agents that regulate the diameter of the structure
D. Oxidizes cholesterol-rich circulating LDLs (low-density lipoproteins)
E. Forms a nonthrombogenic platform that prevents blood clotting

Consider the following case for questions 18 to 19:

A 15-year-old girl presents with nosebleed. She reports that she has been menstruating for the past 16 days, and the bleeding seems to have increased after the 5th day. She also tires easily and has no appetite. Her laboratories came back with reduced hemoglobin level, increased bleeding time (BT) and activated partial thromboplastin time (aPTT), and normal platelet count and prothrombin time (PT). Attached is an electron micrograph of a tissue biopsy obtained from her.

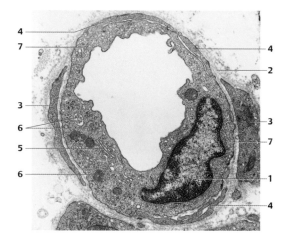

18. Which of the following labeled structures is the source for the defective protein in her?

A. 1

B. 2

C. 3

D. 5

E. 6

19. Which of the following is true for the structures labeled 3?

A. Its cytoplasm lacks actin.

B. Its cytoplasm lacks desmin.

C. Its cytoplasm lacks vimentin.

D. It can be found in a postcapillary venule.

E. It is absent in CNS.

Consider the following case for questions 20 to 21:

A 26-year-old was brought in unconscious following an automobile accident. He had a fractured left tenth rib and presented with severe hypotension, tachycardia, and feeble peripheral pulses. The organ removed at surgery is being examined under the microscope (image). Labels 1 and 2 indicate lumens of two principle blood vessels within the organ.

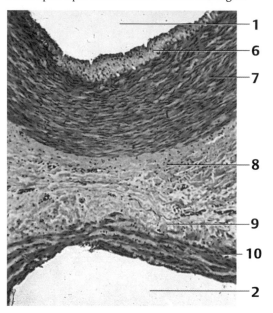

20. Which of the following is true for the vessel indicated by label 1?

A. This is a direct branch from the superior mesenteric artery.

B. This is the primary arterial supply to the head of the pancreas.

C. This is the primary arterial supply to the body and tail of the pancreas.

D. This is a large tributary of the inferior vena cava.

E. This is a large tributary of the hepatic portal vein.

21. Which of the following is true for the vessel indicated by label 2?

A. This is a direct branch from the celiac trunk.

B. This is a direct branch from the superior mesenteric artery.

C. This is a direct branch from the left renal artery.

D. This is a large tributary of the inferior vena cava.

E. This is a large tributary of the hepatic portal vein.

12.2 Answers and Explanations

| Easy | Medium | Hard |

1. Correct: Adjust the rate of blood flowing in an organ by vasoconstriction or vasodilation (B)

Image key:

1 – tunica intima

2 – tunica media

Multiple layers of smooth muscle fibers in the tunica media and the presence of internal elastic lamina confirm the structure as a medium artery, as are most named arteries of the body. The function of such an artery would be to regulate blood flow to an organ.

Arterioles are major contributors to regulate peripheral vascular resistance (**A**) and to regulate the amount of blood flowing into the capillary bed (**C**). These have only 2 to 3 layers of smooth muscle in their walls as opposed to numerous layers of smooth muscles as seen in the wall of the structure in the image. Large, elastic arteries (such as the aorta and pulmonary arteries) buffer pressure against the arterial wall due to their extensive elasticity, and thereby minimize pressure difference during ventricular systole and diastole (**D**). These have several elastic fibers scattered through the tunica media. Veins bring in deoxygenated blood from the periphery to the heart (**E**). Their walls have disproportionately larger tunica adventitia (compared to tunica media) and indistinct internal elastic laminae.

2. Correct: A – Pancreas; B – Liver (D)

Panel A in the image shows a visceral (fenestrated) capillary and Panel B shows a discontinuous sinusoidal capillary.

Image key:

Panel A

1 – capillary lumen

2 – fenestrated endothelium

3 – basal lamina

4 – endocrine gland cells

Panel B

1 – capillary lumen

2 – endothelial cell

3 – space of Disse

4 – hepatocyte

Visceral capillaries are principally present in the small intestine, gallbladder, and endocrine glands (as in pancreas). Sinusoidal capillaries are present in the liver, bone marrow, and spleen. CNS (**A–C**) features continuous or somatic capillaries.

3. Correct: An intact basal lamina surrounds the endothelium. (D)

Visceral capillaries are characterized by large fenestrae between endothelial cells bridged by diaphragms (except in renal glomerulus). The basal lamina is continuous.

Somatic or continuous capillaries have no gaps between the endothelial cells (**A**). These cells present numerous pinocytic vesicles (**C**), and these capillaries are predominantly found in muscle, connective tissue (**E**), lung, CNS, and exocrine glands. Discontinuous or sinusoidal capillaries, shown in panel B, have the largest lumen of all the capillaries (**D**).

4. Correct: Diameter is larger than the blood vessel in panel A. (C)

In discontinuous or sinusoidal capillaries, endothelial cells form a discontinuous layer. Multiple fenestrations between endothelial cells lack diaphragms. The basal lamina is discontinuous. These have the largest lumen among capillaries.

Somatic or continuous capillaries have no gaps between the endothelial cells (**A**). These capillaries are predominantly found in muscle, connective tissue (**E**), lung, CNS, and exocrine glands. Visceral capillaries have fenestrated endothelia bridged by diaphragms (**B**). Both somatic and visceral capillaries have endothelial cells with intact basal laminae (**D**).

5. Correct: Collects fluid from the interstitial space and returns it to the bloodstream (E)

The patient is probably suffering from a desmoid tumor, which develops mostly as an extra-colonic manifestation of familial adenomatous polyposis.

Image key:

1 – lymph vessels

2 – intralymphatic valve

3 – lymphatic endothelial cells

Lymph vessels are lined with endothelial cells, which themselves are covered with delicate connective tissue. These endothelia lack basal lamina. The vessels are equipped with numerous valves. Lymphatic vessels collect tissue fluid from interstitial space and return it to the bloodstream.

Medium muscular arteries adjust the rate of blood flowing in an organ by vasoconstriction or vasodilation (**A**). Their walls have multiple layers of smooth muscle cells in the media and lack valves. Large elastic arteries minimize blood pressure difference during ventricular systole and diastole (**C**). Their walls have multiple layers of elastic fibers in the media and lack valves. Arterioles regulate the amount of blood flowing into the capillary bed (**B**) and are the major contributors to regulate peripheral vascular resistance (**D**). Their walls have 2 to 3 layers of smooth muscles in the media and lack valves.

6. Correct: It could be directly involved with aneurysms in Marfan's syndrome. (D)

Image key:

1 – tunica intima

2 – internal elastic lamina

3 – tunica media

4 – tunica adventitia

Several elastic fibers in the media and presence of internal elastic lamina confirm the structure as a large, elastic artery. Such arteries are exemplified by the aorta and the pulmonary trunk. Thoracic aortic aneurysms are characteristic and frequent findings in patients with Marfan's syndrome.

The posterior circumflex humeral artery (along with the axillary nerve) is injured in a fracture of the humeral neck (**A**). The radial artery is injured with a supracondylar humeral fracture (**B**). The posterior tibial artery is involved in compartment syndrome of the posterior leg (**C**). The appendicular artery (off the ileocolic artery) is involved in ischemia of the vermiform appendix (**E**). All these arteries are medium-sized muscular arteries. These have several layers of smooth muscles in the tunica media, instead of abundant elastic fibers (image).

7. Correct: Minimizes the blood pressure difference during ventricular systole and diastole (D)

Elastic arteries buffer pressure against the arterial wall due to their extensive elasticity and thereby minimize pressure difference during ventricular systole and diastole.

Arterioles are major contributors to regulate peripheral vascular resistance (**A**) and to regulate the amount of blood flowing into the capillary bed (**C**). These have only 2 to 3 layers of smooth muscles in their walls as opposed to a thick tunica media filled with elastic fibers as seen in the wall of the structure in the figure. The regulation of blood flow to an organ (**B**) is a function of the medium, muscular arteries. Their structure is different from the image in having multiple layers of smooth muscle fibers in the tunica media. Veins bring in deoxygenated blood from the periphery to the heart (**E**). Their walls would have disproportionately larger tunica adventitia compared to the media and indistinct internal elastic laminae.

8. Correct: Enables diffusion of O_2 and nutrients to deeper layers (A)

Structure 2 is the internal elastic membrane, which is a thin sheet of elastic material found mostly in muscular arteries. Its fenestrations enable luminal substances (O_2 and nutrients) to reach deeper layers in the vessel wall.

Endothelial cells, in tunica intima, produce vasoactive agents that regulate the diameter of the vessel (**C**), oxidize cholesterol-rich circulating LDLs (**D**), and form a nonthrombogenic platform that prevents blood clotting (**E**). Smooth muscle cells, in tunica media, produce contraction and relaxation that affect the diameter of the artery (**B**).

9. Correct: May contain smaller blood vessels and nerve fibers (E)

Vasa vasorum (small blood vessels that supply the vascular wall themselves) and nervi vasorum (autonomic nerve fibers that control contraction of smooth muscles) are present in the tunica adventitia of larger vessels. Tunica adventitia is disproportionately large in veins (**A**). Smooth muscle cells (**D**) are present in the tunica media that contract to regulate the diameter of the vessel (**B**). Endothelial cells in the tunica intima produce vasoactive substances (**C**) that regulate diameter of the blood vessel.

10. Correct: Reroutes the bloodstream directly from the arterial to venous circulation (B)

Image key:

1 – winding tubules

2 – epithelioid muscle cells

The image presents an arteriovenous shunt—a connection between arterioles and venules bypassing the capillary network. These shunts reroute blood directly from arterial high-pressure to venous low-pressure circulation. A useful example is low capillary flow in the skin, which conserves heat while high flow allows heat dissipation. This is important in thermoregulatory function. The characteristic features of such a shunt are winding tubules with thick walls and narrow lumen. The presence of a strong layer of epithelioid muscle cells deep to the endothelia emphasizes the shunts.

Medium muscular arteries adjust the rate of blood flowing in an organ by vasoconstriction or vasodilatation (**A**). Their walls have several layers of smooth muscles in the media and a prominent internal elastic lamina. Veins bring in deoxygenated blood from the periphery to the heart (**C**). Their walls have a disproportionately large tunica adventitia. Lymphatic vessels collect tissue fluid from interstitial space and return it to the bloodstream (**D**). These are thin-walled structures lined with endothelial cells that lack basal lamina.

11. Correct: A (A)

Proportions of smooth muscle, elastic fibers, and collagen fibers are keys to identifying different vessels.

The pulmonary artery is an example of a large, elastic artery. The large artery (**A**) consists of moderate smooth muscles and maximum elastic fibers in tunica media; moderate type I collagen fibers in tunica adventitia.

12. Correct: C (C)

Proportions of smooth muscle, elastic fibers, and collagen fibers are keys to identifying different vessels.

The popliteal artery is an example of a medium muscular artery. The medium artery (**C**) consists of maximum smooth muscle in tunica media; moderate collagen and elastic fibers in tunica adventitia.

13. Correct: E (E)

Proportions of smooth muscle, elastic fibers, and collagen fibers are keys to identifying different vessels.

The arteriole (**E**) consists of 1 to 3 layers of smooth muscle in the tunica media; few collagen type I fibers in tunica adventitia.

14. Correct: B (B)

Proportions of smooth muscle, elastic fibers, and collagen fibers are keys to identifying different vessels.

The capillary (**B**) consists of a single layer of endothelial cells rolled up in the form of a tube and is devoid of smooth muscle and tunica adventitia

15. Correct: D (D)

Proportions of smooth muscle, elastic fibers, and collagen fibers are keys to identifying different vessels.

The femoral vein is an example of a large vein (**D**). The large vein has disproportionately large tunica adventitia, therefore, it has the maximum collagen type I fibers; moderate smooth muscle in tunica media.

16. Correct: It could be a branch off the axillary artery. (A)

Image key:

2 – tunica media

3 – internal elastic membrane

4 – tunica adventitia

Multiple layers of smooth muscle fibers in the tunica media and the presence of internal elastic lamina confirm the structure as a medium artery. The branches off the axillary artery are all named medium (muscular) arteries.

The aorta arises directly out of the left ventricle (**B**), and the pulmonary trunk arises directly out of the right ventricle (**C**). These are examples of large elastic arteries. Their structure is different from the image because they have several elastic fibers scattered through the media. Draining into the right atrium (**D**) are large veins, and tributaries of the inferior vena cava (**E**) are large and medium veins. Their walls would have disproportionately large tunica adventitia and indistinct internal elastic laminae.

17. Correct: Produces contraction and relaxation that affect the diameter of the structure (B)

Multiple layers of smooth muscle fibers in the tunica media produce a contraction that regulates the diameter of the vessel and blood flow to individual organs.

Endothelial cells affect permeability (**A**) and produce vasoactive agents that regulate the diameter (**C**) of the vessel. These also oxidize cholesterol-rich circulating LDLs (**D**) and form a nonthrombogenic platform that prevents blood clotting (**E**).

18. Correct: 6 (E)

The image is that of a continuous capillary.

Image key:

1 – endothelial cell nucleus

2 – basal lamina

3 – pericyte

4 – endothelial cell process

5 – Golgi apparatus

6 – Weibel Palade bodies

7 - pinocytic vesicles

von Willebrand's disease (vWD) is an inherited hemorrhagic disorder caused by a deficiency or dysfunction of the protein termed von Willebrand factor (vWF). In response to numerous stimuli, vWF is released from storage granules (Weibel Palade bodies) in platelets and endothelial cells. It performs two major roles in hemostasis. First, it mediates the adhesion of platelets to sites of vascular injury. Second, it binds and stabilizes the procoagulant protein factor VIII. Consequently, a defective vWF interaction between platelets and the vessel wall impairs primary hemostasis. A normal platelet count and PT, along with increased BT and aPTT, are suggestive findings in vWD. A confirmatory diagnosis requires measuring the total plasma vWF antigen, vWF function as determined by the ability of plasma to support agglutination of normal platelets by ristocetin (ristocetin cofactor activity), and plasma factor VIII level.

19. Correct: It can be found in a postcapillary venule. (D)

The structures labeled 3 are pericytes. Pericytes line capillaries and postcapillary venules.

Contractile proteins (**A**) such as α-SMA (smooth muscle actin), tropomyosin, and myosin are found in both smooth muscle cells and pericytes. Similar to the smooth muscle cells of larger vessels, pericytes can produce vasoconstriction and vasodilation within capillary beds to regulate vascular diameter and capillary blood flow. Pericytes in capillaries of cardiac muscle, the exocrine pancreas, and the kidney (peritubular capillary) contain both desmin (**B**) and vimentin (**C**).

The highest density of pericytes in the body is found in vessels of the neural tissues, such as the brain (**E**) and the retinas. The reason for this is that endothelial cells in the brain form a continuous endothelium with complex, tight junctions, and they interact with astrocytic pedicels and with numerous pericytes to create the blood-brain barrier (BBB), which protects brain cells from potentially toxic blood-derived factors.

20. Correct: This is the primary arterial supply to the body and tail of the pancreas. (C)

The patient had a splenic rupture following the automobile accident. The spleen lies beneath the left 9th through 11th ribs, and is commonly ruptured following fractures of these ribs. If the intraabdominal bleeding is severe, clinical signs of shock (hypotension, tachycardia, etc.) may manifest. Hypotension in a patient with a suspected splenic injury is a grave sign and a surgical emergency. Splenectomy is usually performed in hemodynamically unstable patients.

Labels '1' and '2' indicate the lumens of splenic artery and vein, respectively. The artery has a thicker media (7) than its adventitia (8), while it is reverse in case of the vein (media – 10, adventitia – 9).

The splenic artery, through its pancreatic branches, is the primary supply to the body and the tail of pancreas. The head of the pancreas (**B**) is supplied by the anastomosis between superior and inferior pancreaticoduodenal vessels, neither of which is derived from the splenic artery. The superior is a continuation of the gastroduodenal artery and the inferior is given off by the superior mesenteric artery. The splenic artery arises from the celiac trunk and not from the superior mesenteric artery (**A**). The splenic artery is not a tributary of the inferior vena cava (D) or the hepatic portal vein (E).

21. Correct: This is a large tributary of the hepatic portal vein. (E)

The splenic vein joins the superior mesenteric vein to form the trunk of the hepatic portal vein behind the neck of pancreas. This is not a tributary of the inferior vena cava (**D**). The splenic vein is not given off from the celiac trunk (**A**), superior mesenteric artery (**B**), or renal artery (**C**).

Chapter 13

Respiratory System Histology

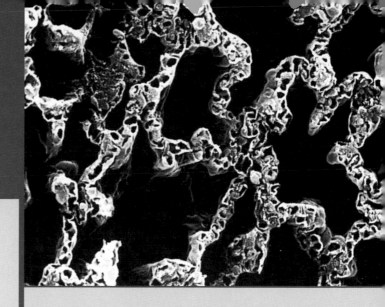

LEARNING OBJECTIVES

▶ Describe the organization of cells (ciliated columnar, olfactory, sustentacular, goblet, brush, granule, Clara, basal, alveolar type I, II, and macrophages) in the respiratory epithelium and evaluate their functions; critique their microstructure in histologic sections.

▶ Describe the basic components of the conducting and respiratory portion of the airway in humans; justify distinctive structural features of each related to functions.

▶ Describe the structure of the olfactory mucosa and correlate it with its functions; critique its microstructure in histologic sections; distinguish it from normal respiratory mucosa.

▶ Describe the microscopic structure of the respiratory tract based on epithelial cell types, glands, cartilage, smooth muscle, and connective tissue fibers present in their walls. Correlate these with their functions.

▶ Describe the etiopathogenesis of tracheomalacia. Correlate this with its clinical features.

▶ Describe the etiopathogenesis of asthma. Correlate this with its clinical features.

▶ Describe the etiopathogenesis of Kartagener's syndrome. Correlate this with its clinical features.

13.1 Questions

Easy	Medium	Hard

1. A 23-year-old male industrial worker presents with a restrictive pattern of pulmonary disease. A biopsy reveals massive necrosis of the alveolar epithelial lining, most likely due to inhalation of toxic fumes. He was advised to stay away from the toxin and report back after 6 weeks. His pulmonary function tests improved substantially by the follow-up visit. Which of the following cells are responsible for the regenerated epithelium in him?

A. Type I pneumocytes

B. Type II pneumocytes

C. Alveolar macrophages

D. Goblet cells

E. Brush cells

F. Clara cells

2. A 23-year-old woman presents with dyspnea and high fever. Physical and laboratory findings indicate a viral infection. Pulse oximetry reveals gradually decreasing oxygen saturation, and severe impairment in gaseous exchange is reckoned. Which of the following organs is most likely to be the primary target of the virus?

A. Trachea

B. Primary bronchus

C. Secondary bronchus

D. Terminal bronchiole

E. Respiratory bronchiole

Consider the following case for questions 3 to 5:

A 16-year-old girl presents with voice changes and anosmia. She has a history of a viral infection that affected her upper respiratory tract over the past 2 weeks. She was treated with antibiotics to prevent secondary infection. A tissue biopsy obtained from her is examined under the electron microscope and is seen in the image.

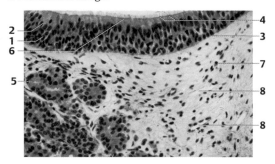

3. Which of the following might be a probable source for the tissue?

A. Maxillary sinus

B. Vocal cord

C. Roof of the nasal cavity

D. Trachea

E. Alveoli

4. Which of the following might be damaged and is responsible for some of her symptoms?

A. Structure 1

B. Structure 2

C. Structure 3

D. Structure 5

E. Structure 7

5. Which of the following is true for the structure labeled 5?

A. These are the primary sensory cells within the structure.

B. These are the primary supporting cells within the epithelium.

C. These are the primary regenerating cells within the epithelium.

D. These are secretory serous cells within the epithelium.

E. These are secretory mucous cells within the epithelium.

6. A 56-year-old man presents with rectal bleeding. He has passed bright red blood with his stool for the previous 2 weeks. A colonic mucosal specimen obtained from him is seen in the image. If the biopsy was obtained from his respiratory tract and you observed the cell indicated by structure 3, which of the following would be the probable location for the tissue?

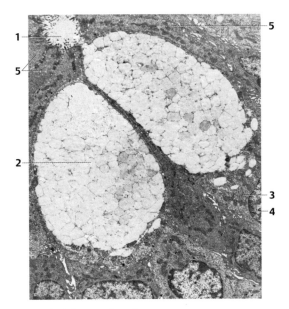

A. Roof of the nasal cavity

B. Floor of the nasal cavity

C. Terminal bronchiole

D. Respiratory bronchiole

E. Alveoli

Consider the following case for questions 7 to 8:

A 9-year-old girl presents with a long history of recurrent respiratory tract infections, accompanied with cough, dyspnea, and occasional wheezing. Examination reveals congenital weakness of the wall of a respiratory organ that lies directly ventral to the esophagus.

7. Which of the following is true for the defective structure in her?

A. It is important in olfaction.

B. It is important in gas exchange.

C. It is important in warming and humidification of air.

D. The muscle in its wall is supplied by the external laryngeal nerve.

E. The defective cartilage in its wall is primarily of elastic type.

8. Which of the following types of epithelium lines the defective structure in her?

A. Simple squamous epithelium

B. Stratified squamous epithelium

C. Simple columnar ciliated epithelium

D. Pseudostratified columnar ciliated epithelium without goblet cells

E. Pseudostratified columnar ciliated epithelium with goblet cells

Consider the following case for questions 9 to 11:

A 25-year-old woman presents with shortness of breath and chest tightness. On examination, she is afebrile, with a heart rate of 82 bpm, blood pressure 110/80 mm Hg, respiration of 18/min, and resting oxygen saturation of 90%. Her lung examination is notable for mild wheezing that is worse with forced expiration. Spirometry revealed reduced FEV_1, $FEV_1/$ FVC, and peak expiratory flow rate (PEFR). Diffusion capacity of the lung for carbon monoxide (DLCO) was increased. A tissue biopsy obtained from her is examined under the light microscope, as shown in the image.

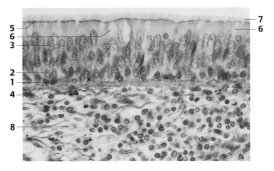

9. Which of the following is the underlying cause for her respiratory symptoms?

A. Emphysema

B. Kyphoscoliosis

C. Asthma

D. Asbestosis

E. Neuromuscular disorder

10. Which of the following might be the source for the tissue?

A. Vocal cord

B. Vestibule of the nose

C. Roof of the nasal cavity

D. Larynx

E. Alveoli

11. Wheezing in her case is caused by a combination of smooth muscle contraction and mucus hypersecretion and retention, resulting in airway caliber reduction and prolonged turbulent airflow. Hyperactivity of which of the following cells is responsible for excessive mucus production in her?

A. Structure 1

B. Structure 2

C. Structure 3

D. Structure 4

E. Structure 5

F. Structure 6

12. A 6-year-old girl presents with a wheeze, recurrent respiratory tract and ear infections, persistent nasal congestion, and obstructive sleep apnea. History, physical and laboratory findings, and imaging concludes the diagnosis of primary ciliary dyskinesia. Which of the following cells in the respiratory system exhibits cilia?

A. Sustentacular cells

B. Olfactory cells

C. Clara cells

D. Brush cells

E. Goblet cells

13. An 18-year-old young man presents with a viral infection that has a predilection for the type of epithelium that lines the oropharynx. Which of the following structures might also be affected in him?

A. Ethmoidal air cells

B. Nasopharynx

C. Terminal bronchiole

D. Vocal cords

E. Alveoli

Consider the following case for questions 14 to 18:

A 25-year-old man presents with complaints of recurrent sneezing, rhinorrhea, productive cough, on-and-off fever, and breathlessness on exertion since childhood. Chest auscultation revealed crepitation and wheezes over bilateral lung fields. Routine blood investigation was significant for increased ESR. A chest X-ray revealed dextrocardia with bronchiectatic changes seen in both lower lung fields. Ultrasound of the abdomen revealed left-sided liver and gallbladder, and right-sided stomach and spleen. A mucosal biopsy obtained from him has been attached.

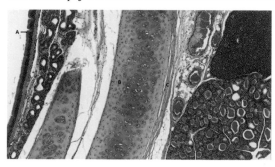

14. Which of the following regions in his body is the source for the tissue?

A. Head

B. Neck

C. Thorax

D. Abdomen

E. Pelvis

15. A defect in which of the following structures is responsible for his symptoms?

A. A

B. B

C. C

D. D

E. E

16. Which of the following additional defects might be expected in him?

A. Anemia

B. Nephrotic syndrome

C. Peptic ulcer

D. Infertility

E. Intestinal malabsorption

17. Which of the following structures might be dysfunctional if this patient also had involuntary cramping spasms of his limb musculature?

A. A

B. B

C. C

D. D

E. E

18. Which of the following is the source of arterial blood for structure D?

A. Vertebral artery

B. Internal carotid artery

C. External carotid artery

D. Thoracic aorta

E. Abdominal aorta

19. During a near-peer teaching session, a second-year medical student describes different types of cells scattered within the respiratory system to her mentee. She mentions a cell that functions primarily in preventing alveoli from collapsing at end expiration. Which of the following statements will also be true for that cell?

A. It is a flat cell that participates in forming the blood-gas barrier.

B. It is located at branching points of the alveolar septum.

C. It produces mucus and humidifies incoming air.

D. It serves as general sensory cells for the respiratory tract.

E. It produces the enzyme elastase which, when uninhibited, breaks down the alveolar wall.

20. A 42-year-old man presents with a low-grade fever and nonproductive cough of about a month's duration. Mucosal biopsies obtained via flexible bronchoscope from different parts of his respiratory tract are being examined under the light microscope. Which of the following is true for structure 1 in the image?

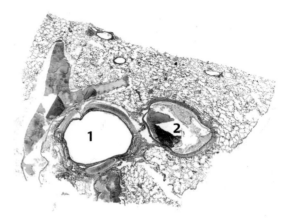

A. It is an important organ for gas exchange.

B. It mostly occupies the superior mediastinum.

C. It contains crisscrossing bundles of smooth muscle in the lamina propria.

D. It is lined extensively by Clara cells, which secrete proteins that protect against oxidative pollutants.

E. It is lined by cells that participate in regeneration of alveolar epithelium following injury.

13.1 Answers and Explanations

Easy	Medium	Hard

1. Correct: Type II pneumocytes (B)

Type II pneumocytes, identified by the presence of lamellar bodies in the cytoplasm, are typically located at a branching point of the alveolar septum. They divide and contribute to a regenerating alveolar epithelium and produce pulmonary surfactant.

Type I pneumocytes (**A**) are flat cells that line the alveoli and form the blood-air barrier across which gas exchange occurs. The alveolar macrophages (**C**, dust cells) phagocytose and remove inhaled particulate matter (carbon etc.) and organisms that gain unwanted access to air spaces. Goblet cells (**D**) are unicellular mucus glands that function in humidifying the inspired air and trapping dust, etc. These are present up to the level of the largest bronchioles. The brush cells (**E**) are nonciliated cells with microvilli. They serve as general sensory cells for the respiratory tract. Clara cells (**F**) are found in the bronchioles. These are nonciliated cells that secrete proteins that protect against oxidative pollutants and inflammation. They detoxify airborne toxins and have a role in producing components of surfactant that prevent distal bronchioles from collapsing at end expiration.

2. Correct: Respiratory bronchiole (E)

The conducting portion of the airway comprises segments of the tract from the nasal cavity through the terminal bronchioles, where air is cleaned, moistened, and warmed. These include the nasal cavity and paranasal sinuses, nasopharynx, larynx, trachea (**A**), bronchi (**B**,**C**), and bronchioles (up to and including terminal bronchioles, **D**). Gas exchange occurs in the respiratory bronchioles, alveolar ducts, alveolar sacs, and alveoli.

3. Correct: Roof of the nasal cavity (C)

Upper respiratory infections, usually viral in nature, are the most common cause of permanent hyposmia or anosmia. Such infections inflict damage to olfactory cells within the olfactory epithelium.

Olfactory epithelium, specialized for smell, lines the roof of the nasal cavity. This region may be recognized by the tall epithelium (ciliated pseudostratified columnar) that lacks goblet cells.

The maxillary sinus (**A**) and trachea (**D**) are lined by respiratory epithelium (ciliated pseudostratified columnar with goblet cells); the vocal cord (**B**) is lined by nonkeratinized stratified squamous epithelium; and alveoli (**E**) are lined by type I (squamous) and type II (cuboidal) cells.

4. Correct: Structure 1 (A)

Anosmia is primarily caused by damage to olfactory cells, identified by the location of their nuclei in the middle tier. Nuclei in the top tier (structure 2, **B**) belong to supporting cells, and those in the bottom tier (structure 3, **C**) belong to the stem cells within the epithelium. Structure 5 is the olfactory (Bowman's) gland (**D**), while structure 7 represents a plasma cell (**E**, activated lymphocyte, component of mucosa-associated lymphoid tissue [MALT]).

5. Correct: These are secretory serous cells with the epithelium. (D)

The structure labeled 5 is a specialized olfactory (Bowman's) gland, secretions from which are serous rather than mucus. The secretions dissolve odorants to facilitate their detection.

6. Correct: Floor of the nasal cavity (B)

Structure 3 is a goblet cell, which can be identified by its extensive apical mucus droplets (structure 2 in the adjacent cell) accumulated toward the lumen (structure 1), and the basal nucleus (structure 4). Goblet cells are present in the respiratory epithelium lining the floor of the nasal cavity.

The roof of the nasal cavity (**A**) features olfactory epithelium (tall ciliated pseudostratified columnar epithelium without goblet cells). Linings for terminal bronchiole (**C**, ciliated simple cuboidal), respiratory bronchiole (**D**, simple cuboidal to simple squamous) or alveoli (**E**, simple squamous) do not contain goblet cells.

7. Correct: It is important in warming and humidification of air. (C)

The trachea is located directly ventral to the esophagus, and the girl is suffering from tracheomalacia. Tracheomalacia results from missing, hypoplastic, or unusually soft tracheal cartilage. Clinical symptoms include stridor, barking cough, wheezing, dyspnea, feeding problems, and recurrent and prolonged respiratory infections.

The trachea belongs to the conducting part of the airway and therefore functions in warming, filtering, and moistening of inhaled air. Olfaction (**A**) is a function of the specialized mucosa located in the roof of the nasal cavity. Gas exchange (**B**) occurs onwards and includes the respiratory bronchiole. The trachea is innervated by the vagus nerve, not by its external laryngeal branch (**D**), which innervates the cricothyroid muscle of the larynx. The tracheal wall contains hyaline cartilage, not elastic (**E**).

8. Correct: Pseudostratified columnar ciliated epithelium with goblet cells (E)

The trachea is lined by pseudostratified ciliated columnar epithelium with goblet cells (respiratory epithelium). Simple squamous (**A**, as in alveoli), stratified squamous (**B**, as in vocal cord), simple columnar ciliated (**C**, as in bronchioles), or pseudostratified columnar ciliated epithelium without goblet cells (**D**, as in olfactory epithelium) does not line the trachea.

9. Correct: Asthma (C)

The patient is suffering from asthma based on her clinical and spirometry findings.

During an asthmatic attack, all indices of expiratory airflow may be reduced, including FEV_1, FEV_1/FVC, and peak expiratory flow rate. FVC may also be reduced as a result of premature airway closure. Diffusion capacity of the lung for carbon monoxide (DLCO) may be increased because of increased lung and capillary blood volume.

Asbestosis (**D**), neuromuscular weakness (**E**), or chest wall disease (**B**) produces restrictive lung disease characterized by reduction in the FVC with a normal or elevated FEV_1/FVC, and reduced DLCO. Emphysema (**A**) produces obstructive lung disease but is also characterized by reduced DLCO.

10. Correct: Larynx (D)

Typical respiratory epithelial lining (pseudostratified columnar ciliated epithelium with goblet cells) of the tissue helps in identifying it as the larynx. Vocal cords (**A**, stratified squamous epithelium), nasal vestibule (**B**, mucocutaneous junction/transition of stratified squamous epithelium into respiratory epithelium, dilated veins), roof of the nasal cavity (**C**, pseudostratified columnar ciliated epithelium without goblet cells or olfactory epithelium), or alveoli (**E**, simple squamous epithelium) are not lined by the respiratory epithelium.

11. Correct: Structure 6 (F)

Structure 6 represents goblet cells that produce mucus. Structure 1 (**A**, basal cells), 2 (**B**, intermediary cells), 3 (**C**, columnar cells), 4 (**D**, basement membrane) or 5 (**E**, basal bodies) does not produce mucus.

12. Correct: Olfactory cells (B)

Sustentacular cells (**A**) are nonciliated with microvilli. These support the olfactory cells and have more apical nuclei within the olfactory epithelium. Clara cells (**C**) are found in the bronchioles. These are nonciliated cells that secrete proteins that protect against oxidative pollutants and inflammation. Brush cells (**D**) are nonciliated cells with microvilli. These serve as general sensory cells for the respiratory tract. Goblet cells (**E**) are unicellular mucus glands which function in humidifying the inspired air and trapping dust, etc. These too are nonciliated.

13. Correct: Vocal cords (D)

The vocal cord, similar to the oropharynx, is lined by nonkeratinized stratified squamous epithelium.

Ethmoidal air cells (**A**) and the nasopharynx (**B**) are lined by pseudostratified columnar ciliated epithelium with goblet cells (respiratory epithelium). Terminal bronchioles (**C**) are lined by ciliated simple cuboidal cells. Alveoli (**E**) are lined by simple squamous cells.

14. Correct: Neck (B)

The patient is suffering from Kartagener's syndrome (KS), which comprises a triad of chronic sinusitis, bronchiectasis, and situs inversus.

Presence of ciliated (structure A) pseudostratified columnar epithelium with goblet cells, hyaline cartilage (structure B), and smooth muscles (structure C) hint toward trachea or bronchus. Presence of thyroid, identified by simple cuboidal cells lining thyroid follicles containing colloid—structure D and parathyroid, identified by numerous chief cells and a few scattered oxyphil cells—structure E glands confirm the section to be from the neck.

15. Correct: A (A)

Image key:
A - cilia
B - hyaline cartilage
C - smooth muscle
D - thyroid gland
E - parathyroid gland

Kartagener's syndrome results from an inherent defect in the ciliary ultrastructure (defective dynein arm), due to which ciliary motility and consequently its function is impaired. Impaired mucociliary clearance, attributed to uncoordinated and inefficient ciliary movements, predisposes the patient to recurrent respiratory infections.

16. Correct: Infertility (D)

In men, infertility is frequently seen in Kartagener's syndrome (KS) because of impaired motility of spermatozoa (structure of sperm tail is identical to that of a motile cilium). None of the other listed features are common in KS.

17. Correct: E (E)

Involuntary cramping of muscles (tetany) is commonly due to severe hypocalcemia. Hypofunctioning of the parathyroid gland could cause profound hypocalcemia and consequent tetany. Although hyperfunction of parafollicular cells of thyroid gland (**D**) could secrete excess calcitonin with consequent hypocalcemia, this is not the case in human (due to other regulatory mechanisms). Dysfunction of other listed structures (**A, B,** and **C**) are not related to hypocalcemia.

18. Correct: External carotid artery (C)

The thyroid gland is supplied by superior (off external carotid) and inferior (off thyrocervical from subclavian) thyroid arteries.

19. Correct: It is located at branching points of the alveolar septum. (B)

Type II pneumocytes produce pulmonary surfactant, which reduces alveolar surface tension and prevents alveoli from collapsing at end expiration. These cells are identified by the presence of lamellar bodies in the cytoplasm, and are typically located at a branching pointd of the alveolar septum.

Type I pneumocytes are flat cells that line the alveoli and form the blood-air barrier across which gas exchange occurs (**A**). Goblet cells are unicellular mucus glands that function in humidifying the inspired air (**C**) and trapping dust, etc. Brush cells serve as general sensory cells for the respiratory tract (**D**). The alveolar macrophages phagocytose and remove inhaled particulate matter (carbon etc.) and organisms that gain unwanted access to air spaces. These cells are the source of elastase (**E**).

20.   Correct: It contains crisscrossing bundles of smooth muscle in the lamina propria. (C)

Structure 1 in the image can be identified as a bronchus because of the presence of cartilage in the walls that appear as discontinuous plates. An important feature for bronchi is the presence of crisscrossing smooth muscle bundles in the lamina propria (not discernible at this magnification).

Gas exchange (**A**) occurs in the respiratory bronchioles, alveolar ducts, alveolar sacs, and the alveoli.

None of these organs are equipped with cartilage in their walls. The trachea occupies the superior mediastinum (**B**). Discontinuous cartilage plates instead of C-shaped cartilage rings (characteristic of trachea) shifts the identification of the organ toward bronchus. Clara cells (**D**) are present in bronchioles, which do not have cartilage in their walls. Type II pneumocytes participate in regeneration of alveolar epithelium following injury (**E**). These line alveoli, which also do not have cartilage in their walls.

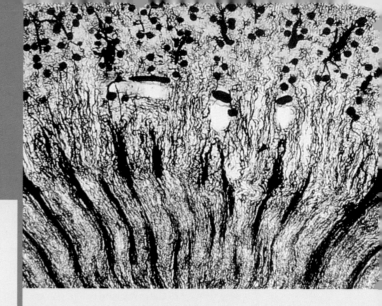

Chapter 14

Urinary System Histology

LEARNING OBJECTIVES

- ▶ Describe the cells of origin, stimulus for secretion, and site and mechanism of action for antidiuretic hormone.
- ▶ Describe the microvasculature of the kidneys. Correlate the structure and distribution of the components with their functions.
- ▶ Describe the microstructure of distal convoluted tubules and correlate it with its functions.
- ▶ Define the role of parathyroid hormone on kidney tubules.
- ▶ Describe the etiopathogenesis of Alport's syndrome. Correlate this with its clinical features.
- ▶ Describe the ultrastructure and function of the filtration barrier.
- ▶ Predict the tonicity of tubular fluid during its passage through the nephron.
- ▶ Describe the microstructure of proximal convoluted tubules and correlate it with their functions.
- ▶ Describe the microstructure of collecting ducts and correlate it with their functions.
- ▶ Describe the etiopathogenesis of nephrotic syndrome. Correlate these with its clinical features.
- ▶ Predict changes in renal plasma flow and glomerular filtration rate due to alteration of structures within the renal corpuscle.
- ▶ Describe the structure, components, and functions of the juxtaglomerular apparatus.
- ▶ Describe the etiopathogenesis of Goodpasture's syndrome. Correlate this with its clinical features.

14.1 Questions

Easy | Medium | Hard

Consider the following case for questions 1 to 2:

A 26-year-old woman participates for the first time in a marathon on a hot and humid Sunday afternoon. She collapses halfway through the race. She has not drunk enough fluids since morning and has passed less urine than regular. A physical examination at the ER reveals tachycardia and severe dehydration.

1. Which of the following is likely to occur in her?

A. Decreased activity of the juxtaglomerular cell in the kidneys

B. Decreased activity of the zona glomerulosa cells in the adrenal gland

C. Decreased activity of the basophils and pars distalis in the pituitary gland

D. Decreased activity of the pars nervosa in the pituitary gland

E. Increased activity of the pars nervosa in the pituitary gland

F. Increased activity of the acidophils and pars distalis in the pituitary gland

2. Which of the following zones within the nephron is directly affected by the altered activity of cells (described in the previous question) in her?

A. Proximal convoluted tubules

B. Proximal straight tubule

C. Thin descending limb of Henle loop

D. Thin ascending limb of Henle loop

E. Distal straight tubule

F. Distal convoluted tubule

G. Collecting duct

Consider the following case for questions 3 to 4:

A 78-year-old man presents with a 2-month history of a pitting edema in the lower extremities. His history is significant for hypertension for the past 12 years. His physical and laboratory exams are within normal range. A renal angiogram is ordered to rule out renal arterial stenosis secondary to atherosclerosis. Consider the following vessels in renal microvasculature:

1–interlobular arteries

2–arteriolae rectae

3–efferent arteriole

4–arcuate artery

5–afferent arteriole

6–interlobar artery

3. Which of the following is the correct order for circulation of dye within the kidneys?

A. 1, 2, 3, 4, 5, 6

B. 6, 1, 4, 5, 3, 2

C. 6, 2, 4, 1, 5, 3

D. 6, 4, 1, 5, 3, 2

E. 1, 4, 6, 5, 2, 3

4. Which of the following vessels might be visible in a section obtained from the renal medulla?

A. 1

B. 2

C. 3

D. 4

E. 5

5. A renal biopsy from a 48-year-old woman indicates a segment of the nephron lined by simple cuboidal epithelium with basal infoldings that contain numerous mitochondria and abundant Na^+-K^+-ATPase within the basolateral membranes. The epithelium lacks a discrete brush border. Which of the following substances might have the most effect on the segment?

A. Angiotensin I

B. Angiotensin II

C. Aldosterone

D. Parathyroid hormone

E. Antidiuretic hormone

Consider the following case for questions 6 to 10:

A 39-year-old man is admitted to the hospital with hematuria. He has no known history of renal, liver, or cardiac disease. His serum creatinine level is slightly elevated, and serum albumin level is slightly reduced. Urinalysis is significant for proteinuria. Genetic testing reveals mutation of *COL4A5*. A renal biopsy obtained from him is seen in the image.

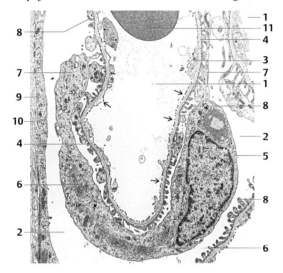

6. Which of the labeled ultra structural features initially impedes the passage of albumin in normal kidneys?

A. Structure 3

B. Structure 4

C. Structure 5

D. Structure 7

E. Structure 8

7. Which of the following areas might have been affected in the individual?

A. Structure 3

B. Structure 4

C. Structure 5

D. Structure 7

E. Structure 8

8. Which of the following might be an associated finding in him?

A. Spontaneous fractures of bones

B. Spontaneous rupture of the aorta

C. Spontaneous rupture of the intestines

D. Sensorineural deafness

E. Hypermobile joints

9. Which of the following is true of the cell indicated by structure 5?

A. Instrumental in secreting renin

B. Instrumental in monitoring the osmolarity of tubular fluid

C. Instrumental in initial filtration of blood

D. Instrumental in contraction of glomerular capillaries

E. A parietal epithelial cell of Bowman's capsule

10. Gaps between which of the following structures might be affected by mutation of the gene encoding for the protein nephrin?

A. Structure 3

B. Structure 4

C. Structure 5

D. Structure 7

E. Structure 8

Consider the following case for questions 11 to 12:

A 48-year-old male farmer passes out on his farm during a hot summer afternoon. He has been working since morning and did not drink any fluids other than a couple of beers. At the ER, he presents with tachycardia and severe dehydration. His serum antidiuretic hormone (ADH) level is several times above normal.

11. Within which of the following nephron segments will the most hypotonic fluid be found in him?

A. Segment that displays juxtaglomerular cells

B. Segment that displays podocytes

C. Segment that is lined by simple cuboidal cells with prominent microvilli

D. Segment that is lined by simple squamous cells

E. Segment that displays macula densa cells

F. Segment that displays cells with maximum concentration of aquaporin 2 receptors

12. Within which of the following nephron segments will most water be absorbed in him?

A. Segment that displays juxtaglomerular cells

B. Segment that displays podocytes

C. Segment that is lined by simple cuboidal cells with prominent microvilli

D. Segment that is lined by simple squamous cells

E. Segment that displays macula densa cells

F. Segment that displays cells with maximum concentration of aquaporin 2 receptors

Consider the following case for questions 13 to 14:

A renal biopsy from a 48-year-old woman indicates a segment of the nephron lined by simple cuboidal epithelial cells, each of which possesses a single central cilium. The epithelium lacks a discrete brush border.

13. Which of the following substances might have the most effect on the segment?

A. Angiotensin II

B. Aldosterone

C. Parathyroid hormone

D. Antidiuretic hormone

E. A and B

F. B and C

G. B and D

H. B, C, and D

14. Which of the following is an important function of the cells that are being examined?

A. Reabsorption of K^+

B. Secretion of K^+

C. Secretion of Na^+

D. Secretion of H^+

E. Secretion of HCO_3^-

Consider the following case for questions 15 to 16:

A 6-year-old boy presents with progressing facial puffiness. Physical examination reveals moderate periorbital edema and bilateral mild pitting edema in both upper and lower extremities. Laboratory investigations reveal severe proteinuria, hypoalbuminemia, and hypercholesterolemia.

15. Which of the following might be an associated finding in him?

A. ↑ renal plasma flow, ↓ glomerular filtration rate

B. ↑ renal plasma flow, ↑ glomerular filtration rate

C. ↓ renal plasma flow, ↓ glomerular filtration rate

D. ↓ renal plasma flow, ↑ glomerular filtration rate

16. Which of the following might have occurred in him?

A. Dilatation of afferent glomerular arterioles

B. Constriction of afferent glomerular arterioles

C. Dilatation of efferent glomerular arterioles

D. Constriction of efferent glomerular arterioles

Consider the following case for questions 17 to 19:

A 26-year-old woman sustained a significant crush injury to her left lower limb while on the job at a local construction site. On the second hospital day, her urine output dropped. Her laboratories came back significant for increased serum creatinine and serum creatine kinase. A renal biopsy obtained from her is seen in the image.

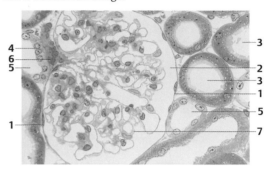

17. Which of the following primarily functions in monitoring the osmolarity of tubular fluid?

A. 1

B. 2

C. 3

D. 4

E. 5

F. 6

18. Which of the following is true for structures labeled 3?

A. Site of action of angiotensin I

B. Site of action of angiotensin II

C. Site of action of parathyroid hormone

D. Site of action of aldosterone

E. Site of action of antidiuretic hormone

19. Which of the following structures are component(s) of the juxtaglomerular apparatus?

A. 3 and 5

B. 1, 3, and 5

C. 4 and 6

D. 1, 4, and 6

E. 2, 3, 4, and 6

20. A 42-year-old woman was treated for repeated episodes of hemoptysis, hematuria, and proteinuria. Her lung biopsy showed evidence of intra-alveolar hemorrhage. Autoantibodies directed against specific components of the lungs and kidneys were detected using an enzyme-linked immunosorbent assay (ELISA) and were suggested as the pathogenic agents. Which of the following might be the other target of such an antibody?

A. Epiphyseal cartilage on the femur

B. Respiratory cartilage in the bronchus

C. Vitreous body in the eye

D. Lens fibers in the eye

E. Anchoring fibrils, basement membrane

14.2 Answers and Explanations

Easy	Medium	Hard

1. Correct: Increased activity of the pars nervosa in the pituitary gland (E)

When water intake is reduced, urine flow is less. Obligatory water loss still occurs through the lungs (↓ plasma volume), and this is not accompanied by the loss of solutes. Retention of sodium tends to concentrate the extracellular fluid (↑ plasma osmolarity).

Antidiuretic hormone (ADH) is released from the pars nervosa of the posterior pituitary in response to increased plasma osmolarity (detected by osmoreceptors in the anterolateral hypothalamus) and/or a decrease in plasma volume (detected by baroreceptors in the cardiac atria). Activity within the pars nervosa, therefore, should increase and not decrease (D) in severe dehydration.

A decrease in extracellular fluid volume will increase renin (A, from juxtaglomerular cells) and consequently aldosterone (B, from zona glomerulosa cells) activity.

Basophils in the anterior pituitary (C) synthesize corticotropin, thyrotropin, and gonadotropins. Acidophils in the anterior pituitary (F) synthesize somatotropin and prolactin. Their activities are not dependent on plasma osmolarity or volume.

2. Correct: Collecting duct (G)

In the kidney, aquaporin 1 is constitutively active in all water-permeable segments of the proximal and distal tubules, whereas ADH-regulated aquaporins 2, 3, and 4 in the inner medullary collecting duct promote rapid water permeability. All other listed choices are not directly affected by ADH.

3. Correct: 6, 4, 1, 5, 3, 2 (D)

The gold standard in detecting renal artery occlusive disease remains renal angiography because it provides maximum information about the vascular architecture as well as an opportunity for intervention if hemodynamically significant lesions are found.

Blood enters each kidney via a renal artery, which then divides into interlobar arteries. The arcuate arteries arise from the interlobar arteries and run along the corticomedullary junction. The arcuate arteries give rise to the interlobular arteries, which then supply the glomeruli via afferent arterioles. Efferent arterioles of glomeruli in the outer cortex form the peritubular plexus, which surrounds proximal and distal tubules. Efferent arterioles of glomeruli in the deeper cortex contribute to the adjacent peritubular plexus and also form the vasa recta (arteriolae rectae and venae rectae), which accompany the loop of Henle into the medulla.

4. Correct: 2 (B)

Vasa recta accompany the loop of Henle into the medulla. Interlobular arteries (A) and afferent (E) and efferent (C) arterioles are found in the cortex. Arcuate arteries (D) are found in the corticomedullary junction.

5. Correct: Parathyroid hormone (D)

The indicated nephron segment is the distal convoluted tubule, which is the site of the parathyroid hormone (PTH)-regulated Ca²⁺ reabsorption. PTH directly stimulates Ca²⁺ reabsorption, phosphate excretion, and the activity of 1α-hydroxylase (enzyme responsible for formation of the active form of vitamin D).

Angiotensin I (A) does not have any biologic activity. Angiotensin II (B) acts on proximal convoluted tubules, the epithelium of which resembles that of a distal convoluted tubule but will additionally have a pronounced brush border (microvilli).

Aldosterone (C) and antidiuretic hormone (E) act primarily on principal cells of collecting ducts. These light-staining simple cuboidal cells are equipped with a single, central cilium and lack prominent basal infoldings.

6. Correct: Structure 3 (A)

Image key:

1 Capillary lumen

2 Bowman's space

3 Endothelium with pores (black arrow)

4 Glomerular basement membrane

5 Podocyte

6 Golgi apparatus

7 Primary podocyte process

8 Secondary podocyte processes (pedicels) and filtration slits

9 Parietal lamina of Bowman's capsule

10 Subepithelial connective tissue fibers

11 Erythrocyte

Endothelial cells, including their fenestrations, are covered on the capillary side by a thick glycocalyx coat composed of glycoproteins and negative-charged glycosaminoglycans (GAGs). These are initial structures to repel negatively charged proteins (as albumin) in normal kidneys.

Structure 4 (**B**) is the lamina densa of the basement membrane consisting primarily of type IV collagen. Particle discrimination on the basis of molecular size and configuration occurs here. While lamina rarae externa and interna contain heparan sulfate (GAG) and repel negative-charged proteins, they are next in line to the endothelial cells (and their fenestrations).

Podocytes and their processes (**C, D,** and **E**) do not repel albumin.

7. Correct: Structure 4 (B)

The patient is suffering from Alport's syndrome, which is a progressive nephropathy caused by mutations in type IV collagen, the predominant collagenous constituent of glomerular basement membranes (GBM).

Classically, patients with Alport's syndrome develop thinning and splitting of the GBMs.

8. Correct: Sensorineural deafness (D)

Mutations in type IV collagen result in critical defects in the structure and function of glomerular, cochlear, and ocular basement membranes. Sensorineural deafness is an associated finding. Some patients develop lenticonus of the anterior lens capsule.

Spontaneous fractures of bones (**A**) are seen in mutations of type I collagen (as in osteogenesis imperfecta). Spontaneous ruptures of aorta (**B**) and intestines (**C**) are seen in mutations of type III collagen (as in vascular Ehlers-Danlos syndrome). Hypermobile joints (**E**) are seen in various subtypes of Ehlers-Danlos syndromes but are not common in or specific for mutations of type IV collagen.

9. Correct: Instrumental in initial filtration of blood (C)

Podocytes are initial parts of the nephron involved in filtration. These cells have long primary processes, from which arise interdigitating foot processes (pedicels) that adhere tightly to the fused capillary-podocyte basal lamina. Gaps between pedicels are filtration slits that form important components of the filtration barrier.

Juxtaglomerular cells, which are differentiated smooth muscle cells in the walls of the afferent arterioles, secrete renin (**A**). Macula densa, which consists of specialized thick ascending limb epithelial cells, monitors osmolarity of tubular fluid (**B**). Contraction of mesangial cells (intraglomerular) regulates surface area available for glomerular filtration (**D**). Podocytes line the inner visceral, but not the parietal, wall of Bowman's capsule (**E**).

10. Correct: Structure 8 (E)

Filtration slits are bridged by diaphragms that are composed of a single layer of transmembrane protein, nephrin. Mutation of the gene encoding nephrin would affect the filtration slits (gaps between pedicels).

11. Correct: Segment that displays macula densa cells (E)

During dehydration, ADH will cause water retention by acting on principal cells of the collecting duct.

Tubular fluid will be most hypotonic at the junction of the distal straight tubule (also known as pars recta of distal convoluted tubule or thick ascending limb of the loop of Henle) and the distal convoluted tubule. This segment displays macula densa cells and produces dilute fluid by remaining impermeable to water while allowing transport of solutes.

The afferent arteriole (**A**, segment that displays juxtaglomerular cells), urinary space within Bowman's capsule (**B**, lined by podocytes), and proximal convoluted tubules (**C**, lined by simple cuboidal cells with prominent microvilli) contain isotonic fluid.

Tubular fluid is hypertonic in the thin segments of the loop of Henle (**D**, lined by simple squamous cells) due to the high osmolarity of medullary interstitium (countercurrent mechanism).

Permeability of water is re-established in the collecting ducts (with ADH acting on cells with maximum concentration of aquaporin 2 receptors (**F**)). Water is reabsorbed, thereby increasing the tonicity of the tubular fluid compared with that in the proximal distal convoluted tubule.

12. Correct: Segment that is lined by simple cuboidal cells with prominent microvilli (C)

While water reabsorption increases within the collecting ducts (**F**, cells with maximum concentration of aquaporin 2 receptors) under the influence of ADH, maximum (≈ 65%) tubular reabsorption of water at any given time is still from the proximal convoluted tubules (**C**, lined by simple cuboidal cells with prominent microvilli).

Water reabsorption does not occur in the afferent arteriole (**A**, segment that displays juxtaglomerular cells), in the urinary space within Bowman's capsule (**B**, lined by podocytes), or at the junction of the distal straight tubule and the distal convoluted tubule (**E**, segment that displays macula densa cells). Approximately 25% water is absorbed in the thin segments of the loop of Henle (**D**, lined by simple squamous cells) and 10% each within the distal convoluted tubules and collecting ducts (in the absence of ADH).

13. Correct: B and D (G)

Cells being examined are principal (light) cells of the collecting ducts.

Aldosterone (**B**) and the antidiuretic hormone (**D**) act primarily on principal cells of collecting ducts. Angiotensin II (**A**) acts on proximal convoluted tubules. The site of the parathyroid hormone (**C**) regulation of Ca^{2+} reabsorption is the distal tubules. Both proximal and distal tubules are lined by simple cuboidal epithelial cells with basal infoldings that contain numerous mitochondria and abundant Na^+-K^+-ATPase within the basolateral membranes. Proximal convoluted tubules, in addition, have a prominent brush border.

14. Correct: Secretion of K⁺ (B)

Principal cells express an abundance of cytoplasmic mineralocorticoid receptors that are primary targets for aldosterone action. This results in reabsorption of Na^+ (**C**) and secretion of K^+ (**A**). Secretion of H^+ (**D**) and HCO_3^- (**E**) are functions of α– and β– intercalated (dark) cells found within the collecting duct, respectively.

15. Correct: ↓ Renal plasma flow, ↓ glomerular filtration rate (C)

The boy is suffering from nephrotic syndrome. It classically presents with heavy proteinuria, minimal hematuria, hypoalbuminemia, hypercholesterolemia, edema, and hypertension. If left undiagnosed or untreated, some of these syndromes will progressively damage enough glomeruli to cause a fall in GFR, producing renal failure.

Patients with nephrotic syndrome have hypoalbuminemia and profoundly decreased plasma oncotic pressures because of the loss of serum proteins in the urine. This leads to intravascular volume depletion and consequently a decrease in both renal plasma flow and GFR.

16. Correct: Constriction of afferent glomerular arterioles (B)

In this case, both renal plasma flow (RPF) and glomerular filtration rate (GFR) are reduced. Constriction of afferent arterioles will increase vascular resistance. This will decrease RPF. Also, constriction of afferent arterioles will decrease glomerular capillary hydrostatic pressure. This will decrease GFR.

Dilatation of afferent arterioles (**A**) will decrease vascular resistance (thereby increasing RPF) and increase glomerular capillary hydrostatic pressure (thereby increasing GFR).

By comparable mechanisms, dilatation of efferent arterioles (**C**) will increase RPF but decrease GFR, and their constriction (**D**) will decrease RPF but increase GFR.

17. Correct: 4 (D)

Image key:

1 – Bowman's capsule, parietal layer

2 – Bowman's (urinary) space

3 – Proximal tubule

4 – Macula densa

5 – Distal tubule

6 – Extraglomerular mesangial cells

Macula densa, identified by the tall, narrow, and closely packed nature of the epithelial cells at the junction of the thick ascending limb and the distal convoluted tubule, monitors the osmolarity of tubular fluid and transmits the information to juxtaglomerular cells.

18. Correct: Site of action of angiotensin II (B)

Structures labeled 3 can be identified as proximal tubules by the presence of a simple cuboidal epithelial lining and prominent brush border. Angiotensin II acts on proximal convoluted tubules.

Angiotensin I (**A**) does not have any biologic activity. The site of parathyroid hormone (**C**) regulation of Ca^{2+} reabsorption is the distal tubules. Aldosterone (**D**) and antidiuretic hormone (**E**) act primarily on principal cells of collecting ducts.

19. Correct: 4 and 6 (C)

Juxtaglomerular apparatus is made up of 3 cell types: juxtaglomerular (granular) cells, which are differentiated smooth muscle cells in the walls of the afferent arterioles; extraglomerular mesangial cells (structure 6); and macula densa cells (structure 4), which are specialized epithelial cells of the thick ascending limb.

20. Correct: Lens fibers in the eye (D)

The patient is suffering from Goodpasture's syndrome, which consists of a triad of pulmonary hemorrhage, rapidly progressive glomerulonephritis, and anti–glomerular basement membrane (anti-GBM) antibodies. The autoantibodies are directed against the Goodpasture antigen, which is part of the non-collagenous domain of the α 3(IV) collagen chain. Lens fibers are the only structures from the list that contain type IV collagen and therefore can be affected by the antibody.

Epiphyseal (hyaline) cartilage of the bones (**A**), respiratory (hyaline) cartilage of the bronchus (**B**), and the vitreous body of the eye (**C**) primarily contain type II collagen. Anchoring fibrils within the basement membrane (**E**) are primarily composed of type VII collagen.

Chapter 15

Endocrine System Histology

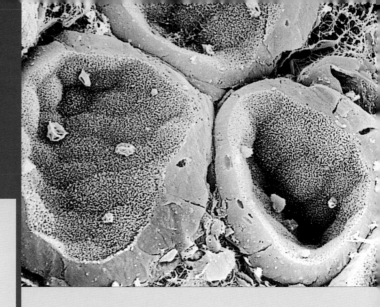

LEARNING OBJECTIVES

► Describe the microstructure of the pituitary gland; correlate it with its functions.

► Define the role of hypothalamic neurosecretion in the function of the neurohypophysis and in the regulation of the adenohypophysis.

► Describe the blood supply to the pituitary gland.

► Describe the microstructure of the adrenal gland; correlate it with its functions.

► Describe the blood supply to the adrenal gland.

► Describe the microstructure of the thyroid and parathyroid glands.

► Describe the etiopathogenesis of hyperthyroidism, hypothyroidism, hyperparathyroidism, and hypoparathyroidism. Correlate these with their clinical features.

► Describe the blood supply of the thyroid gland.

► Describe the etiopathogenesis of hypercalcemia and hypocalcemia. Correlate these with their clinical features.

► Describe the etiopathogenesis of Sheehan's syndrome. Correlate this with its clinical features.

15.1 Questions

Easy	Medium	Hard

Consider the following case for questions 1 to 2:

An endocrinology intern is reviewing normal histology slides prior to his boards. He comes across the figure, which demonstrates a sagittal section through an important gland. He consults his senior to review his understanding of the basic sciences related to the gland.

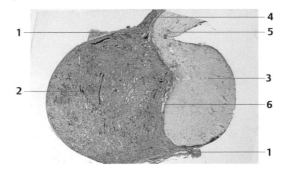

1. Which of the following is a true statement regarding the structures labeled 3 in the accompanying image?

A. It synthesizes a hormone that stimulates milk ejection by the mammary glands.

B. It synthesizes a hormone that stimulates milk production in the mammary glands.

C. It is primarily connected to magnocellular hypothalamic neurons.

D. It is primarily connected to parvocellular hypothalamic neurons.

E. It is developed from oral ectoderm.

2. Which of the following is a true statement regarding the structure labeled 6?

A. It contains the primary capillary plexus for the organ.

B. It contains the principal portal vessels for the organ.

C. It contains cysts derived from endoderm.

D. It contains basophilic cells that mostly secrete gonadotrophs.

E. It contains basophilic cells that mostly secrete β–MSH.

3. A pathologist is studying some cells under the electron microscope obtained from a biopsy specimen of a 56-year-old man who presented with a headache, palpitation, and hypertension. He observes that most of the cells have abundant smooth endoplasmic reticulum, plenty of mitochondria, and lots of large lipid droplets, giving them a vacuolated appearance. Which of the following regions is most likely being examined?

A. Pars distalis in the pituitary gland

B. Pars nervosa in the pituitary gland

C. Zona fasciculata in the adrenal gland

D. Zona glomerulosa in the adrenal gland

E. Thyroid gland

Consider the following case for questions 4 to 7:

A 16-year-old girl was operated on for a cyst associated with the upper pole of the gland depicted in panel X of the figure below. Panel Y in the figure depicts an electron micrograph obtained by zooming in the zone described by the blue rectangle in panel X.

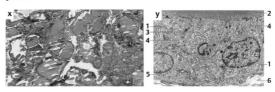

4. Which of the following might be a complication consequent to inadvertent nerve injury while clamping a vessel during surgical removal of the cyst?

A. Loss of abduction of her shoulder

B. Loss of abduction of the vocal cord

C. Loss of tension of the vocal cord

D. Loss of sensation over the laryngotracheal junction

E. Loss of sensation over the skin of the anterior neck

5. Which of the following germ layers might have suffered from a developmental defect if structure 5 was absent in her?

A. Ectoderm

B. Neuroectoderm

C. Splanchnic mesoderm

D. Endoderm

E. Neural crest

6. Which of the following might be a presenting feature (theoretically) in her if structure 5 was absent?

A. Cold intolerance

B. Prolongation of the QTc interval in EKG

C. Tachycardia

D. Kidney stones

E. Increased appetite

7. Which of the following germ layers might have suffered from a developmental defect if structures 1, 3, and 4 were dysfunctional in a newborn?

A. Ectoderm

B. Endoderm

C. Splanchnic mesoderm

D. Neuroectoderm

E. Neural crest

Consider the following case for questions 8 to 15:

A 72-year-old woman presented to the ER with hypertension, headache, palpitation, and diaphoresis. She was diagnosed with multiple endocrine neoplasia type 2A and died on the second day after admission due to sudden cardiac arrest. Endocrine organs from her were being examined for pathology at autopsy.

Case 1: Photomicrograph of one such organ is seen in the following image. Panel Y in the figure demonstrates a magnified area indicated by the blue rectangle in panel X. Refer to this for questions 8–11.

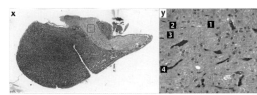

8. Which of the following is true for structure 1?

A. It is the cell body of a neuron that synthesizes the hormone responsible for the milk ejection reflex.

B. It is the cell body of a neuron that supports axons of neurons that synthesize the hormone responsible for the milk ejection reflex.

C. It is the axon terminal of a neuron that synthesizes the hormone responsible for the milk ejection reflex.

D. It is the unmyelinated axon of a neuron that synthesizes the hormone responsible for the milk ejection reflex.

E. It is a capillary fed primarily by the superior hypophyseal artery.

F. It is a capillary fed primarily by the inferior hypophyseal artery

9. Which of the following is true for structure 2?

A. It is the cell body of a neuron that synthesizes the hormone responsible for the milk ejection reflex.

B. It is the cell body of a neuron that supports axons of neurons that synthesize the hormone responsible for the milk ejection reflex.

C. It is the axon terminal of a neuron that synthesizes the hormone responsible for the milk ejection reflex.

D. It is the unmyelinated axon of a neuron that synthesizes the hormone responsible for the milk ejection reflex.

E. It is a capillary fed primarily by the superior hypophyseal artery.

F. It is a capillary fed primarily by the inferior hypophyseal artery

10. Which of the following is true for structure 3?

A. It is the cell body of a neuron that synthesizes the hormone responsible for the milk ejection reflex.

B. It is the cell body of a neuron that supports axons of neurons that synthesize the hormone responsible for the milk ejection reflex.

C. It is the axon terminal of a neuron that synthesizes the hormone responsible for the milk ejection reflex.

D. It is the unmyelinated axon of a neuron that synthesizes the hormone responsible for the milk ejection reflex.

E. It is a capillary fed primarily by the superior hypophyseal artery.

F. It is a capillary fed primarily by the inferior hypophyseal artery

11. Which of the following is true for structure 4?

A. It is the cell body of a neuron that synthesizes the hormone responsible for the milk ejection reflex.

B. It is the cell body of a neuron that supports axons of neurons that synthesize the hormone responsible for the milk ejection reflex.

C. It is the axon terminal of a neuron that synthesizes the hormone responsible for the milk ejection reflex.

D. It is the unmyelinated axon of a neuron that synthesizes the hormone responsible for the milk ejection reflex.

E. It is a capillary fed primarily by the superior hypophyseal artery.

F. It is a capillary fed primarily by the inferior hypophyseal artery

Case 2: Photomicrograph of another organ obtained from here is shown below. Refer to this image for questions 12 to 15.

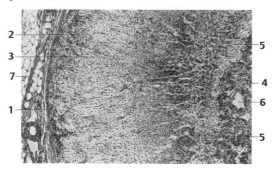

12. Which of the following statements is true for the organ?

A. It is primarily retroperitoneal.

B. It is secondarily retroperitoneal.

C. It is related to the anterior abdominal wall.

D. It is supplied by branches from the lumbar plexus of nerves.

E. It is primarily supplied by vessels serving the foregut.

13. If cancer cells spread through veins, which of the following vessels would initially lodge such cells, if the right gland was affected?

A. Renal vein

B. Superior mesenteric vein

C. Inferior mesenteric vein

D. Inferior vena cava

E. Splenic vein

14. Which of the following vessels would need to be ligated for surgical procedures on the organ?

A. Abdominal aorta, inferior phrenic artery, and celiac trunk

B. Abdominal aorta, renal artery, and celiac trunk

C. Abdominal aorta, superior and inferior phrenic arteries

D. Abdominal aorta, renal artery, and inferior phrenic artery

E. Abdominal aorta, superior and inferior mesenteric arteries

15. From which of the following sources did cells in zones 4 and 5 develop?

A. 4, ectoderm; 5, endoderm

B. 4, mesoderm; 5, endoderm

C. 4, mesoderm; 5, neural crest

D. 4, ectoderm; 5, neural crest

E. 4 and 5, neural crest

F. 4 and 5, mesoderm

Consider the following case for questions 16 to 18:

A laboratory technician, during the course of a usual super busy day, forgets to tag the biopsy specimen (accompanying image) obtained from a 23-year-old woman.

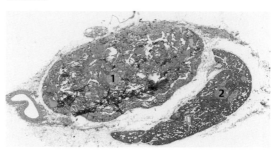

16. From which of the following locations in her body has the tissue been obtained?

A. Head

B. Neck

C. Thorax

D. Abdomen

E. Pelvis

17. Which of the following would be a presenting feature for her due to hyperfunctioning of the structure labeled 1?

A. Weight gain

B. Increased appetite

C. Slowing of heart rate

D. Cold intolerance

E. Delayed relaxation of deep tendon reflex

18. Which of the following might be a presenting feature for her due to hypofunctioning of the structure labeled 2?

A. Protruding eyeballs

B. Spontaneous fractures of fragile bones

C. Prolongation of the QTc interval in EKG

D. Heat intolerance

Consider the following case for questions 19 to 20:

A 42-year-old female presents in the ER with shock, due to postpartum hemorrhage, following a normal delivery at home. Her blood pressure was undetectable, pulse rate was 130 per minute, and extremities were cold. Immediate care involved vascular expansion with colloids via a central venous catheter, followed by transfusion of packed red cells. The short-term evolution was marked by lactation failure, profuse sweats, agitation, and convulsions. The medium-term evolution was marked by prolonged amenorrhea, fatigue, and apathy.

19. Which of the following is an expected finding in her?

A. Elevated estrogen and elevated follicle stimulating hormone (FSH)

B. Low estrogen and elevated FSH

C. Low thyroxine (T4) and low thyroid stimulating hormone (TSH)

D. Low T4 with elevated TSH

E. Low cortisol with elevated adrenocorticotropic hormone (ACTH)

20. Which of the following structures is primarily responsible for her symptoms?

A. The organ that develops from ectoderm of Rathke's pouch

B. The organ that develops from a neuroectodermal outgrowth from the diencephalon

C. The organ that develops from an endodermal outgrowth from the foramen cecum

D. The organ that develops from an endodermal outgrowth from the foregut

E. The organ that develops from the intermediate mesoderm

15.2 Answers and Explanations

Easy	Medium	Hard

1. Correct: It is primarily connected to magnocellular hypothalamic neurons. (C)

The image is a section through the pituitary gland.

Image key:

1 – Capsule

2 – Pars distalis, anterior pituitary

3 – Pars nervosa, posterior pituitary

4 – Pars tuberalis, anterior pituitary

5 – Infundibulum, median eminence

6 – Pars intermedia, anterior pituitary

The structure labeled 3 is the pars nervosa of the neurohypophysis. Axons arising from groups of hypothalamic neurons (e.g., the magnocellular neurons of the supraoptic and paraventricular nuclei) terminate in the neurohypophysis. They form the neurosecretory hypothalamohypophysial tract and terminate near the sinusoids of the pars nervosa.

Some smaller parvocellular neurons (**D**) in the periventricular zone of hypothalamus have shorter axons and end in the median eminence and infundibular stem among the primary capillary plexus of the portal circulation. These small neurons produce releasing and inhibitory hormones, which control the secretory activities of the adenohypophysis.

Oxytocin (**A**) stimulates milk ejection by the mammary glands and is synthesized primarily by cells of the paraventricular nucleus in the hypothalamus. Prolactin (**B**) stimulates milk production in the mammary glands and is synthesized by mammotrophs primarily in the pars distalis of adenohypophysis. Neurohypophysis develops from an outgrowth from the floor of the diencephalon (neuroectoderm), while adenohypohysis develops from the oral ectoderm (**E**).

2. Correct: It contains basophilic cells that mostly secrete β–MSH. (E)

The structure labeled 6 is the pars intermedia of the pituitary gland, which contains scattered clumps and cords of basophilic cells, or melanotrophs, which secrete the melanocyte-stimulating hormone (β-MSH).

The primary capillary plexus (**A**) lies in the upper infundibular stalk and lower median eminence; it extends into the pars tuberalis. The plexus receives blood from superior hypophyseal arteries and drains into the hypophyseal portal veins.

Hypophyseal portal vessels (**B**) lie mainly in the middle and lower infundibular stalk and in parts of the pars tuberalis. They receive blood from the primary capillary plexus and carry it directly to the secondary capillary plexus in the pars distalis.

The pars intermedia contains Rathke's cysts—small, irregular, colloid-containing cavities lined with cuboidal epithelium that are the remnants of Rathke's pouch (derived from oral ectoderm, not from endoderm [**C**]). Histologically, pars tuberalis resembles pars distalis but contains mostly gonadotrophs (**D**).

3. Correct: Zona fasciculata in the adrenal gland (C)

Presence of abundant smooth endoplasmic reticulum, mitochondria, and large lipid droplets indicate these to be steroid-synthesizing cells. Adrenal cortex, testis, and ovaries are some of the organs that will exhibit such cells. Cells in the zona fasciculata extensively contain large lipid droplets and are referred to as spongiocytes.

Cells of pars distalis (**A**) or thyroid gland (**E**) synthesize hormones that are structurally either glycoproteins or polypeptides; these cells have abundant rough endoplasmic reticula and well-developed Golgi complexes. Cells present in pars nervosa (**B**) are mostly pituicytes, which are glial cells with a protein-synthesizing ultrastructure. While cells in the zona glomerulosa (**D**) have abundant smooth endoplasmic reticulum and mitochondria, they have few small lipid droplets (an important differentiating feature from cells in the zona fasciculata).

4.   Correct: Loss of tension of the vocal cord (C)

Panel X depicts the thyroid gland, identified by colloid-filled follicles lined by simple cuboidal follicular cells. Panel Y depicts three follicular cells (1, 3, and 4) lining the colloid-filled follicle (2), and a parafollicular cell (5, identified by its location and calcitonin-containing secretory granules).

The superior thyroid artery needs to be clamped during operating on the upper pole of the thyroid. The artery is accompanied by the external laryngeal nerve (for a considerable course) that supplies the cricothyroid muscle. The cricothyroid muscle is a tensor of the vocal cord.

Loss of abduction of the shoulder [**A**, supraspinatus (suprascapular nerve) and deltoid (axillary nerve)], loss of abduction of the vocal cord [**B**, posterior cricoarytenoid (recurrent laryngeal nerve)], and loss of sensation over laryngotracheal junction (**D**, recurrent laryngeal nerve) or skin of the anterior neck (**E**, cervical plexus) are not common complications following such surgery.

5.   Correct: Neural crest (E)

Parafollicular cells derive from migrating neural crest cells that populate the ultimopharyngeal body (derived from the 4th pharyngeal pouch).

6.   Correct: Kidney stones (D)

Parafollicular cells synthesize calcitonin, which is a hypocalcemic peptide hormone that acts as an indirect antagonist to the calcemic actions of parathyroid hormone. Absence of calcitonin could technically cause hypercalcemia, kidney stones being one of its characteristic features. This, however, is not the usual case for humans, beause decreased levels of calcitonin in the blood usually do not alter serum calcium concentration (due to other regulatory mechanisms).

Cold intolerance (**A**, hypothyroidism), tachycardia and increased appetite (**C** and **E**, hyperthyroidism), or prolongation of QTc interval in EKG (**B**, hypocalcemia) are not associated with calcitonin deficiency.

7.   Correct: Endoderm (B)

Follicular cells lining the thyroid follicles develop from endodermal outgrowth from the foramen cecum.

8.   Correct: It is an axon terminal of the neuron that synthesizes the hormone responsible for the milk ejection reflex. (C)

The image is of the pituitary gland. Panel Y demonstrates a magnified view of the pars nervosa of the neurohypophysis. Oxytocin, synthesized by hypothalamic neurons, is responsible for the milk ejection reflex. The cell bodies of the unmyelinated neurosecretory axons are located in the hypothalamus. ADH and oxytocin are sent down the nerves (structure 4, unmyelinated axons) via axonal transport. The secretory products sometimes accumulate at the termination of the fibers and are referred to as Herring bodies (structure 1). These appear as small globs of eosinophilic material. These can be distinguished from blood capillaries (structure 3) because of their lighter eosinophilic stain and more spherical shape.

9.   Correct: It is a cell body of the neuron that supports axons of neurons that synthesize the hormone responsible for the milk ejection reflex. (B)

The nuclei (structure 2) seen in this section of the neurohypophysis belong to the supportive cells (pituicytes, which are the most abundant cell type in neurhypophysis).

10.   Correct: It is a capillary fed primarily by the inferior hypophyseal artery. (F)

Structure 3 can be identified as a capillary vessel. The inferior hypophyseal arteries form an arterial ring around the infundibulum. Fine branches from this circular anastomosis enter the neurohypophysis to supply its capillary bed. The superior hypophyseal arteries supply the primary capillary plexus (median eminence and infundibulum) and, via the portal vessels, the secondary capillary plexus (pars distalis).

11.   Correct: It is an unmyelinated axon of the neuron that synthesizes the hormone responsible for milk ejection reflex. (D)

The cell bodies of the unmyelinated neurosecretory axons, responsible for oxytocin synthesis, are located in the hypothalamus. ADH and oxytocin are sent down the nerves (structure 4, unmyelinated axons) via axonal transport.

12.   Correct: It is primarily retroperitoneal. (A)

The image is from the adrenal gland, identified by the three distinct cortical zones and the medulla.

Image key:

1 – capsule

2 – zona glomerulosa

3 – zona reticularis

4 – zona fasciculata

5 – medulla

6 – medullary vein

The adrenal gland is a primary retroperitoneal organ, related to the posterior abdominal wall (**C**). Secondary retroperitoneal organs (**B**, duodenum, pancreas, ascending and descending colon, for example) refer to those that obtained their positions due to a developmental process (gut rotation, for example). The lumbar plexus (**D**) provides somatic nerves and does not supply viscera. Vessels supplying the foregut are celiac arteries (**E**). These do not supply the adrenal glands.

13. Correct: Inferior vena cava (D)

The right adrenal gland drains directly to the inferior vena cava (IVC), while the left gland drains in the IVC via the renal vein (**A**). The superior mesenteric (**B**), inferior mesenteric (**C**), and splenic (**E**) veins drain in the portal vein and do not drain the adrenal gland.

14. Correct: Abdominal aorta, renal artery, and inferior phrenic artery (D)

Superior, middle, and inferior suprarenal arteries branch from the inferior phrenic artery, abdominal aorta, and renal arteries, respectively. The celiac (**A, B**), superior phrenic (**C**), and superior and inferior mesenteric (**E**) arteries do not supply the adrenal glands.

15. Correct: 4, mesoderm; 5, neural crest (C)

The cortex and medulla of the adrenal gland develop from the intermediate mesoderm and neural crest, respectively. Ectoderm and endoderm do not contribute to developing adrenal.

16. Correct: Neck (B)

Structure 1 can be identified as the thyroid gland from the colloid-filled follicles. Structure 2 can be identified as the parathyroid gland, given its vicinity to the thyroid and the typical cellular disposition (numerous chief cells and a few scattered oxyphil cells).

The tissue, therefore, has been obtained from her neck.

17. Correct: Increased appetite (B)

Weight loss associated with increased appetite is a common presenting feature for hyperthyroid-ism. Weight gain (**A**), bradycardia (**C**), cold intolerance (**D**), and delayed relaxation of deep tendon reflex (**E**, Woltman sign) are classic features of hypothyroidism.

18. Correct: Prolongation of the QTc interval in EKG (C)

Hypoparathyroidism presents with hypocalcemia. The EKG hallmark of hypocalcemia is prolongation of the QTc interval because of lengthening of the ST segment, which is directly proportional to the degree of hypocalcemia. Protruding eyeballs (**A**, Graves' disease), spontaneous fractures of fragile bones and kidney stones (**B** and **E**, hyperparathyroidism), and heat intolerance (**D**, hyperthyroidism) are not usual associations for hypoparathyroidism.

19. Correct: Low T4 and low TSH (C)

The patient is suffering from Sheehan's syndrome, which is characterized by partial or complete pituitary insufficiency due to postpartum necrosis of the adenohypophysis in women with severe blood loss and hypotension during delivery. The pituitary gland is physiologically enlarged in pregnancy and is therefore very sensitive to the decreased blood flow caused by massive hemorrhage and hypovolemic shock. Women with Sheehan's syndrome have varying degrees of hypopituitarism, ranging from panhypopituitarism to only selective pituitary deficiencies. Lactation failure and amenorrhea indicate prolactin deficiency. Hypoglycemia (marked by profuse sweats, agitation, and convulsions), fatigue and apathy can result from ACTH deficiency.

Elevated FSH (**A, B**), elevated TSH (**D**), or elevated ACTH (**E**) will not be seen in pituitary failure.

20. Correct: The organ that develops from ectoderm of Rathke's pouch (A)

Clinical features of Sheehan's syndrome arise largely due to insufficiency of the adenohypophysis. The anterior pituitary is more susceptible to damage than the posterior pituitary (**B**) in Sheehan's syndrome.

The thyroid gland (**C**), pancreas (**D**), and adrenal cortex (**E**) are secondarily involved in this disorder consequent to panhypopituitarism.

Chapter 16

Male Reproductive System Histology

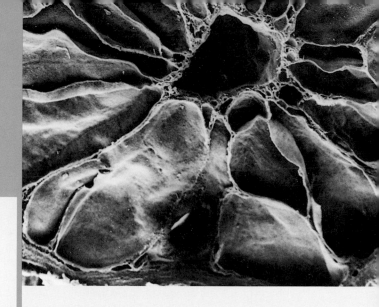

LEARNING OBJECTIVES

- ▶ Describe the organization of the spermatic cord. Critique its microstructure in histologic sections.
- ▶ Describe the etiopathogenesis of torsion of the spermatic cord. Correlate this with its clinical features.
- ▶ Describe the organization of the penis. Critique its microstructure in histologic sections.
- ▶ Describe the blood supply and lymphatic drainage of the penis.
- ▶ Describe the organization of the testis. Critique its microstructure in histologic sections.
- ▶ Describe the blood supply and lymphatic drainage of the testis.
- ▶ Describe the organization of the prostate gland. Critique its microstructure in histologic sections.
- ▶ Describe the organization of the epididymis. Critique its microstructure in histologic sections.
- ▶ Describe the etiopathogenesis of acute epididymitis. Correlate this with its clinical features.

16.1 Questions

Easy	Medium	Hard

Consider the following case for questions 1 to 7:

An 18-year-old young man presents with acute onset of severe left scrotal pain that awoke him from sleep. The pain is constant and does not change with position. There is no history of trauma. He has no dysuria, fever, chills, nausea, or vomiting. A physical examination reveals a mildly edematous and erythematous left hemiscrotum. There is marked tenderness on palpation. Doppler ultrasound scanning of the scrotum demonstrates absence of blood flow to the left testicle and epididymis. A micrograph for cross section of the affected structure in him is seen in the figure.

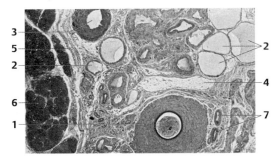

1. Which of the following is a true statement for structure 1?

A. It is a direct branch from the abdominal aorta.

B. It drains directly into the inferior vena cava.

C. It is lined by pseudostratified columnar epithelium with stereocilia.

D. It is innervated by branches from the lumbar plexus.

E. It develops from primitive sex cords of the gonadal ridge.

2. Which of the following is a true statement for the structures labeled 2?

A. These are branches from the abdominal aorta.

B. These drain directly into the renal veins.

C. These drain directly into the internal iliac veins.

D. These drain directly into the inferior vena cava.

E. These are lined by pseudostratified columnar epithelium with stereocilia.

3. Which of the following is a true statement for structure 3?

A. It is a direct branch from the abdominal aorta.

B. It is a direct branch from the internal iliac artery.

C. It drains directly into the inferior vena cava.

D. 1It is lined by pseudostratified columnar epithelium with stereocilia.

E. It is innervated by branches from the lumbar plexus.

4. Which of the following is a true statement for structure 4?

A. It is a branch from the abdominal aorta.

B. It drains directly into the renal vein.

C. It drains into the internal iliac vein.

D. It drains into the cisterna chyli.

E. It is lined by pseudostratified columnar epithelium with stereocilia.

5. Which of the following is a true statement for structure 5?

A. It sheds structures passing through the superficial inguinal ring.

B. It sheds structures passing through the deep inguinal ring.

C. It is derived from the abdominal external oblique muscle.

D. It is derived from the abdominal internal oblique muscle.

E. It is derived from the cremaster muscle.

6. Which of the following is a true statement for structure 6?

A. It is primarily innervated by sympathetic fibers from the T10 spinal segment.

B. It is primarily innervated by parasympathetic fibers from the vagus nerve.

C. It is primarily innervated by parasympathetic fibers from the pelvic splanchnic nerves.

D. It is primarily innervated by sympathetic fibers from the superior hypogastric plexus.

E. It is primarily innervated by branches from the lumbar plexus.

7. Which of the following is a true statement for structure 7?

A. It is a direct branch from the abdominal aorta.

B. It is a direct branch from the superior vesical artery.

C. It is a direct branch from the internal iliac artery.

D. It drains directly into the inferior vena cava.

E. It is innervated by branches from the lumbar plexus.

Consider the following case for questions 8 to 11:

A first-year-medical student has obtained several sections from a donor, who featured generalized lymphadenopathy. One of the sections is attached below.

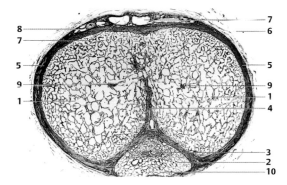

8. Which of the following is the direct source of arterial blood for structure 1?

A. Internal iliac artery

B. External iliac artery

C. Internal pudendal artery

D. External pudendal artery

E. Abdominal aorta

9. If metastatic cells were to spread via lymphatics, which of the following lymph nodes would initially be affected in case of malignancy affecting structure 1?

A. Superficial inguinal lymph nodes

B. Deep inguinal lymph nodes

C. External iliac lymph nodes

D. Internal iliac lymph nodes

E. Lateral aortic lymph nodes

10. If metastatic cells were to spread via lymphatics, which of the following lymph nodes would initially be affected in case of malignancy affecting structure 6, given the biopsy has been obtained from the anterior third of the organ?

A. Superficial inguinal lymph nodes

B. Deep inguinal lymph nodes

C. External iliac lymph nodes

D. Internal iliac lymph nodes

E. Lateral aortic lymph nodes

11. Which of the following is the epithelial lining for structure 3?

A. Simple squamous

B. Stratified squamous

C. Simple columnar

D. Stratified columnar

E. Transitional

Consider the following case for questions 12 to 16:

A 28-year-old man presents with right flank pain. Computed tomography shows a mass located between his aorta and inferior vena cava. His serum levels of lactate dehydrogenase and α-fetoprotein are extremely high. Ultrasonography reveals multiple low echoic lesions in an organ. A histologic section of that organ is seen in the figure. He is diagnosed with cancer involving the organ.

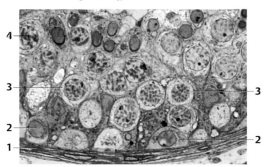

12. Which of the following lymph nodes will initially be involved, if metastatic cells travel via the lymphatics?

A. External iliac

B. Internal iliac

C. Superficial inguinal

D. Deep inguinal

E. Lumbar

13. Which of the following veins will initially be involved, if metastatic cells travel via veins?

A. Renal vein

B. Suprarenal vein

C. Internal iliac vein

D. External iliac vein

E. Inferior vena cava

14. Which of the following is true for structure 2?

A. It produces testosterone.

B. It produces androgen-binding protein.

C. It undergoes mitotic cell division.

D. It undergoes meiotic cell division.

E. It contains a haploid number of chromosomes.

15. Which of the following is true for structure 3?

A. It produces testosterone.

B. It produces androgen-binding protein.

C. It undergoes mitotic cell division.

D. It undergoes meiotic cell division.

E. It contains a haploid number of chromosomes.

16. Which of the following is true for structure 4?

A. It produces testosterone.

B. It produces androgen-binding protein.

C. It undergoes mitotic cell division.

D. It undergoes meiotic cell division.

E. It contains a haploid number of chromosomes.

Consider the following case for questions 17 to 18:

A 62-year-old man presents with urinary hesitancy, weak stream, and incomplete emptying. The organ responsible for the symptoms in the patient was surgically removed via a transurethral approach. A biopsy from the specimen is seen in the figure.

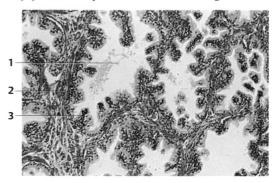

17. Which of the following is the most unlikely location within the organ from where the biopsy could have been obtained?

A. Central zone

B. Peripheral zone

C. Transition zone

D. Anterior zone

18. Which of the following is the developmental origin for structure 1?

A. Ectoderm

B. Endoderm

C. Neural crest

D. Paraxial mesoderm

E. Intermediate mesoderm

Consider the following case for questions 19 to 21:

A 27-year-old man presents with gradual onset of pain that is localized to the posterior left scrotum. The pain radiates to the lower abdomen and is relieved with scrotal elevation. Physical examination reveals erythema, swelling, and tenderness of the left scrotum. The cremasteric reflex is intact. An ultrasound with color Doppler reveals thickening of and increased blood flow to the organ. A histologic section of the organ is seen in the figure.

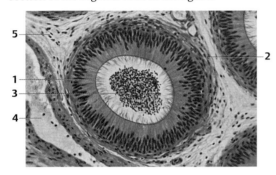

19. Which of the following is the most likely diagnosis in him?

A. Acute orchitis

B. Acute epididymitis

C. Testicular torsion

D. Testicular malignancy

20. Which of the following is true for structure 1?

A. The core is composed of microtubules in a 9+2 arrangement.

B. The core is composed of microtubules in a 9+0 arrangement.

C. The core is comprised of actin microfilaments.

D. Its primary function is to propel tubular content forward.

E. It is widely distributed in the jejunum.

21. Which of the following is true for structure 2?

A. It is stimulated primarily by pudendal nerve fibers.

B. It is stimulated primarily by genitofemoral nerve fibers.

C. It is stimulated primarily by ilioinguinal nerve fibers.

D. It is stimulated primarily by sympathetic nerve fibers.

E. It is stimulated primarily by parasympathetic nerve fibers.

16.2 Answers and Explanations

Easy	Medium	Hard

1. Correct: It is lined by pseudostratified columnar epithelium with stereocilia. (C)

The patient is suffering from torsion of the left spermatic cord, leading to an ischemic testicle. Detorsion of the left testis followed by fixation of both testes to scrotal walls is recommended. A cross section of the left spermatic cord can be seen in the figure.

Image key:

1 – vas deferens

2 – veins of the pampiniform plexus

3 – testicular artery

4 – lymph vessels

5 – internal spermatic fascia

6 – cremaster muscle

7 – branches of the artery of the ductus deferens

The ductus deferens can be identified by a thick three-layered muscular wall (greatest muscle-to-lumen ratio of any hollow viscus in the body). It is lined by pseudostratified columnar epithelium with nonmotile cilia, develops from the mesonephric duct, and is richly innervated by sympathetic fibers derived from the pelvic plexus.

2. Correct: These drain directly into the renal veins. (B)

Veins of the pampiniform plexus can be identified from their thinner walls and larger lumens. These form testicular veins, which, from the left side, drain directly into the left renal veins. These vessels are lined by simple squamous endothelial cells.

3. Correct: It is a direct branch from the abdominal aorta. (A)

The testicular artery can be identified by the intermediate thickness of its wall (between the ductus deferens and the veins), and a lumen smaller than the veins. It is lined by simple squamous endothelial cells and is innervated by sympathetic nerve fibers.

4. Correct: It drains into the cisterna chyli. (D)

Lymphatic vessels can be identified by the thinnest wall and the largest lumen. Lined by simple squamous endothelial cells, these drain into the cisterna chyli via the left lumbar trunk (from the lateral aortic lymph nodes).

5.   Correct: It sheds structures passing through the deep inguinal ring. (B)

Given its position deep to the cremaster muscle, this can be identified as the internal spermatic fascia. Derived from fascia transversalis, it sheds structures that pass through the deep inguinal ring. External spermatic fascia derives from external oblique abdominal muscle and sheds structures that pass through the superficial inguinal ring. Cremasteric muscle and fascia derive from the abdominal internal oblique muscle.

6.   Correct: It is primarily innervated by branches from the lumbar plexus. (E)

Cremaster muscle is innervated by the genital branch of the genitofemoral nerve, derived from the lumbar plexus. This is a skeletal muscle and therefore has no autonomic innervation.

7.   Correct: It is a direct branch from the superior vesical artery. (B)

Arteries to the ductus can be identified by their presence within the outer adventitial layer of the ductus deferens, and the proportional thickness of their walls to their lumen. These are usually branches from the superior vesical artery and are primarily innervated by sympathetic nerve fibers.

8.   Correct: Internal pudendal artery (C)

The image represents a cross section from the penis.
Image key:

1 – corpora cavernosa

2 – corpus spongiosum

3 – penile urethra

4 – penile septum

5 – tunica albuginea

6 – superficial fascia

7 – dorsal vein (paired in this specimen)

8 – dorsal artery

9 – deep artery

10 – thin tunica albuginea of the corpus spongiosum

The corpora cavernosa are primarily supplied by the deep penile artery, which is off the common penile branch of the internal pudendal artery.

9.   Correct: Internal iliac lymph nodes (D)

Lymphatics from the erectile tissue and penile urethra pass to the internal iliac lymph nodes. The penile and perineal skin (and the superficial fascia) are drained by the lymphatic vessels to the superficial inguinal nodes. Lymphatics from the glans penis (tip of the organ) pass to the deep inguinal and external iliac nodes. Lateral aortic lymph nodes drain the abdominal walls, kidneys, adrenal glands, gonads, pelvic walls and viscera, and the lower limbs.

10.   Correct: Superficial inguinal lymph nodes (A)

The penile and perineal skin (and the superficial fascia) is drained by the lymphatic vessels to the superficial inguinal nodes.

Lymphatics from the glans penis (tip of the organ) pass to the deep inguinal and external iliac nodes, and those from the erectile tissue and penile urethra pass to the internal iliac nodes. Lateral aortic lymph nodes drain the abdominal walls, kidneys, adrenal glands, gonads, pelvic walls and viscera, and the lower limbs.

11.   Correct: Stratified columnar (D)

Penile urethra is lined by stratified columnar epithelium. The urethra is lined by transitional epithelium till its prostatic part (to the colliculus seminalis, to be precise). Membranous and cavernous (penile) parts of it are lined by stratified or pseudostratified columnar epithelium. It is lined by stratified squamous epithelium at its tip at the navicular fossa.

12.   Correct: Lumbar (E)

The patient is suffering from right testicular cancer with retroperitoneal lymph node metastasis.
Image key:

1 – basal lamina

2 – spermatogonium

3 – primary spermatocyte

4 – mature spermatid

Lymph from the testis drains into the lumbar (para-aortic/lateral aortic) lymph nodes. From here it makes its way to the cisterna chyli via the right lumbar trunk.

13.   Correct: Inferior vena cava (E)

Venous drainage from the right testis is directly into the inferior vena cava, while that from the left one is through the left renal vein.

14.   Correct: It undergoes mitotic cell division. (C)

A spermatogonium can be identified by its location adjacent to the basal lamina of the seminiferous epithelium and the round nucleus. These are diploid (**E**) cells that divide by mitosis (**D**) to maintain their own population and also to generate primary spermatocytes. Interstitial cells of Leydig produce testosterone (**A**), while Sertoli cells produce androgen-binding protein (**B**).

15.   Correct: It undergoes meiotic cell division. (D)

Primary spermatocytes are identified by their intermediate location between the basal lamina and the lumen and their large nuclei with distinct chromatin structure. These have a diploid chromosome number (**E**) and a tetraploid DNA content and undergo meiosis I (**D**) to generate secondary spermatocytes. Interstitial cells of Leydig produce testosterone (**A**), while Sertoli cells produce androgen-binding protein (**B**).

16. Correct: It contains a haploid number of chromosomes. (E)

Spermatids can be identified by their location close to the lumen and their dense round nuclei. The darker-stained acrosomal caps of the spermatid nuclei are clearly discernible. Secondary spermatocytes rapidly undergo meiosis II to form haploid spermatids. Spermatids do not undergo nuclear division (**C, D**) but undergo cytoplasmic maturation (spermiogenesis) to transform into spermatozoa. Interstitial cells of Leydig produce testosterone (**A**), while Sertoli cells produce androgen-binding protein (**B**).

17. Correct: Anterior zone (D)

The patient is suffering from benign prostatic hyperplasia (BPH), which clinically manifests with urinary hesitancy, weak stream, and incomplete emptying. BPH causes bladder outlet obstruction by spasm of the urethral muscles and mechanical compression of the urethra due to the enlarged prostate. The biopsy seen in the figure has been obtained from the prostate gland.

Image key:

1 – prostatic gland (tubuloalveolar)

2 – fibromuscular stroma

3 – epithelial plicae

Glandular tissue within the prostate gland can be divided into three distinct zones: peripheral (70%), central (25%), and transitional (5%). Glands are absent and fibromuscular stroma predominates in the anterior zone.

18. Correct: Endoderm (B)

Prostatic glands develop from outgrowths of the prostatic urethra and are, therefore, endodermal in origin. Fibromuscular stroma develops from the surrounding mesoderm.

19. Correct: Acute epididymitis (B)

The patient is suffering from acute epididymitis. Men with epididymitis typically present with a gradual onset of scrotal pain and symptoms of lower urinary tract infection, including fever. Typical physical findings include a swollen, tender epididymis or testis located in the normal anatomic position with an intact ipsilateral cremasteric reflex. Ultrasound usually reveals an enlarged, thickened epididymis with increased blood flow on color Doppler. The diagnosis can be confirmed by identifying the figure as epididymis. Keys to identification are pseudostratified columnar epithelium with stereocilia (structure 1), lamina propria comprising 2 to 3 layers of smooth muscle cells (structure 2), and spermatozoa (structure 3) within the lumen. Structure 4 is a sectioned vein.

Orchitis (**A**) usually occurs when the inflammation from the epididymis spreads to the adjacent testicle. The onset of pain is abrupt. Ultrasound reveals swollen testicles with hypoechoic and hypervascular areas. Testicular torsion (**C**) presents with acute and severe pain. Pain is not relieved (actually aggravated) with testicular elevation. There is an abnormal cremasteric reflex. Decreased blood flow can be seen with color Doppler. Testicular cancer (**D**) patients could present with a painless testicular mass, scrotal heaviness, a dull ache, acute pain, infertility, or metastasis. Ultrasonography should detect an intra-testicular mass.

20. Correct: Their core is composed of actin microfilaments. (C)

Stereocilia are nonmotile and function to resorb testicular fluid; similar to microvilli, their core contains actin microfilaments.

The core of motile cilia comprise microtubules in a 9+2 arrangement (**A**). These propel tubular content forward (**D**). The core of a primary cilium or monocilium comprises microtubules in a 9+0 arrangement (**B**). Microvilli, but not stereocilia, are widespread in the jejunum (**E**).

21. Correct: It is stimulated primarily by sympathetic nerve fibers. (D)

The primary function of autonomic innervation of the epididymis is to mediate neuromuscular events required for the transport of spermatozoa. Contraction of smooth muscles of the epididymis for antegrade propulsion of spermatozoa is achieved primarily by sympathetic stimulation.

Epididymis, being an organ, is devoid of somatomotor supply (**A–C**). Parasympathetics (**E**) have no stimulatory function for the epididymis.

Chapter 17

Female Reproductive System Histology

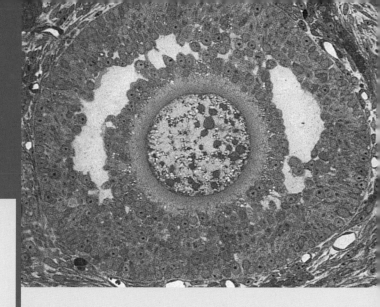

LEARNING OBJECTIVES

- ▶ Describe the organization of the ovary. Critique its microstructure in histologic sections.
- ▶ Describe the blood supply and lymphatic drainage of the ovary.
- ▶ Describe the organization of uterine tubes. Critique their microstructure in histologic sections. Correlate this with their functions.
- ▶ Describe the etiopathogenesis of acute salpingitis. Correlate these with its clinical features.
- ▶ Describe the organization of the uterus. Critique its microstructure in histologic sections. Correlate it with its functions.
- ▶ Analyze the changes in the levels of hormones that occur through a regular menstrual cycle. Correlate it with their functions.
- ▶ Describe the organization of the vagina. Critique its microstructure in histologic sections. Correlate it with its functions.
- ▶ Describe the etiopathogenesis of ectopic pregnancy. Correlate this with its clinical features.

17.1 Questions

Easy	Medium	Hard

Consider the following case for questions 1 to 7:

A 42-year-old woman presents with vague lower abdominal pain. She has regular menstrual periods with a 28-day cycle. Laboratory exams are significant for an elevated serum CA 125. Transvaginal ultrasonography reveals a right adnexal mass. She is diagnosed with cancer and subsequently treated with surgical resection of the organ from which the figure has been obtained.

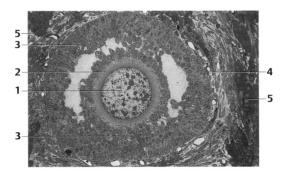

1. Which of the following ligaments, containing neurovasculature supply for the organ, would have been clamped during its surgical removal?

A. Broad ligament

B. Round ligament of the uterus

C. Proper ovarian ligament

D. Suspensory ovarian ligament

E. Mackenrodt's ligament

2. Which of the following is the primary and direct source of arterial blood for the resected organ?

A. Internal iliac artery

B. External iliac artery

C. Internal pudendal artery

D. External pudendal artery

E. Abdominal aorta

3. If metastatic cells were to spread via lymphatics, which of the following groups of lymph nodes would initially be affected in her case?

A. External iliac

B. Internal iliac

C. Lumbar

D. Superficial inguinal

E. Deep inguinal

4. Which of the following veins would initially be involved, if metastatic cells travel via veins?

A. Renal vein

B. Suprarenal vein

C. Internal iliac vein

D. External iliac vein

E. Inferior vena cava

5. In which of the following divisional stages is structure 1?

A. Prophase, meiosis I

B. Metaphase, meiosis I

C. Anaphase, meiosis I

D. Prophase, meiosis II

E. Metaphase, meiosis II

6. Which of the following is secreted by structure 4?

A. Estrogen

B. Progesterone

C. Aromatase

D. Androstenedione

E. Luteinizing hormone

7. On which of the following days during her cycle was the surgery (and hence the biopsy) probably done?

A. 3

B. 7

C. 10

D. 14

E. 21

Consider the following case for questions 8 to 10:

A 26-year-old woman presents with dull lower abdominal and pelvic pain, fever, and yellowish malodorous vaginal discharge. She has regular menstrual periods with a 28-day cycle. A physical exam is significant for a tender and swollen left adnexa. Laboratory exams are significant for an elevated ESR. Transvaginal ultrasonography reveals a left adnexal mass. She was diagnosed with inflammation of the organ from which the panels in the figure have been obtained.

Panel **b** is a 400X magnified area around structure 1 from panel **a**.

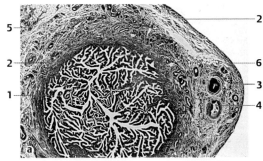

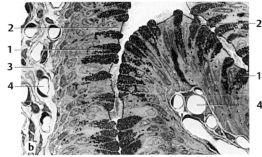

8. Which of the following is the diagnosis for her?

A. Acute oophoritis

B. Left ovarian cyst

C. Acute salpingitis

D. Acute endometritis

E. Acute appendicitis

9. Which of the following is true for structure 1 from panel **b**?

A. This is involved in secretion and has an extensive Golgi apparatus.

B. This is involved in absorption and has apical modifications that contain actin microfilaments in their core.

C. This is involved in fluid movement and has apical modifications that contain actin microfilaments in their core.

D. This is involved in fluid movement and has apical modifications that contain microtubules in their core.

E. This is found predominantly during the proliferative phase of the menstrual cycle.

10. Which of the following is true for structure 2 from panel **b**?

A. This is involved in secretion and has an extensive Golgi apparatus.

B. This is involved in absorption and has apical modifications that contain actin microfilaments in their core.

C. This is involved in fluid movement and has apical modifications that contain actin microfilaments in their core.

D. This is found predominantly during the proliferative phase of the menstrual cycle.

E. This is found predominantly during the secretory phase of the menstrual cycle.

Consider the following case for questions 11 to 15:

A 39-year-old woman presents with infertility. She has regular menstrual periods with a 28-day cycle, and she bleeds heavily for the first 3 days. Her physician explains that she will need a thorough examination of hormonal levels and endometrial features spanning through the entire menstrual cycle. Endometrial biopsies (all micrographs with same magnification) obtained from her through the cycle are seen in the figure.

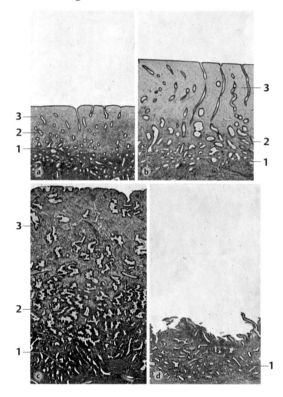

11. Which of the images above were obtained earliest from when she started to bleed?

A. a

B. b

C. c

D. d

12. Levels of which of the following hormones in her circulation is expected to be highest while panel a was obtained?

A. Estrogen

B. Progesterone

C. Follicle-stimulating hormone

D. Luteinizing hormone

13. Levels of which of the following hormones in her circulation is expected to be highest when panel **b** was obtained?

A. Estrogen

B. Progesterone

C. Follicle-stimulating hormone

D. Luteinizing hormone

14. Levels of which of the following hormones in her circulation is expected to be highest when panel **c** was obtained?

A. Estrogen

B. Progesterone

C. Follicle-stimulating hormone

D. Luteinizing hormone

15. Levels of which of the following hormones in her circulation is expected to be highest when panel d was obtained?

A. Estrogen

B. Progesterone

C. Follicle-stimulating hormone

D. Luteinizing hormone

Consider the following case for questions 16 to 17:

A 52-year-old diabetic patient presents with white vaginal discharge accompanied by severe itching. Physical examination reveals vulvovaginal erythema and a thick, curdy, nonmalodorous vaginal discharge. A local biopsy obtained from her is seen in the image.

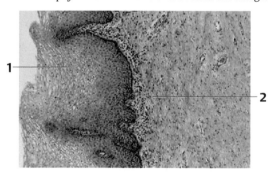

16. Which of the following is the source for the image?

A. Fallopian tube

B. Endocervical canal

C. Vagina

D. Labia minora

E. Perineal skin

17. Which of the following areas in humans would also exhibit structure 1?

A. Epidermis

B. Trachea

C. Vocal cord

D. Stomach

E. Follicles of thyroid gland

Consider the following case for questions 18 to 20:

A 32-year-old woman presents to the ER with acute and severe abdominal pain, and vaginal bleeding preceded by amenorrhea for 3 months. She has never been pregnant and has a history of regular menstrual periods with a 28-day cycle. She smokes ~ 5 to 6 cigarettes per day (for the past 6 years) and drinks socially. A physical exam is significant for an extremely tender left lower abdominal quadrant and tachycardia. The figures show normal sections from her various reproductive structures.

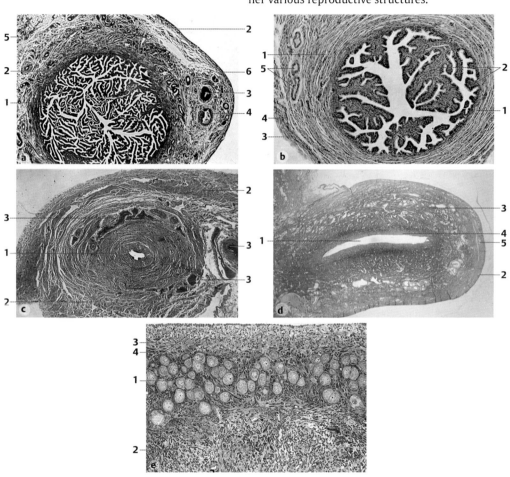

18. Which of the following is the probable diagnosis for her?

A. Endometriosis

B. Ruptured ectopic pregnancy

C. Acute salpingitis

D. Acute endometritis

E. Ovarian torsion

19. Which of the following is an expected finding in her?

A. ↑ Serum α-fetoprotein (AFP)

B. ↑ Amniotic fluid α-fetoprotein (AFP)

C. ↑ Elevated blood pressure

D. ↑ Serum β-human chorionic gonadotropin (hCG)

E. ↑ Serum carcinoembryonic antigen (CEA)

20. Which of the panels in the figure demonstrates the structure that was most likely involved in the abnormal process in the patient?

A. a

B. b

C. c

D. d

E. e

17.2 Answers and Explanations

Easy	Medium	Hard

1.   Correct: Suspensory ovarian ligament (D)

The patient was diagnosed with ovarian cancer and underwent an oophorectomy. Most women with either benign or malignant ovarian neoplasms either are asymptomatic or experience only mild nonspecific gastrointestinal symptoms or pelvic pressure. Serum CA 125 is elevated in 80% of women with epithelial ovarian cancer. The figure shows a secondary (antral) follicle within the ovarian cortex.

Image key:

   1 – primary oocyte

   2 – zona pellucida

   3 – granulosa cells

   4 – theca interna

   5 – interstitial gland cells

   Ovarian neurovasculature is transmitted to and fro between the ovaries and the lateral pelvic wall through the suspensory ligament of the ovary.

   The broad ligament (**A**) is a double layer of peritoneum that extends from lateral walls of the uterus to the pelvic walls. This contains uterine vessels. The round ligament of the uterus (**B**) is the distal remnant of the ovarian gubernaculum that extends from the uterine cornu to the labia majora. The proper ovarian ligament (**C**) is the proximal remnant of the ovarian gubernaculum that attaches the ovary to the uterine cornu. Mackenrodt's ligament (**E**), also termed transverse cervical ligament or cardinal ligament, inserts into the paracervical fascia medially and into the muscular side walls of the pelvis laterally. This forms the thick base of the broad ligament.

2.   Correct: Abdominal aorta (E)

Ovaries are primarily supplied by the ovarian arteries that are given off as direct branches from the abdominal aorta.

3.   Correct: Lumbar (C)

Lymph from ovaries drains into the lumbar (para-aortic/lateral aortic) lymph nodes. From here it makes its way to the cisterna chyli via the right lumbar trunk.

4.   Correct: Inferior vena cava (E)

Venous drainage from the right ovary is directly into the inferior vena cava, while that from the left one is through the left renal vein.

5.   Correct: Prophase, meiosis I (A)

Structure 1 is the primary oocyte of an antral follicle, which stays arrested in the diplotene stage of the prophase of its first meiotic division. It will complete the first meiotic division only prior to ovulation.

   Primordial germ cells populate the indifferent gonad during the 4th gestational week and differentiate into oogonia. Oogonia give rise to primary oocytes by mitotic division. Primary oocytes, formed by the 5th gestational month, enter meiosis I and stay arrested in prophase till prior to ovulation. At ovulation, a primary oocyte converts into a haploid secondary oocyte, which in turn, stays arrested in the metaphase of meiosis II (**E**) until fertilization.

6.   Correct: Androstenedione (D)

The theca cells surrounding the follicle are highly vascularized and use cholesterol, derived primarily from circulating lipoproteins, as the starting point for the synthesis of androstenedione under the control of LH. Androstenedione is transferred across the basal lamina to the granulosa cells, which are particularly rich in aromatase (**C**) and, under the control of FSH, produce estradiol, the primary ovarian steroid secreted during the follicular phase and the most potent estrogen (**A**). The large luteinized granulosa cells are the main source of progesterone (**B**) production in the ovary. Luteinizing hormone (**E**) is synthesized and secreted by the gonadotrophs located within the anterior pituitary gland.

7.   Correct: 10 (C)

A single dominant follicle emerges from the growing follicle pool within the first 5 to 7 (**A, B**) days of a regular menstrual cycle, while the majority of follicles fall off their growth trajectory and become atretic. The dominant follicle undergoes rapid expansion during the 5 to 6 days prior to ovulation (day 14), reflecting granulosa cell proliferation and accumulation of follicular fluid (thereby turning to a secondary or antral follicle). The dominant follicle would have turned into a graafian follicle at day 14 (**D**) and could be identified by a large antrum occupying most of the follicle, and arrangement of granulosa cells into corona radiata and cumulus oophorus. At day 21 (**E**), a corpus luteum would have developed that could be identified by granulosa lutein and theca lutein cells and highly vascularized surrounding connective tissue.

8. Correct: Acute salpingitis (C)

The patient is suffering from acute salpingitis.

Image key:

Panel **a**

1 – mucosa fold

2 – smooth muscle

3 – artery

4 – vein

5 – mesosalpinx

6 – tunica serosa

Panel **b**

1 – secretory (peg) cells

2 – ciliated cells

3 – lamina propria

4 – capillaries

The micrograph in panel **a** can be identified as the ampulla of the uterine tube by noting the extensive branching pattern of the mucosa that rises to high longitudinal folds. This is surrounded by irregularly arranged smooth muscle bundles.

9. Correct: This is involved in secretion and has an extensive Golgi apparatus. (A)

Peg cells secrete substances needed to provide nutrition and protection for the ovum and to activate the sperm. They lack cilia (**D**) or microvilli (**B**). These cells are particularly prominent from day 14 onward of the menstrual cycle, i.e., during the secretory phase (not proliferative phase, **E**). Structures that are involved in fluid movement (e.g., cilia) do not have apical modifications that contain actin microfilaments in their core (**C**).

10. Correct: This is predominant during the proliferative phase of the menstrual cycle. (D)

Apical surfaces of these simple columnar cells are ciliated, which help to move the fluid away from the ovary toward the uterus, thus moving the ovum toward the uterus. These cells are predominant during the proliferative phase of the menstrual cycle.

11. Correct: d (D)

Panel **a** was obtained during the early proliferative phase (days 6–9), **b** during the late proliferative phase (days 12–14), **c** during the mid-secretory phase (days 20–23), and **d** during the menstrual phase (days 1–3) of the menstrual cycle.

Image key:

1 – zona basalis

2 – zona spongiosa of functionalis

3 – zona compacta of functionalis

Endometrium is thinnest and comprises only the basal layer in panel **d**. The entire functional layer has been sloughed out. Hence this biopsy was obtained during the menstrual phase, i.e., during days 1 to 3 of her cycle.

12. Correct: Estrogen (A)

The intermediate thickness of the endometrium, appearance of the functional zone, and increased number of glands indicate the biopsy in panel **a** to have been obtained during the early proliferative phase (days 6–9) of the menstrual cycle. It corresponds to the follicular phase of the ovarian cycle, when estrogen is the predominant hormone (secreted from the ovarian follicles).

13. Correct: Luteinizing hormone (D)

Thicker endometrium (compared with panels **a** and **d**), expansion of zona compacta, and lengthening of glands that begin to coil (as seen in panel **b**) indicate the late proliferative phase (days 12–14) of the menstrual cycle. While the level of estrogen is still high, a surge in the levels of luteinizing hormone (LH) occurs during the periovulatory period (positive feedback by estrogen). LH, secreted from the anterior pituitary, is the predominant hormone during this period; it stimulates completion of first meiosis of the oocyte and ovulation.

14. Correct: Progesterone (B)

Thickest endometrium, dense population of undulating glands with saw-toothed acini and luminal secretion (as seen in panel **c**) indicate the secretory phase (days 15–27) of the menstrual cycle. This corresponds to the luteal phase of the ovarian cycle, when progesterone, secreted from the corpus luteum, is the predominant hormone.

15. Correct: Follicle-stimulating hormone (C)

Endometrium is thinnest and is found only in the basal layer, indicating the desquamation phase (days 1–5) of the menstrual cycle (as seen in panel **d**). FSH, secreted from the anterior pituitary, is the predominant hormone (negative feedback by estrogen) during this period and promotes folliculogenesis.

16. Correct: Vagina (C)

The patient is suffering from vulvovaginal candidiasis. The figure has been obtained from the vagina.

Image key:

1 – nonkeratinized stratified squamous epithelium

2 – lamina propria

The vagina is lined by nonkeratinized stratified squamous epithelium, and the mucosa is devoid of any glands.

The fallopian tube (**A**) is lined by simple columnar epithelium with alternating ciliated and secretory (peg) cells. The endocervical canal (**B**) is lined by simple columnar epithelium with long, branched mucus glands. Both labia minora (**D**) and perineal skin (**E**) will feature keratinized stratified squamous epithelium and plenty of sebaceous glands.

17. Correct: Vocal cord (C)

Vocal cords, like the vagina, are lined by nonkeratinized stratified squamous epithelium.

Epidermis (**A**, keratinized stratified squamous), trachea (**B**, pseudostratified columnar, ciliated), stomach (**D**, simple columnar, pits), and follicles of the thyroid gland (**E**, simple cuboidal) are lined by various distinct epithelia.

18. Correct: Ruptured ectopic pregnancy (B)

An ectopic pregnancy should be considered in any woman of child-bearing age who presents with the classic triad of symptoms (abdominal pain, amenorrhea, and vaginal bleeding). Risk factors should be included in the history, including prior ectopic pregnancy, history of pelvic inflammatory disease, smoking, use of intrauterine contraceptive devices, progestin-only birth control pills, and implanted progestin contraception. After the ectopic pregnancy has ruptured, the patient will experience sudden, continuous, and severe unilateral abdominal or pelvic pain.

Patients with endometriosis (**A**) usually have a history of dysmenorrhea and previous cyclic attacks of cramps and pains in the lower abdomen and possibly in the flank. Pain is worse with menses. Patients with both acute salpingitis (**C**) and acute endometritis (**D**) typically report a gradual onset of pelvic and lower abdominal pain frequently with associated foul-smelling vaginal discharge and/or bleeding. A history of amenorrhea is unlikely. Torsion of the ovary (**E**) is characterized by sudden unilateral lower abdominal or pelvic pain of moderate or severe intensity that is often made worse by a change in position. Amenorrhea or vaginal bleeding is unlikely.

19. Correct: ↑ Serum β-human chorionic gonadotropin (hCG) (D)

A quantitative serum β-hCG is positive in almost all cases of ectopic pregnancy. Hypotension (not hypertension, **C**) or shock may be found on initial examination. Serum AFP (**A, B**) and serum CEA (**E**) levels are not altered in ectopic pregnancy.

20. Correct: A (A)

Nearly all ectopic pregnancies (> 95%) occur in the fallopian tube (tubal pregnancy); it includes ampullary (70%), isthmic (12%), fimbrial (11%), and interstitial (2%). The ampullary portion of the uterine tube can be identified by noting the extensive branching pattern of the mucosa (structure 1) that rises to high longitudinal folds. This is surrounded by irregularly arranged smooth muscle (structure 2) bundles.

The isthmus of the uterine tube (**B**) can be identified by relatively wide mucosal folds (structure 2) that rarely branch. Also, thickness of the muscle layer (structure 1) increases from that of the ampullary part.

The intramural (uterine) part of the uterine tube (**C**) can be identified by a thick muscular layer (structure 1) that encases the narrow lumen, with complete lack of mucosal plicae.

Panel **d** is a sagittal section through the uterus identified by its cavity (structure 1) and the layers (endometrium is structure 4, myometrium is structure 3, and perimetrium is structure 2).

Panel **e** is a section through the ovary, featuring the cortex (lodging several follicles [structure 1]) and the medulla (structure 2).

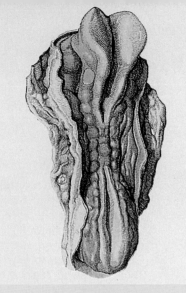

Chapter 18
General Embryology

LEARNING OBJECTIVES

- ▶ Analyze the pathogenesis, clinical presentation, diagnosis, and complications of hydatidiform mole (gestational trophoblastic disease).
- ▶ Describe the derivatives of neural crest cells in the adult human.
- ▶ Analyze the pathogenesis, clinical presentation, diagnosis, and complications of ruptured tubal pregnancy.
- ▶ Define the role of syncytiotrophoblasts during early development.
- ▶ Analyze the pathogenesis, clinical presentation, diagnosis, and complications of teratomas.
- ▶ Describe the timeline of events or stages in embryology and their unique vulnerabilities during early development.
- ▶ Analyze the pathogenesis, clinical presentation, diagnosis, and complications of Kartagener's syndrome.
- ▶ Define the contributions of individual germ layers to the future organs and systems.
- ▶ Describe the formation and composition of the bilaminar germ disk during early development.
- ▶ Analyze the pathogenesis, clinical presentation, diagnosis, and complications of mandibulofacial dysostosis (Treacher Collins' syndrome).
- ▶ Define the role of the prechordal plate in early development.
- ▶ Analyze the pathogenesis, clinical presentation, diagnosis, and complications of sirenomelia.
- ▶ Describe the important stages of the preimplantation phase. Outline the fundamental mechanisms of implantation.

18. 1 Questions

Easy	Medium	Hard

Consider the following case for questions 1 to 2:

A 33-year-old primigravida presents with vaginal bleeding and hyperemesis during the 10th week of her pregnancy. Physical examination reveals a uterine size much larger than expected for her gestational age, and a fetal heart sound cannot be located. Laboratory confirms abnormally elevated β-hCG levels in both serum and urine. Ultrasound demonstrates multiple hypoechoic areas suggestive of intrauterine mass, absence of gestational sac, and absent fetus. *PHLDA2* (a paternally imprinted, maternally expressed gene) staining of the evacuated mass is negative.

1. Proliferation of which of the following structures might be responsible for her symptoms?

A. Amnioblast

B. Cytotrophoblast

C. Syncytiotrophoblast

D. Cytotrophoblast and syncytiotrophoblast

E. Cytotrophoblast, syncytiotrophoblast, and amnioblast

2. Which of the following statements might be true for the patient?

A. A karyotype of the evacuated mass is likely to reveal a triploid pattern, commonly 69, XXX.

B. Chorionic villi within the evacuated mass are likely to contain proliferating blood vessels, which might have been the primary cause of her problems.

C. Serum thyroxine hormone (T$_4$) levels are most likely to be normal for her, and it would be a waste of resources to order her thyroid profile.

D. Ovarian cysts are highly unlikely in her case, and ultrasound examination should primarily focus inside the uterus.

E. She might secrete abnormal levels of protein in her urine during the first trimester, which should be adequately treated.

3. An embryologist develops fluorescent antibodies that bind to neural crest cells. Which of the following structures might be identified in a growing embryo employing these antibodies?

A. An organ that forms the roof of the 4th ventricle

B. A structure that forms the outermost layer of facial skin

C. An organ that stores antidiuretic hormone synthesized in the hypothalamus and releases it into circulation on stimulation

D. A cell that secretes hydrochloric acid within the gastrointestinal tract

E. A cell that myelinates peripheral spinal nerves

Consider the following case for questions 4 to 6:

A 20-year-old woman presents at the emergency department with severe abdominal pain on the right side, vaginal bleeding, and syncope. She indicates that she has been sexually active without contraception and missed her last menstrual period. A physical examination reveals diffuse abdominal tenderness, hypotension, feeble pulses, and tachycardia. β-hCG levels in both her serum and urine are positive for pregnancy.

4. Which of the following might the attending physician suggest as the immediate next step?

A. Reassure her, administer intravenous diazepam, and ask her to return to the ER if she misses her next menstrual period.

B. Reassure her, advise oral diazepam, and ask her to return for laboratories the next morning.

C. Reassure her and advise oral diethylstilbestrol.

D. Resuscitate and schedule her for a laparotomy the next morning.

E. Resuscitate, plan for immediate laparotomy.

5. Which of the following is true of the structure of the pathological organ (most likely) in her case?

A. It is lined by nonkeratinized stratified squamous epithelium.

B. It is lined by keratinized stratified squamous epithelium.

C. It is lined by simple cuboidal epithelium.

D. It is lined by nonciliated simple columnar epithelium.

E. It is lined by ciliated simple columnar epithelium.

6. Which of the following is true of the blood supply to the pathological organ (most likely) in her case?

A. It will suffer from ischemic necrosis because of blockage of the inferior mesenteric artery.

B. It will suffer from ischemic necrosis because of blockage of the superior mesenteric artery.

C. It will suffer from ischemic necrosis because of blockage of the abdominal aorta immediately proximal to the origin of the renal artery.

D. It will suffer from ischemic necrosis because of blockage of the abdominal aorta immediately proximal to the origin of the inferior mesenteric artery.

E. It will suffer from ischemic necrosis because of blockage of the uterine artery.

7. A family physician explains the mechanism by which over-the-counter pregnancy tests work to a 20-year-old woman. She mentions that these measure a hormone that appears in the urine and blood once the woman is pregnant. The cells that secrete the hormone are also responsible for which of the following?

A. Secreting amniotic fluid

B. Forming the anterior visceral endoderm

C. Forming the notochord

D. Invading the uterine endometrium during implantation

E. Initiating gastrulation

8. A 3-day-old newborn undergoes surgical correction of a spinal mass located at the caudal aspect of the spinal cord. Examination of the mass reveals adipose tissue, neural tissue, pancreatic endocrine tissue, skin, and skeletal muscle. Which of the following is the most likely origin of this mass?

A. Ectoderm

B. Endoderm

C. Mesoderm

D. Primitive streak

E. Notochord

9. A 26-year-old pregnant woman at 20 weeks gestation comes to her OB/GYN for a scheduled prenatal examination. Ultrasound reveals a cardiac septation defect in the fetus due to defective neural crest cell migration. During which weeks of gestation did this defect most likely occur?

A. 1 to 2 weeks

B. 4 to 6 weeks

C. 9 to 11 weeks

D. 12 to 15 weeks

E. 16 to 19 weeks

Consider the following case for questions 10 to 11:

A 34-year-old nonsmoking man presents with a chronic upper respiratory tract infection. On auscultation, bilateral wheeze and right basal crackles were audible, with heart sounds best heard on the right side of the chest. A chest X-ray PA view revealed a cardiac apex and an aortic arch on the right side. An ultrasound of the abdomen revealed a normal liver and gallbladder on the left side and a normal spleen on the right side.

10. Which of the following defects during embryonic development might be the underlying cause of his defect?

A. Persistence of primitive streak

B. Ineffective gastrulation

C. Ciliary dysfunction

D. Defective neural crest cell migration

E. Defective neurulation

11. Which of the following might be an associated finding in his case?

A. Peptic ulcer

B. Obstructive jaundice

C. Infertility

D. Pancreatitis

E. Cholelithiasis

12. A male newborn suffers a complex of congenital defects involving malformation of the urinary and genital ducts. Examination of his family history reveals several members sharing a similar background of genitourinary problems spanning three generations. These issues may be related to a genetic defect that is expressed in which of the following embryonic sites?

A. Surface ectoderm

B. Yolk sac endoderm

C. Intermediate mesoderm

D. Paraxial mesoderm

E. Neural crest

Consider the following case for questions 13 to 14:

An anxious 18-year-old woman rushes to the clinic as soon as she misses her menstrual period. She has a history of unprotected sexual intercourse through the previous month. She also reports that her menstrual cycles have otherwise been very regular. In the clinic, her urine tests positive for pregnancy.

13. In which week of embryonic development is she most likely in?

A. Start of week 1

B. Start of week 2

C. Start of week 3

D. Start of week 4

E. Start of week 5

14. Which of the following, most likely, is the composition of her embryo at the current stage?

A. Epiblast

B. Epiblast and hypoblast

C. Ectoderm

D. Ectoderm and mesoderm

E. Ectoderm, mesoderm, and endoderm

15. A 10-year-old girl presents with the chief complaint of decayed teeth. An examination revealed downward slanting of eyes, depressed zygomatic arches, sunken cheekbones, deformed external ears, coloboma of the lower eyelid, and a deviated nasal septum. Genetic testing revealed a mutation of the treacle (*TCOF1*) gene, which encodes a serine/alanine-rich nucleolar phosphoprotein responsible for the craniofacial development. Which of the following embryonic tissue is the most affected by this mutation?

A. Endoderm

B. Ectoderm

C. Mesoderm

D. Neural crest cells

E. Notochord

16. During early development, the prechordal plate (or anterior visceral endoderm) functions as an important signaling center in patterning the cranial end of the neural tube (forebrain). Which of the following cells gives rise to the prechordal plate?

A. Epiblast

B. Hypoblast

C. Amnioblast

D. Cytotrophoblast

E. Syncytiotrophoblast

Consider the following case for questions 17 to 18:

A routine sonogram at the 27th gestational week in a 23-year-old primigravida revealed a single fetus with bilateral renal agenesis and fused lower extremities. A full-term infant, small for its age and of undetermined sex, was born to the mother by spontaneous vaginal delivery. The infant had sacral agenesis, hypoplastic pelvis, fused lower extremities with paired femurs and tibias, but an absent fibula. The infant expired within 1 hour after delivery.

17. Which of the following might have been associated with the mother during pregnancy?

A. Elevated serum α-fetoprotein

B. Markedly elevated serum β-hCG

C. Diabetes

D. Polyhydramnios

E. Hyperemesis

18. Which of the following should be an invariable postmortem finding for the infant?

A. Single umbilical artery

B. 45, XO karyotype

C. Fusion of the upper limbs

D. Fusion of the cervical vertebrae

E. Fusion of the upper ribs

19. A 28-year-old pregnant woman undergoes chemotherapy with an antimitotic drug during the second through fifth gestational weeks. Which of the following layers might directly be affected by the drug, hindering implantation of the blastocyst?

A. Amnioblast

B. Epiblast

C. Hypoblast

D. Cytotrophoblast

E. Syncytiotrophoblast

20. A 23-year-old first-year medical student finds out that she is 4 weeks pregnant. It upsets her that she can't hear fetal heart sounds at least until 10 weeks' gestation. Which of the following is true for the embryo at the current stage?

A. Gastrulation is yet to begin.

B. Somites are yet to be formed.

C. The amniotic cavity is yet to be formed.

D. Neurulation may be complete.

E. The heart is yet to start developing.

18.2 Answers and Explanations

Easy	Medium	Hard

1. Correct: Cytotrophoblast and syncytiotrophoblast (D)

The patient is suffering from hydatidiform mole (diagnosed from classic symptoms, signs, and ultrasound findings).

These tumors are unique in that they develop from an aberrant fertilization event and therefore arise from fetal tissue within the maternal host. They are composed of both syncytiotrophoblastic (**C**) and cytotrophoblastic (**B**) cells. Amnioblasts (**A, E**) do not contribute to the formation of hydatidiform moles.

2. Correct: She might secrete abnormal levels of protein in her urine during the first trimester, which should be adequately treated. (E)

p57 immunohistochemistry staining can be used to stain for *PHLDA2*, a paternally imprinted, maternally expressed gene product, which is absent in complete moles but present in partial moles. Cytogenetic studies demonstrate that complete moles are usually euploid, paternal in origin, and 46, XX (90%) or 46, XY (10%). They arise when an empty ovum (with absent or inactivated nucleus/chromosomes) is fertilized by a haploid sperm (that duplicates its chromosomes), or by two haploid sperms. Partial moles, on the other hand, are triploid (**A**)—69, XXY (70%), 69, XXX (27%), or 69, XYY (3%). These arise when an ovum with an active nucleus is fertilized by a duplicated sperm or two haploid sperms.

Microscopically, moles may be identified by three classic findings: edema of the villous stroma, avascular villi (**B**), and nests of proliferating trophoblastic elements surrounding the villi.

Bilateral theca lutein cysts (**D**) are found in 15 to 30% of patients with complete moles, and their presence indicates a greater likelihood of developing malignant sequelae of gestational trophoblastic neoplasia.

Preeclampsia in the first trimester is pathognomonic for molar pregnancy. This is much more common with complete moles. A diagnosis of preeclampsia is made based on two criteria: (1) elevated maternal blood pressure of ≧140 mm Hg systolic or ≥ 90 mm Hg diastolic on 2 occasions 6 hours apart, and (2) proteinuria ≥ 300 mg in a 24-hour urine specimen (**E**).

Hyperthyroidism (**C**) from stimulation of thyrotropin receptors by hCG can also occur in 10% of patients. Again, this is much more frequent in patients with complete rather than partial moles.

3. Correct: A cell that myelinates peripheral spinal nerves (E)

Schwann cells, derived from the neural crest, myelinate the peripheral nerves.

The cerebellum forms the roof of the 4th ventricle (**A**). It forms from the rhombic lip of the metencephalon; thus it is derived from neuroectoderm. Epidermis forms the outermost layer of the skin (**B**). It is derived from surface ectoderm. The neurohypophysis (posterior pituitary) stores antidiuretic hormone synthesized in the hypothalamus (**C**). It forms from a downgrowth from the diencephalon; thus it is derived from neuroectoderm. Parietal cells, lining the fundic glands in the stomach, secrete hydrochloric acid within the gastrointestinal tract (**D**). These are derived from endoderm.

4. Correct: Resuscitate, plan for immediate laparotomy. (E)

She is most likely suffering from a ruptured ectopic pregnancy (diagnosed by secondary amenorrhea followed by first trimester vaginal bleeding, positive pregnancy test, and abdominal pain).

This is a hemodynamically compromised patient (diagnosed by hypotension, feeble pulses, tachycardia, and syncope). Immediate surgery is indicated, and exploratory laparotomy is preferred because it can provide rapid access to control intra-abdominal hemorrhage. Delaying surgery (**A–D**) will lead to uncontrolled internal hemorrhage and eventual maternal death. Ectopic pregnancy is the leading cause of pregnancy-related death in the first trimester and accounts for 4 to 10% of all pregnancy-related deaths.

5. Correct: It is lined by ciliated simple columnar epithelium. (E)

Nearly all ectopic pregnancies (> 95%) occur in the fallopian tube (tubal pregnancy). The fallopian tube is lined by ciliated simple columnar epithelium.

6. Correct: It will suffer from ischemic necrosis because of blockage of the abdominal aorta immediately proximal to the origin of the renal artery. (C)

Nearly all ectopic pregnancies (> 95%) occur in the fallopian tube (tubal pregnancy). The fallopian tube is supplied by branches from the uterine artery (off the internal iliac) and ovarian artery (branches off from the abdominal aorta at the level of the L2 vertebra).

The superior (**B**) and inferior (**A**) mesenteric arteries supply the gastrointestinal tract derived from the midgut and hindgut, respectively. The inferior mesenteric artery comes off the abdominal aorta at the level of the L3 vertebra. Blockage of the aorta immediately proximal to its origin (**D**) will not affect the ovarian artery; therefore, the fallopian tubes will not be necrosed. Blockage of the uterine arteries (**E**) will not affect the ovarian artery, so the fallopian tubes will not be necrosed.

7.   Correct: Invading the uterine endometrium during implantation (D)

Over-the-counter pregnancy kits measure human chorionic gonadotrophin (hCG) in the urine and serum of mothers, and hCG is produced by syncytiotrophoblasts. Syncytiotrophoblasts are also responsible for invading the uterine endometrium during implantation.

Early in the 2nd week, an amniotic cavity develops within the cells of the epiblast. Amnioblasts proliferate from the edges of the epiblast and secrete amniotic fluid (**A**).

An anterior visceral endoderm (**B**) is formed from hypoblast cells at the cranial end of the embryonic disc. It is an important signaling center to establish craniocaudal axis of the embryo and produces head-forming genes.

The notochord (**C**), a median cellular cord of the mesoderm extending from the primitive node to the prechordal plate, also acts as an embryonic organizer.

Gastrulation is the process that establishes the three definitive germ layers of the embryo. It is first indicated by formation of the primitive streak (day 15), caused by proliferation of epiblast cells (**E**).

8.   Correct: Primitive streak (D)

The newborn, most likely, had a sacrococcygeal teratoma. This germ cell tumor, originating from remnants of the primitive streak, consists of derivatives of all germ layers. Presence of adipose tissue and skeletal muscle (mesoderm, **C**), neural tissue (neuroectoderm, **A**), skin (surface ectoderm, **A**), and pancreatic endocrine tissue (endoderm, **B**) in the tumor confirms this to be a teratoma.

Chordomas are rare malignant tumors that arise from abnormal embryonic notochordal remnants (**E**). Other germ layer derivatives would not be found in such a tumor.

9.   Correct: 4 to 6 weeks (B)

The embryonic period (weeks 4–8) is most vulnerable to teratogens. Also, cardiac septation begins during the end of the 4th week and is almost complete by the end of the 5th week.

The germinal period (**A**, weeks 1–3) is characterized by a high rate of spontaneous abortions, chromosomal abnormalities being the leading cause. Weeks 9 through 19 (**C–E**) are not considered to be as vulnerable to teratogens as the embryonic period. These are times when most organ systems grow and mature, rather than form.

10.   Correct: Ciliary dysfunction (C)

The patient is suffering from Kartagener's syndrome (KS), which is an autosomal recessive ciliary motility disorder involving the triad of situs inversus, chronic sinusitis, and bronchiectasis.

The fibroblast growth factor (secreted by the primitive node) causes NODAL (also secreted by the node) to be concentrated to the left side of the developing embryo by the action of nodal cilia. This initiates a cascade of gene expression on that side, culminating in expression of the transcription factor *PITX2*, which is the master gene for establishing left-sidedness. Ciliary dysfunction causes laterality defects, such as dextrocardia (cardiac malrotation in which the heart is situated on the right side of the body with the apex pointing to the right) and situs inversus (transposition of thoracic or abdominal viscera). Also, ciliary movements propel fluid or particulate matter in one direction over the epithelial surface. Dysfunctional cilia lead to impaired mucociliary clearance with subsequent recurrent respiratory tract infections.

Persistence of primitive streak (**A**) can cause sacrococcygeal teratoma. Ineffective gastrulation (**B**) might cause caudal dysgenesis (sirenomelia). Defective neural crest cell migration (**D**) causes various abnormalities (cardiac septation defects, gastrointestinal tract motility defects, nerve conduction defects, etc.), and defective neurulation (**E**) can lead to structural defects within the central nervous system.

11.   Correct: Infertility (C)

The basic problem in KS lies in the defective movement of cilia, leading to recurrent chest infections, ear/nose/throat symptoms, and infertility. Infertility in male KS patients is due to diminished sperm motility. None of the other clinical features (**A–B** and **D–E**) are related to KS.

12.   Correct: Intermediate mesoderm (C)

Intermediate mesoderm primarily develops into genitourinary organs.

Surface ectoderm (**A**) develops into epidermis of the skin. Yolk sac endoderm (**B**) provides the first blood cells and the germ cells (eggs and sperm) for the embryo. Paraxial mesoderm (**D**) differentiates into somites and primarily develops into axial skeleton and skeletal muscles of the head and neck. Major derivatives of the neural crest cells (**E**) include spinal, cranial, and autonomic ganglia; Schwann and satellite cells; pia and arachnoidea mater; adrenal medulla, melanocytes; conotruncal septum (heart); and parafollicular cells of the thyroid gland.

13. Correct: Start of week 3 (C)

Embryonic age starts at fertilization. Fertilization occurs shortly after ovulation, which occurs at the 14th day of a normal menstrual cycle.

The woman notices her first missed period after a complete menstrual cycle (28 days), or at least after 2 completed weeks post-fertilization. Therefore, the embryo should be at the end of the 2nd week when she misses her first period.

14. Correct: Epiblast and hypoblast (B)

As noted earlier, the embryo should be at the end of the 2nd week when she misses her first period. Beginning at 2 weeks, the inner cell mass or embryoblast differentiates into the dorsal epiblast (**A**) and ventral hypoblast (bilaminar germ disk). The epiblast will form all three germ layers (ectoderm, mesoderm, and endoderm) by gastrulation during the 3rd week (**C–E**).

15. Correct: Neural crest cells (D)

The girl is suffering from Treacher Collins' syndrome (TCS), otherwise known as mandibulofacial dysostosis, which is an autosomal dominant disorder of craniofacial development. Mutation of *TCOF1* results in failure of neural crest cells to migrate into the first and second branchial arches, which may affect the size and shape of the ears, eyelids, cheekbones, and jaws. Endoderm (**A**), ectoderm (**B**), mesoderm (**C**), and notochord (**E**) do not contribute to the defective bone and cartilages in the child.

16. Correct: Hypoblast (B)

Prechordal plate cells are modified tall columnar cells located at the cranial end of the hypoblast. The epiblast will form all three germ layers (ectoderm, mesoderm, and endoderm) by gastrulation during the 3rd week (**A**). Amnioblasts proliferate from the edges of the epiblast and secrete amniotic fluid (**C**). Cytotrophoblast (**D**) and syncytiotrophoblast (**E**) form placental structures.

17. Correct: Diabetes (C)

The fetus suffered from sirenomelia, which is a lethal condition characterized by fusion of the lower limbs and severe malformations of the urogenital and lower gastrointestinal tracts. Other anomalies associated with this condition are defects in the lumbar and sacral vertebrae, renal agenesis, imperforate anus, and agenesis of the internal genital structures except the testes and ovaries.

Sirenomelia is most frequently observed among infants of diabetic mothers.

Serum α-fetoprotein (**A**) and β-hCG (**B**) are not elevated in sirenomelia. Renal agenesis is complicated by oligohydramnios, not polyhydramnios (**D**). Hyperemesis (**E**) has no known significant association with sirenomelia.

18. Correct: Single umbilical artery (A)

Sirenomelia, invariably accompanied by a single umbilical artery, may be caused by abnormalities that affect the distribution of blood to the caudal region of the fetus. The vascular steal theory indicates that a single large artery assumes the function of the umbilical arteries, thus diverting blood flow from the caudal portion of the embryo to the placenta.

Fetal karyotype is usually normal (46, XY) in sirenomelia (**B**). Bones of the upper limbs and thorax are usually normal in sirenomelia (**C–E**), since ineffective gastrulation/inadequate blood supply chiefly affects the lower body.

19. Correct: Cytotrophoblast (D)

Trophoblast differentiates into cytotrophoblast and syncytiotrophoblast early in the 2nd week. The cells of the cytotrophoblast are mitotically active and continuously contribute to the syncytiotrophoblast. Cells within the syncytiotrophoblast (**E**) are responsible for invading the uterine endometrium during implantation, but do not divide. Amnioblast (**A**), epiblast (**B**), and hypoblast (**C**) do not directly participate in blastocyst implantation.

20. Correct: Neurulation may be complete. (D)

Neurulation is the process by which the neural plate forms the neural tube. It initiates during the 3rd week and concludes at the end of the 4th week (with closure of the posterior neuropore, day 28).

Gastrulation establishes the three germ layers for the embryo by the 3rd week (**A**). The first pair of somites forms in the occipital region of the embryo at around the 20th day (**B**). The amniotic cavity develops within the cells of epiblast early in the 2nd week (**C**). The heart begins to form late in the 3rd week and starts to beat by the 4th week (**E**).

Chapter 19

Musculoskeletal and Integumentary System Embryology

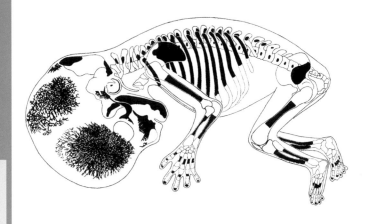

LEARNING OBJECTIVE

- ▶ Analyze the etiopathogenesis, clinical features, and diagnosis of hypohidrotic ectodermal dysplasia.
- ▶ Describe the embryological derivation of the skin and its appendages.
- ▶ Describe the embryological derivation of cells within the epidermis. Correlate their microstructure with their functions.
- ▶ Analyze the etiopathogenesis, clinical features, and diagnosis for Duchenne's muscular dystrophy.
- ▶ Discuss the embryological derivation of skeletal muscles.
- ▶ Analyze the etiopathogenesis, clinical features, and diagnosis of piebaldism.
- ▶ Discuss the embryological derivation of intervertebral disk.
- ▶ Analyze the etiopathogenesis, types, clinical features, and diagnosis of epidermolysis bullosa.
- ▶ Analyze the etiopathogenesis, clinical features, and diagnosis of osteogenesis imperfecta.
- ▶ Analyze the etiopathogenesis, clinical features, and diagnosis of Hirschsprung's disease.

19.1 Questions

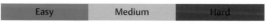

| Easy | Medium | Hard |

Consider the following case for questions 1 to 2:

An 8-year old boy presents due to lack of teeth as well as speech and mastication problems. Physical examination revealed a prominent forehead, sparse and very fine scalp hair and eyebrows, depressed nasal bridge, protuberant lips, large chin, and soft, dry, light-colored skin. An intraoral examination revealed complete absence of primary and permanent teeth.

1. Which of the following might be responsible for his defects?

A. Antibodies against hemidesmosomal proteins

B. Antibodies against anchoring fibrils in the basement membrane zone

C. Mutation in the *KIT* proto-oncogene

D. Defective enzyme tyrosinase

E. Mutation in the gene ectodysplasin

2. A histopathological slide obtained from him might show normal growth of which of the following structures?

A. Epidermis

B. Hair papillae

C. Sweat glands

D. Sebaceous glands

E. Lacrimal glands

3. A 26-year-old 4-week pregnant mother presents with a viral fever. The virus has a known predilection for the bone marrow. Which of the following functions might be affected in the newborn?

A. Attachment between the epidermal cells

B. Attachment of the epidermis to the underlying dermis

C. Coloration of the skin

D. Processing of invading pathogens

E. Tactile two-point discrimination

Consider the following case for questions 4 to 9:

A 3-year-old boy is brought to the physician because of difficulty rising to stand and an unstable gait. He falls frequently and has difficulty keeping up with friends when playing. Family history for similar symptoms is negative for his parents or his elder sister (who is 5 years old), but is positive for his maternal grandfather. On getting up from the floor, he uses his hands to climb up himself. A physical examination revealed bulging of the calf area. No sensory or other neurological deficits could be demonstrated. Laboratory findings were significant for an elevated serum creatine kinase.

4. Which of the following is the seat of the defect in him?

A. Chromosome 21

B. Chromosome 13

C. Chromosome 18

D. X chromosome

E. Y chromosome

5. Which of the following proteins is defective in him?

A. Actin

B. Myosin

C. Titin

D. Troponin

E. Dystrophin

6. Which of the following muscles will initially be affected in him?

A. Sternocleidomastoid

B. Rectus femoris

C. Pronator teres

D. Orbicularis oculi

E. Pectoralis major

7. Which of the following is an almost invariable complication of the disease?

A. Anemia

B. Cardiomyopathy

C. Stroke

D. Pathologic fractures

E. Seizure disorders

8. Extensions of the hip and knee are severely compromised with progression of the disease. Which of the following embryonic sources accounts for the structures defective for the movements?

A. Paraxial mesoderm

B. Intermediate mesoderm

C. Visceral mesoderm

D. Parietal mesoderm

E. Neural crest

9. Which of the following is a usual cause of death from the disease?

A. Cardiac arrhythmia

B. Congestive cardiac failure

C. Left ventricular failure

D. Respiratory failure

E. Renal failure

Consider the following case for questions 10 to 12:

A 20-month-old girl presented with white patches over the ventral surfaces of the mid-trunk and over mid-portions of the ventral surfaces of the lower extremities. The patches were asymptomatic and did not show any progression after their appearance. A well-circumscribed white forelock in the mid-frontal region with a depigmented macule on the middle of the forehead was also seen. She had no obvious ocular, hearing, or neurological defects.

10. Which of the following is the probable diagnosis for her?

A. Oculocutaneous albinism type 1 (OCA1)

B. Oculocutaneous albinism type 2 (OCA2)

C. Vitiligo

D. Piebaldism

E. Waardenburg's syndrome

11. Which of the following might be responsible for her defects?

A. Antibody-mediated destruction of epidermal melanocytes

B. Mutation in the *OCA2* gene

C. Mutation in the *KIT* proto-oncogene

D. Mutation in the *TYR* gene

E. Mutation in gene coding for ectodysplasin

12. Defect in which of the following embryonic germ layers is responsible for the features in the child?

A. Surface ectoderm

B. Neuroectoderm

C. Neural crest cells

D. Mesoderm

E. Endoderm

13. A 33-year-old woman presents with progressive low back pain and severe, radiating pain in the right lower extremity of 2 months' duration. She also reports associated numbness and weakness in her right lower extremity. Physical examination revealed positive sciatic nerve stretch testing and weakness in her lower limb muscles, particularly below the knee. An MRI revealed a herniated structure compressing the roots of the right sciatic nerve. Which of the following embryonic sources accounts for the structure(s) that is/are most likely defective in her?

A. Notochord

B. Paraxial mesoderm

C. Lateral plate mesoderm

D. A and B

E. A, B, and C

Consider the following case for questions 14 to 15:

A male neonate was born with large areas of skin damage and erosion and was admitted to the hospital several hours after birth. Areas primarily affected were bilateral lower limbs below the knee joint and bilateral upper limbs below the elbow joints. The oral cavity, conjunctiva, cornea, nails, scalp, and genitalia were normal. He eventually developed multiple blisters followed by skin peeling and erosion, but no scarring, mostly when subject to friction. Bacterial cultures obtained from the skin lesions were negative. An electron micrograph of the histopathology specimen obtained from the lesions showed disruption of the dermoepidermal basement membrane zone. Immunomapping studies with antibodies to a hemidesmosomal protein and a lamina densa protein reveal both localizing at the floor of the blister.

14. Defect in which of the following is the possible diagnosis for the neonate?

A. Bullous pemphigoid

B. Pemphigus vulgaris

C. Junctional epidermolysis bullosa

D. Dystrophic epidermolysis bullosa

E. Epidermolysis bullosa simplex

15. Which of the following proteins is most likely defective or absent in her case?

A. Keratin 5

B. Integrin β4

C. Laminin 5

D. Collagen type XVII

E. Collagen type VII

Consider the following case for questions 16 to 18:

A male newborn is brought in with a swelling and deformity of the right lower extremity. He is screaming relentlessly and is in obvious pain. An X-ray reveals multiple fractures of the right femur and tibia with reduced bone density. Family history is notable for multiple childhood fractures following trivial trauma in his mother and maternal grandfather that got better as they grew into adulthood.

16. Which of the following is the most likely diagnosis for the newborn?

A. Rickets

B. Paget's disease

C. Osteomyelitis

D. Osteoporosis

E. Osteogenesis imperfecta

17. Which of the following tissues predominantly contains the structure that is defective in the newborn?

A. Hyaline cartilage

B. Fibrous cartilage

C. Vitreous body of the eye

D. Papillary layer of the dermis

E. Glomerular basement membrane

18. Which of the following clinical features might be expected in his maternal grandfather?

A. Osteoarthritis

B. Cataract

C. Deafness

D. Hematuria

E. Proteinuria

Consider the following case for questions 19 to 20:

A 33-year-old woman delivers a full-term infant. After 3 days and several feeding sessions, the baby has still not passed stool. Over the next 8 hours, the baby wets his diaper, has a bulge in the abdomen, but still has not had his first stool. Auscultation reveals normal peristaltic sounds in the upper abdomen and almost absent sounds in the lower abdomen. A per-rectal exam came back normal with meconium-covered gloved fingers.

19. Which of the following might be an associated defect in the neonate?

A. Attachment between the epidermal cells

B. Attachment of the epidermis to the underlying dermis

C. Coloration of the skin

D. Processing of invading pathogens

E. Dysfunctional barrier in the skin to prevent water loss

20. Which of the following germ layers might be the seat of the defects for the neonate?

A. Endoderm

B. Mesoderm

C. Neuroectoderm

D. Neural crest

E. Surface ectoderm

19.2 Answers and Explanations

Easy	Medium	Hard

1. Correct: A mutation in the gene ectodysplasin (E)

Hypohidrotic ectodermal dysplasia (HED) is a hereditary disorder that occurs as a consequence of disturbances in the ectoderm of the developing embryo. The triad of nail dystrophy (onychodysplasia), alopecia or hypotrichosis (scanty, fine, and light hair on the scalp and eyebrows), and palmoplantar hyperkeratosis is usually accompanied by a lack of sweat glands (hypohidrosis) and a partial or complete absence of primary and/or permanent dentition.

Ectodysplasin belongs to the tumor necrosis factor family and plays a role in regulation of the formation of ectodermal structures. HED results from alterations in the gene for ectodysplasin.

Antibodies against hemidesmosomal proteins (**A**, junctional epidermolysis bullosa) or anchoring fibrils (**B**, dystrophic epidermolysis bullosa) are not seen in HED. These are blistering skin diseases and will not present with generalized involvement of ectodermal derivatives.

Mutation of the *KIT* proto-oncogene (**C**, piebaldism) or loss of function of the enzyme tyrosinase (**D**, oculocutaneous albinism type 1) will present with hypopigmentation. Again, generalized involvement of ectodermal derivatives will be absent.

2. Correct: Hair papillae (B)

Hair papillae are mesodermal invagination within the hair bulbs infiltrated by neurovascular structures.

Skin (**A**, epidermis) and its appendages—the sebaceous glands (**D**), the hair and sweat glands (**C**), the teeth and salivary glands, the lacrimal glands (**E**), and the mammary glands—all are ectodermal derivatives. Loss of function of ectodysplasin would affect all of these.

3. Correct: Processing of invading pathogens (D)

Langerhans cells arise from hematopoietic cells in the bone marrow and function as antigen-presenting cells within the epidermis.

Attachment between epidermal cells (**A**) is primarily mediated by desmosomes of keratinocytes within the stratum spinosum. Attachment between the epidermis and dermis (**B**) is primarily achieved by hemidesmosomes of keratinocytes within the stratum basale. Keratinocytes derive from surface ectoderm.

Melanocytes derive from the neural crest and migrate to the epidermis during embryogenesis. Synthesized by melanocytes, melanin contributes to skin, eye, and hair color (**C**).

Merkel cells function as mechanoreceptors and are important in fine touch sensation for two-point discrimination (**E**). These derive from ectoderm.

4. Correct: X chromosome (D)

The boy is suffering from Duchenne's muscular dystrophy (DMD), which is an X-linked recessive disorder that presents with progressive muscle weakness. While present at birth, it becomes apparent by the age of 3 to 5 years. On getting up from the floor, the patient uses his hands to push himself up to a standing position (Gowers maneuver)—a pathognomonic sign for the disease. Pseudohypertrophy of the calf muscles (replacement of muscle fibers by fibrous tissue) is another characteristic finding.

The defective gene, dystrophin, is localized to the short arm of the X chromosome at Xp21. Also, following the pedigree, this patient is the nonfounding son of two unaffected parents. Therefore, the disease must be X-linked recessive.

5. Correct: Dystrophin (E)

DMD is caused by a mutation of the gene that encodes dystrophin, a protein localized to the inner surface of the sarcolemma of the muscle fiber. Mutation of the dystrophin gene weakens the sarcolemma, causing membrane tears and a cascade of events leading to muscle fiber necrosis.

6. Correct: Rectus femoris (B)

Loss of muscle strength is progressive, with predilection for the proximal limb muscles and the neck flexors. Lower extremity involvement is more severe than upper extremity. Rectus femoris is the only proximal limb muscle listed.

7. Correct: Cardiomyopathy (B)

Virtually all survivors of DMD develop dilated cardiomyopathy, which often is the primary feature of the disease. None of the other listed features are constant associations with DMD.

8. Correct: Paraxial mesoderm (A)

Extension for both hip and knee is mediated by skeletal muscles. All skeletal muscles in humans develop from paraxial mesoderm. The limb (abaxial) muscles develop from myogenic cells from the ventrolateral region of the dermomyotome that migrate into the adjacent parietal layer of the lateral plate mesoderm.

9. Correct: Respiratory failure (D)

Joint contractures and progressive scoliosis often develop in DMD. The chest deformity with scoliosis impairs pulmonary function, which is already diminished by muscle weakness. By age 16 to 18 years, patients are predisposed to serious, sometimes fatal pulmonary infections. Respiratory failure is the usual cause of death in these individuals. A cardiac cause of death is uncommon despite the presence of cardiomyopathy in almost all patients.

10. Correct: Piebaldism (D)

Piebaldism is an autosomal dominant disorder characterized by the congenital absence of melanocytes in affected areas of the skin and hair. Affected individuals present at birth with a white forelock and relatively stable, persistent depigmentation of the skin with a characteristic distribution. A white forelock of hair arising from a midline, depigmented macule on the forehead is invariably associated. Other characteristic distribution of depigmented macules includes the anterior abdomen extending to the chest and the mid-extremities, sparing the hands and feet.

Ocular nystagmus and reduced visual acuity are important features of albinism (**A–B**) that distinguish albinism from other congenital disorders of pigmentation. Vitiligo (**C**) is characterized by progressive autoimmune-mediated destruction of epidermal melanocytes. A congenital presentation is uncommon, and it often demonstrates a predilection for sun-exposed regions, body folds, and periorificial areas. While Waardenburg's syndrome (**E**) might present with a white hair forelock, congenital deafness and pigmentary disturbances (heterochromia) of the iris are diagnostic features.

11.   Correct: Mutation in the *KIT* proto-oncogene (C)

Piebaldism is due to mutations of the *KIT* proto-oncogene that encodes tyrosine kinase (transmembrane receptor for the mast/stem cell growth factor). Vitiligo is characterized by progressive autoimmune-mediated destruction of epidermal melanocytes (**A**). Oculocutaneous albinism type 1 (OCA1) is caused by the loss of function of the melanocytic enzyme tyrosinase resulting from mutations of the *TYR* gene (**D**). Mutation in the *OCA2* gene (**B**) causes the OCA2 phenotype. Mutation in the ectodysplasin gene (**E**) causes hypohidrotic ectodermal dysplasia, in which ectodermal derivatives (skin, hair, nail, teeth, etc.) are affected.

12.   Correct: Neural crest cells (C)

Mutation in the *KIT* proto-oncogene affects differentiation and migration of melanoblasts from the neural crest during embryonic life. Other listed germ layers are not involved in the pathogenesis of piebaldism.

13.   Correct: A and B (D)

The patient is suffering from a right-sided L5-S1 extruded disk herniation. Each intervertebral disk is made up of a strong outer ring of fibers (anulus fibrosus) and a soft, gel-like center (nucleus pulposus). Herniation of a disk occurs when the anulus fibrosus tears and the nucleus pulposus moves out of its normal position and into the spinal canal. The displaced disk may compress nearby spinal nerves (such as the sciatic) or exert pressure on the spinal cord. The notochord (**A**) contributes to the nucleus pulposus, while the anulus fibrosus is formed from sclerotome (**B**, paraxial mesoderm) cells.

14.   Correct: Epidermolysis bullosa simplex (E)

Epidermolysis bullosa (EB) is a heterogeneous group of hereditary disorders characterized by skin fragility with blistering. Epidermolysis bullosa is classified according to the level of dermal–epidermal basement membrane zone (BMZ) separation on transmission electron microscopy into simplex (EBS), junctional (JEB), and dystrophic (DEB) subtypes.

The neonate is suffering from localized EBS. Blistering activity usually follows areas of trauma, with the hands and feet being the most common. Milia and scarring as a rule are absent following blister healing.

Bullous pemphigoid (**A**) is an autoimmune (antibodies directed against hemidesmosomal proteins) subepidermal blistering disease of the elderly. Lesions are usually distributed over the lower abdomen, groin, and flexor surface of the extremities.

Pemphigus vulgaris (**B**) is an antibody-mediated (antibodies directed against desmosomal proteins) mucocutaneous blistering disease that is predominant in patients over the age of 40 years. It typically begins on mucosal surfaces and often progresses to involve the skin. Involvement of the mouth, scalp, face, neck, axilla, groin, and trunk is characteristic.

JEB (**C**) is characterized by generalized and often extensive blistering at birth, with a distinct predilection for periorificial areas around the mouth, eyes, and nares. Nails are usually severely affected—presence of nail involvement with periungual hypertrophic granulation tissue during the neonatal period is a clue to the diagnosis.

DEB (**D**) is characterized by blisters that heal with scarring and milia formation. Nail dystrophy or nail loss with atrophic scarring of the distal digits is common.

15.   Correct: Keratin 5 (A)

Immunomapping with antibodies to a hemidesmosomal protein (BP230) and a lamina densa protein (type IV collagen) can distinguish EBS, JEB, and DEB.

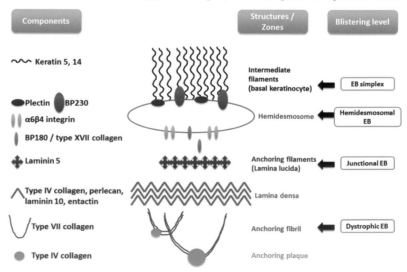

As is evident from the figure:

- In case of mutations in genes coding for keratin 5, as in EBS, both antibodies localize to the floor of the blister.

- In case of mutations in genes coding for β4 integrin (**B**), laminin 5 (**C**), collagen XVII (**D**), as in JEB, BP230 localizes to the roof of the blister, while type IV collagen localizes to the floor.

- In case of mutations in genes coding for collagen type VII (**E**) as in DEB, both antibodies localize to the roof of the blister.

16. Correct: Osteogenesis imperfecta (E)

The newborn is suffering from osteogenesis imperfecta (OI), which is an inherited collagen disorder that might present in the neonate with multiple pathological fractures. The family history (involving a female, and a member from every generation) suggests an autosomal dominant inheritance pattern.

Rickets (**A**) is a dietary deficiency of vitamin D that interferes with skeletal ossification. Abnormal mineralization in growing bone affects the transformation of cartilage into bone. This is highly unlikely to present with multiple pathological fractures in the newborn, and it should not have an autosomal dominant inheritance pattern.

Paget's disease of the bone (**B**) is characterized by excessive abnormal bone remodeling. It usually presents in persons older than 55 years.

Osteomyelitis (**C**) is an infectious process that usually starts in the spongy or medullary bone and extends into compact or cortical bone. In the infant (younger than age 1 year), there is direct vascular communication with the epiphysis across the growth plate. Bacterial spread occurs from the metaphysis to the epiphysis and into the joint. Multiple neonatal bone affection is extremely unlikely, let alone fractures.

Osteoporosis (**D**) is a metabolic skeletal disease defined as a reduction of bone mass that presents as homogeneously osteolytic lesions. Primary osteoporosis occurs in postmenopausal women or in older men and women due to age-related factors. Secondary osteoporosis results from specific clinical disorders, such as endocrinopathies, trauma, or inflammation.

17. Correct: Fibrous cartilage (B)

Osteogenesis imperfecta is a disease of type I collagen, which constitutes the major extracellular protein in the body. More than 90% of cases are caused by mutations of the *COL1A1* or *COL1A2* genes, which encode the subunits of type I collagen, pro-α-1 (I) and pro-α-2 (I). Fibrous cartilage predominantly contains type I collagen.

Hyaline cartilage (**A**) and vitreous body (**C**) primarily contain type II collagen. Collagen fibers are primarily of type III and type IV for the papillary layer of dermis (**D**) and glomerular basement membrane (**E**), respectively.

18. Correct: Deafness (C)

The fracture incidence in OI decreases after puberty and the main features in adult life are mild short stature, conductive hearing loss, and occasionally dentinogenesis imperfecta. Hearing loss usually begins during the second decade of life and occurs in more than 50% of individuals over age 30. The loss can be conductive, sensorineural, or mixed, and it varies in severity. The middle ear usually exhibits maldevelopment, deficient ossification, and abnormal calcium deposits.

The pathologic hallmark of osteoarthritis (**A**) is hyaline articular cartilage (type II collagen) loss. It is not directly related to OI. The lens capsule is primarily made up of type IV collagen. Cataract (**B**) is not a known association for OI. Proteinuria (**D**) and hematuria (**E**) can occur in diseases affecting the glomerular basement membrane (type IV collagen).

19. Correct: Coloration of the skin (C)

Not passing stool for the first 3 days raises the suspicion of a lower GI motility disorder or an imperforate anus. A normal per-rectal exam rules out the possibilities of imperforate anus or anal atresia. The clinical feature is consistent with Hirschsprung's disease, which results from a lack of ganglia in the distal colon due to a defect in migration of neural crest cells.

Melanocytes derive from the neural crest and migrate to the epidermis during embryogenesis. Synthesized by melanocytes, melanin contributes to skin, eye, and hair color.

Attachment between epidermal cells (**A**) is primarily mediated by desmosomes of keratinocytes within stratum spinosum. Attachment between the epidermis and dermis (**B**) is primarily achieved by hemidesmosomes of keratinocytes within stratum basale. Keratinocytes in the stratum corneum provide mechanical protection to the skin and form a barrier to water loss and permeation of soluble substances from the environment (**E**). Keratinocytes derive from surface ectoderm.

Langerhans cells arise from hematopoietic cells (mesoderm) in the bone marrow and function as antigen-presenting cells within the epidermis (**D**).

20. Correct: Neural crest (D)

Defective migration of neural crest cells during embryogenesis is the underlying pathogenic mechanism in Hirschsprung's disease.

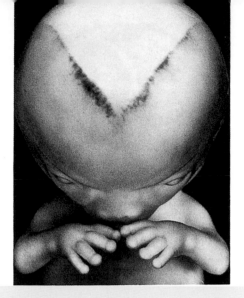

Chapter 20

Head and Neck Embryology

LEARNING OBJECTIVES

► Describe various structures involved in formation of the face; determine how these contribute to formation of the lip and palate.

► Analyze the pathogenesis, clinical features, and differential and definitive diagnoses of congenital midline and lateral neck masses.

► Describe the development of the pharyngeal pouches and their derivatives.

► Analyze the pathogenesis, clinical features, and differential and definitive diagnoses of recurrent laryngeal nerve palsy.

► Describe the development of the pharyngeal arches and their derivatives.

► Analyze the pathogenesis and clinical features of glossopharyngeal nerve palsy.

► Describe the exit pathways for cranial nerves through the skull base.

► Describe the innervation of the tongue and relate this to its development.

► Differentiate between pharyngeal arch, pouch, cleft, and membrane; determine their relationships with each other.

► Analyze the pathogenesis, clinical features, and differential and definitive diagnoses of laryngomalacia and tracheomalacia.

► Analyze the pathogenesis and clinical features of facial nerve palsy.

► Analyze the pathogenesis, clinical features, and differential and definitive diagnoses of thymoma.

► Analyze the pathogenesis, clinical features, and differential and definitive diagnoses of superior laryngeal nerve palsy.

► Analyze the pathogenesis and clinical features of trigeminal nerve palsy.

► Analyze the pathogenesis and clinical features for Treacher Collins' syndrome.

20.1 Questions

Easy	Medium	Hard

1. A 10-month-old male child presents with a lateral cleft lip affecting the left side. There are no abnormalities of the baby's palate. Which of the following developmental defects accounts for this occurrence?

A. Failure of the left maxillary prominence to unite with the left lateral nasal prominence

B. Failure of the left maxillary prominence to unite with the left medial nasal prominence

C. Failure of the primary palate to fuse with the secondary palate

D. Failure of the right and left medial nasal prominences to fuse

E. Failure of the right and left lateral palatine processes to fuse

Consider the following case for questions 2 to 3:

A 12-year-old boy presents with a palpable left-sided asymptomatic neck mass. Physical examination revealed a soft, mobile, and nontender mass located in the left anteroinferior part of the neck. His serum ionic calcium and thyroid and parathyroid hormone levels were normal. An ultrasound revealed a cystic structure contiguous with the lower pole of the left lateral thyroid lobe. Fine needle aspiration revealed crystal-clear fluid from the cyst.

2. Which of the following is the most probable diagnosis for him?

A. Infected branchial cleft cyst

B. Thyroid toxic adenoma

C. Thyroglossal duct cyst

D. Parathyroid gland cyst

E. Parathyroid carcinoma

3. Which of the following structures gives rise to the pathological organ in the patient?

A. First pharyngeal pouch

B. Second pharyngeal pouch

C. Third pharyngeal pouch

D. Fourth pharyngeal pouch

E. Sixth pharyngeal pouch

Consider the following case for questions 4 to 5:

A 15-day-old infant presents with dyspnea, stridor, and intercostal retractions. He was born post-term by a difficult forceps delivery. During a flexible laryngeal endoscopic examination, the right vocal cord was found to be paralyzed and in the paramedian line. Stretching of a specific nerve during forceps application was suggested to be the underlying cause.

4. Which of the following muscle groups, most likely, might suffer due to this iatrogenic injury?

A. Those derived from the 1st pharyngeal arch

B. Those derived from the 2nd pharyngeal arch

C. Those derived from the 3rd pharyngeal arch

D. Those derived from the 4th pharyngeal arch

E. Those derived from the 6th pharyngeal arch

5. Which of the following could be an associated finding in the infant?

A. Paralysis of the sternothyroid muscle

B. Paralysis of the cricothyroid muscle

C. Paralysis of the thyrohyoid muscle

D. Anesthesia of the laryngeal inlet

E. Anesthesia of the laryngotracheal junction

Consider the following case for questions 6 to 7:

An 18-year-old man was involved in a motor vehicle crash. A high resolution CT scan of the cranial base detected a fracture rim encroaching on the left jugular foramen.

6. Which of the following might be a likely consequence in him?

A. Anesthesia of the tip of the tongue

B. Absent taste sensation from the filiform papillae

C. Absent taste sensation from the entire tongue

D. Anesthesia of the pharyngeal part of the tongue

E. Inability to protrude the tongue

7. Derivatives from which of the following pharyngeal arches might be affected in him?

A. 1st and 3rd

B. 1st, 2nd, and 3rd

C. 3rd and 4th

D. 4th and 6th

E. 3rd, 4th, and 6th

8. A 30-year-old woman with an ongoing, long-term history of alcoholism becomes pregnant. The embryo suffers from a defective neural crest cell migration to the second pharyngeal arch during the critical period of development. Which of the following structures is most likely to be affected as a result of this condition?

A. Cricoid cartilage

B. Glossopharyngeal nerve

C. Maxillary bones

D. Orbicularis oris muscle

E. Superior parathyroid gland

Consider the following case for questions 9 to 10:

A 45-year-old woman reports a painful swelling located below the left side of the angle of the mandible. The mass was just anterior and deep to the sternocleidomastoid muscle. On palpation it was soft in consistency, fluctuant, and painful. Serum ionic calcium and thyroid and parathyroid hormone levels were normal. A contrast-enhanced CT scan revealed a cystic and enhancing mass in the neck. Needle aspiration revealed pus-like material within a cystic cavity lined by epithelium. Her physician determined the pathology to be congenital in origin.

9. Which of the following is the most likely diagnosis?

A. Persistent thyroglossal duct

B. Parathyroid adenoma

C. Infected pharyngeal cyst

D. Thyroid toxic adenoma

E. Thymoma

10. Which of the following lines the pathological structure in her?

A. Ectoderm

B. Endoderm

C. Ectoderm and endoderm

D. Mesoderm

E. Neural crest

Consider the following case for questions 11 to 12:

A 6-month-old infant is brought to the clinic for a 2-week history of noisy breathing that worsens in the supine position. The patient's history was significant for delivery at 34 weeks secondary to premature rupture of the membranes. On examination, the patient had mild inspiratory stridor and did not appear to be in any distress.

11. Which of the following is the most probable diagnosis for her?

A. Tracheomalacia

B. Laryngomalacia

C. Bronchiolitis

D. Bronchial asthma

E. Cystic fibrosis

12. Which of the following structures might have suffered from defective development in her?

A. Pharyngeal arch 1

B. Pharyngeal arch 2

C. Pharyngeal arch 3

D. Pharyngeal arch 5

E. Pharyngeal arch 6

13. A 26-year old soccer player sustained a head injury while contesting a ball in the air. He transiently lost his consciousness and remained dizzy for about an hour. A CT scan revealed a fracture line passing through the stylomastoid foramen. Which of the following might be found in him?

A. Paralysis of all muscles that develop from the 1st pharyngeal arch

B. Paralysis of all muscles that develop from the 2nd pharyngeal arch

C. Loss of taste sensation from the tip of the tongue

D. Loss of taste sensation from the vallate papillae

E. Loss of general sensation over a small part of the external acoustic meatus

14. A newborn presents with a mesenchymal defect affecting his medial nasal processes. Which of the following might be malformed in him?

A. Lower lip

B. Primary palate

C. Secondary palate

D. Bridge of the nose

E. Alae of the nose

Consider the following case for questions 15 to 16:

A 25-year-old woman noticed an inability to perform certain yoga positions and was more easily fatigued and had decreased stamina for exercise. She soon developed diplopia and facial and proximal limb muscle weakness with difficulty lifting her arms above her head and difficulty climbing stairs. Her condition deteriorated with difficulty chewing, swallowing, and increasing weakness. Routine laboratory studies were unrevealing, with the exception of acetylcholine receptor antibodies. A chest CT scan showed a large anterior mediastinal heterogeneous mass with solid and cystic components and invasion of the pericardium.

15. Which of the following is the most likely diagnosis?

A. Persistent thyroglossal duct

B. Parathyroid adenoma

C. Pharyngeal cyst

D. Thyroid toxic adenoma

E. Thymoma

16. Which of the following might be the embryological source for the pathological organ?

A. First pharyngeal cleft

B. Second pharyngeal cleft

C. Third pharyngeal pouch

D. Fourth pharyngeal pouch

E. Endodermal invagination from the foramen cecum

Consider the following case for questions 17 to 18:

A 48-year-old man presents with a low and gruff voice for the past two months following an anterior cervical diskectomy. He reports that his voice has slowly improved over the last month but has then plateaued. A laryngoscopy, other than a vibratory phase asymmetry, revealed subtle non-specific changes. A laryngeal electromyography revealed no weakness for the posterior cricoarytenoid muscle.

17. Which of the following could be an associated finding in the patient?

A. Paralysis of the sternothyroid muscle

B. Paralysis of the thyrohyoid muscle

C. Paralysis of the thyroarytenoid muscle

D. Anesthesia of the laryngeal inlet

E. Anesthesia of the laryngotracheal junction

18. The injured nerve supplies a specific pharyngeal arch during fetal development. Which of the following muscles arises from the same arch?

A. Tensor tympani

B. Tensor veli palatini

C. Levator veli palatini

D. Transverse arytenoid

E. Stylopharyngeus

19. A 9-year-old girl presents with the chief complaint of decayed teeth. An examination revealed downward slanting of eyes, depressed zygomatic arches, sunken cheekbones, and deviated nasal septum. Genetic testing revealed a mutation of the treacle (*TCOF1*) gene. What additional structure would most likely be involved in the girl?

A. Greater horn of the hyoid bone

B. Lesser horn of the hyoid bone

C. Mandible bone

D. Superior constrictor muscle of the pharynx

E. Thyroid cartilage

20. A 9-year-old male child presents with deviation of the jaw to the left side on attempted protrusion. Electrodiagnostic studies reveal changes indicative of peripheral neuropathy. Which of the following muscles is most likely to be involved in the course of time?

A. Orbicularis oris

B. Orbicularis oculi

C. Tensor veli palatini

D. Levator veli palatini

E. Stylopharyngeus

20.2 Answers and Explanations

Easy	Medium	Hard

1. Correct: Failure of the left maxillary prominence to unite with the left medial nasal prominence (B)

Fusion of the maxillary and medial nasal prominences forms the lateral portion of the upper lips. Failure in fusion will result in a unilateral cleft lip (the most common congenital facial anomaly).

Failure of the maxillary prominence to unite with the lateral nasal prominence (**A**) will result in an oblique facial cleft. Failure of the right and left medial primary palate to fuse with the secondary palate (**C**) results in an anterior palatal cleft. Failure of the right and left medial nasal prominences to fuse (**D**) will lead to a midline cleft lip and anterior cleft palate. Failure of the right and left lateral palatine processes to fuse (**E**) will lead to a posterior palatal cleft.

2. Correct: Parathyroid gland cyst (D)

The patient presents with classical features of a benign parathyroid cyst, and the crystal-clear fluid content of the cyst is highly suggestive of the diagnosis.

Infected branchial cleft cysts (**A**) appear as tender, inflammatory masses located at the anterior border of the sternocleidomastoid muscle. Aspirated fluid commonly appears to be pus.

A solitary, autonomously functioning thyroid nodule is referred to as toxic adenoma (**B**). Laboratory studies usually reveal suppressed TSH and elevation in serum T_3 levels. Symptoms of weight loss, weakness, shortness of breath, palpitations, tachycardia, and heat intolerance are noted.

Thyroglossal cysts (**C**) arise from remnants of the thyroglossal duct and present as midline neck masses. A pathognomonic sign on physical examination is vertical motion of the mass with swallowing and tongue protrusion, demonstrating the intimate relation to the hyoid bone.

Most patients with parathyroid carcinoma (**E**) are symptomatic and have moderate to severe hypercalcemia. Parathyroid hormone levels are generally five times the normal.

3. Correct: Third pharyngeal pouch (C)

Ultrasound findings suggest the cyst affects the left inferior parathyroid gland. The inferior parathyroids and the thymus develop from pharyngeal pouch 3.

Derivatives of the first pharyngeal pouch (**A**) are the middle ear cavity and the auditory tube. Derivatives of the second pharyngeal pouch (**B**) are the tonsillar fossa and the crypts. Derivatives of the fourth pharyngeal pouch (**D**) are superior parathyroid glands and the parafollicular cells of the thyroid gland. A sixth pharyngeal pouch (**E**) never develops in humans.

4. Correct: Those derived from the 6th pharyngeal arch (E)

Congenital vocal cord paralysis is the second most common cause of congenital stridor, frequently consequent to birth trauma.

The infant is most likely suffering from right recurrent laryngeal nerve palsy. The nerve supplies the 6th pharyngeal arch.

Muscles of the first (**A**, by trigeminal nerve), second (**B**, by facial nerve), and third (**C**, by glossopharyngeal nerve) pharyngeal arches are not supplied by nerves related to the vocal cord.

Muscles of the 4th pharyngeal arch (**D**) are supplied by the external laryngeal nerve. Damage to this nerve (supplying the cricothyroid) is not very common during childbirth and will cause hoarseness of voice due to uneven tension of the vocal cord. Laryngoscopy findings are subtle and nonspecific.

5. Correct: Anesthesia of the laryngotracheal junction (E)

The recurrent laryngeal nerve provides sensory fibers to part of the larynx below the vocal cord and upper trachea. Hence the laryngotracheal junction will be anesthetized by its palsy.

The sternothyroid (**A**) muscle is supplied by the ansa cervicalis of the cervical plexus receiving fibers from the ventral rami of the C1-C3 spinal nerves. The cricothyroid muscle (**B**) is supplied by the external laryngeal branch of the superior laryngeal nerve. The thyrohyoid muscle (**C**) is supplied by a branch from the anterior ramus of the C1 spinal nerve. Sensation to the laryngeal inlet (**D**) is provided by the internal laryngeal branch of the superior laryngeal nerve.

6. Correct: Anesthesia of the pharyngeal part of tongue (D)

Cranial nerves IX (glossopharyngeal), X (vagus), and XI (accessory) exit the skull through the jugular foramen.

The pharyngeal part (posterior third) of the tongue develops from the ventral part of the hypobranchial eminence (3rd pharyngeal arch). This section of the tongue is innervated (both general and taste) by the glossopharyngeal nerve, which will be damaged consequent to jugular foramina fracture.

Mucosa of the oral part (**A**, anterior two-thirds) of the tongue develops from lateral lingual swellings (proliferation of mesenchymal cells in the first pharyngeal arches). Sensory innervation of this part, therefore, is done by the lingual branch of the mandibular division of the trigeminal nerve (exits skull through foramen ovale, not jugular foramen).

Filiform papillae (**B**), which populate the entire dorsal surface of the tongue, are not equipped with taste buds. The dorsal surface of the most anterior part (**C**) is covered with fungiform papillae, which are innervated by the chorda tympani branch of the facial nerve (exits skull through petrotympanic fissure, not jugular foramen).

Protrusion of the tongue (**E**) results from the action of skeletal muscles (primarily the genioglossus) that are supplied by the hypoglossal nerve. The nerve exits the skull through the hypoglossal canal and not the jugular foramen.

7. Correct: 3rd, 4th, and 6th (E)

Cranial nerves IX, X, and XI exit the cranium through the jugular foramina and will be affected by this fracture. CN IX supplies the 3rd and CN X supplies the 4th (via external laryngeal branch) and 6th (via recurrent laryngeal branch) pharyngeal arches. Nerves supplying the 1st (CN V) and the 2nd (CN VII) pharyngeal arches do not pass through the jugular foramen.

8. Correct: Orbicularis oris muscle (D)

Derivatives of the second pharyngeal arch include muscles of facial expression (e.g., orbicularis oris) and are supplied by the facial nerve. Cricoid cartilage (**A**) is derived from the 6th pharyngeal arch. The glossopharyngeal nerve (**B**) is related to the 3rd pharyngeal arch. Maxillary bones (**C**) derive from the 1st pharyngeal arch. Superior parathyroid glands (**E**) derive from the 4th pharyngeal pouch.

9. Correct: Infected pharyngeal cyst (C)

If a portion of the embryonic branchial cleft fails to involute completely, the entrapped remnant forms an epithelium-lined cyst. These cysts most frequently present in late childhood or early adulthood, when they become infected—usually following an upper respiratory tract infection. An infected branchial cleft cyst appears as a tender, inflammatory mass located along the anterior border of the sternocleidomastoid muscle. Aspirated fluid commonly appears to be pus.

Thyroglossal cysts (**A**) arise from remnants of the thyroglossal duct and present as midline neck masses. A pathognomonic sign on physical examination is vertical motion of the mass with swallowing and tongue protrusion, demonstrating the intimate relation to the hyoid bone. Parathyroid adenomas (**B**) commonly present with hypercalcemia, and aspiration typically reveals crystal-clear fluid. A solitary, autonomously functioning thyroid nodule is referred to as toxic adenoma (**D**). Laboratory studies usually reveal suppressed TSH and elevation in serum T_3 levels. Symptoms of weight loss, weakness, shortness of breath, palpitations, tachycardia, and heat intolerance are noted. Location of the tumor in this patient is highly unlikely for thymoma (**E**), which normally manifests as an anterior mediastinal mass with or without local invasion.

10. Correct: Ectoderm (A)

Branchial cleft cysts commonly arise from a failure of obliteration of the second branchial cleft in embryonic development. The second arch grows caudally and, ultimately, covers the third and fourth arches. The buried clefts become ectoderm-lined cavities, which normally involute around week 7 of development. Pharyngeal pouches are endoderm-lined (**B**, **C**) with internal indentations between the arches. Mesoderm (**D**) or neural crest (**E**) does not line pharyngeal clefts.

11. Correct: Laryngomalacia (B)

The infant is suffering from laryngomalacia, which is defined as the collapse of supraglottic structures during inspiration. It is the most common cause of inspiratory stridor (hallmark symptom) in infants.

Tracheomalacia (**A**), bronchiolitis (**C**), asthma (**D**), and cystic fibrosis (**E**) patients present with wheezing (noisy expiration), but not stridor.

History of an infant with tracheomalacia (**A**, flaccid tracheal cartilage) includes wheezing that does not improve with bronchodilator therapy. Unlike infants with bronchiolitis (**C**), asthma (**D**), or cystic fibrosis (**E**), these infants maintain normal oxygenation.

12. Correct: Pharyngeal arch 6 (E)

Laryngomalacia results from malformed laryngeal cartilages due to defective neural crest cell migration within the 6th pharyngeal arches. Skeletal elements primarily derived from the 1st pharyngeal arches (**A**) are facial bones. Skeletal elements primarily derived from the 2nd pharyngeal arches (**B**) are the stapes and the lesser cornu and upper part of the body of the hyoid. Skeletal elements primarily derived from the 3rd pharyngeal arches (**C**) are the greater cornu and lower part of the body of the hyoid. A 5th pharyngeal arch (**D**) never develops in humans.

13. Correct: Loss of general sensation over a small part of the external acoustic meatus (E)

The facial nerve exits the skull through the stylomastoid foramen. As the nerve exits the stylomastoid foramen, it gives off a sensory branch that supplies part of the external acoustic meatus and tympanic membrane. It then gives off motor branches that supply muscles of facial expression.

Muscles that develop from the 1st pharyngeal arch (**A**) are supplied by the trigeminal nerve.

The stapedius is a muscle derived from the 2nd pharyngeal arch. It is supplied by a branch of the facial nerve given off from its mastoid segment (course from pyramidal eminence to stylomastoid foramen), which is proximal to the stylomastoid foramen. Therefore, the stapedius will not be affected by the fracture (**B**).

Taste fibers for the tip of the tongue (**C**) are supplied by the chorda tympani branch of the facial nerve, which is also given off from its mastoid segment and hence will be unaffected by the fracture.

Taste fibers for the vallate papillae (**D**) are supplied by the glossopharyngeal nerve. It exits the skull through the jugular, but not the stylomastoid, foramen.

14. Correct: Primary palate (B)

Structures formed from the medial nasal process (prominence) are the crest and tip of the nose (columella), the philtrum and lateral portion of the upper lip, primary palate, and upper incisors.

The lower lip (**A**) is formed from the mandibular prominence. The secondary palate (**C**) is formed by fusion of the right and left palatine processes, off the respective maxillary prominences. The bridge of the nose (**D**) is formed from the frontonasal prominence. Alae of the nose (**E**) are formed from the lateral nasal prominence.

15. Correct: Thymoma (E)

The patient presents with classic features of myasthenia gravis (MG), which is a neuromuscular junction disease caused in most cases by acetylcholine receptor antibodies.

Thymoma refers to a malignancy arising from epithelial cells of the thymus. One half of cortical thymoma patients develop MG. When MG occurs together with a thymoma, MG is considered as a paraneoplastic disease caused by the presence of the thymoma.

Thyroglossal cysts (A), parathyroid adenomas (B), pharyngeal cysts (C), and toxic thyroid adenomas (D) commonly present as neck masses, and are not associated with MG.

16. Correct: Third pharyngeal pouch (C)

The thymus and inferior parathyroid glands develop from the third pharyngeal pouch. The external auditory meatus develops from the first pharyngeal cleft (A). The second pharyngeal cleft (B) normally obliterates. The superior parathyroid glands develop from the fourth pharyngeal pouch (D). The thyroid gland develops from endodermal invagination from the foramen cecum (E).

17. Correct: Anesthesia of the laryngeal inlet (D)

The patient is most likely suffering from an iatrogenic superior laryngeal nerve (SLN) injury. It is difficult to establish diagnosis of SLN palsy on laryngoscopy alone due to subtle findings and high variability. Laryngeal electromyography has been the gold standard in diagnosis due to the capability to detect signs of denervation.

The SLN branches from the vagus and divides into an external and an internal laryngeal branch. The external innervates the cricothyroid muscle, which controls longitudinal tension of the vocal folds and voice pitch. The internal supplies sensory fibers to part of the larynx above the vocal cord, hence the laryngeal inlet.

The sternothyroid (A) muscle is supplied by the ansa cervicalis of the cervical plexus receiving fibers from the ventral rami of C1-C3 spinal nerves. The thyrohyoid muscle (B) is supplied by a branch from anterior rami of C1 spinal nerve. Paralysis of the thyroarytenoid muscle (C) and anesthesia of the laryngotracheal junction (E) would result from recurrent laryngeal nerve palsy. This is ruled out in the patient by finding an intact posterior cricoarytenoid muscle, which is supplied by the recurrent laryngeal nerve.

18. Correct: Levator veli palatini (C)

The superior laryngeal nerve supplies the 4th pharyngeal arch. Muscles derived from the arch are the cricothyroid, levator veli palatini, and constrictors of pharynx.

The tensor tympani (A) and tensor veli palatini (B) derive from the 1st pharyngeal arch. The transverse arytenoid (D), an intrinsic muscle of the larynx, derives from the 6th pharyngeal arch. Stylopharyngeus (E) derives from the 3rd pharyngeal arch.

19. Correct: Mandible bone (C)

The girl is suffering from Treacher Collins' syndrome (TCS), otherwise known as mandibulofacial dysostosis, which is an autosomal dominant disorder of craniofacial development. Mutation of TCOF1 results in failure of neural crest cells to migrate into the first (primarily affected) and second (less commonly affected) pharyngeal arches, which may affect the size and shape of the ears, eyelids, cheek bones, and jaws. The mandible develops from the 1st pharyngeal arch, and mandibular hypoplasia is a common finding in the syndrome.

Greater (A, 3rd pharyngeal arch derivative) and lesser (B, 2nd pharyngeal arch derivative) horns of hyoid bone are not commonly affected; constrictors of the pharynx (D) or thyroid cartilage (E), both being 4th pharyngeal arch derivatives, are not affected either.

20. Correct: Tensor veli palatini (C)

The child is suffering from paralysis of the left lateral pterygoid muscle, consequent to a neuropathy affecting the mandibular division of the trigeminal nerve. The right and left lateral pterygoid muscles function together to cause symmetrical anterior movement of the mandible during opening of the mouth. In unilateral lateral pterygoid muscle palsy, the jaw deviates toward the paralyzed side. Because the trigeminal nerve supplies the 1st pharyngeal arch, all muscles (including tensor veli palatini) derived from the arch would eventually undergo degeneration.

Orbicularis oris (A) and orbicularis oculi (B) are derived from the 2nd pharyngeal arch, hence supplied by the facial nerve. Levator veli palatini (D) is derived from the 4th pharyngeal arch, hence supplied by the vagus nerve. Stylopharyngeus (E) is derived from the 3rd pharyngeal arch, hence supplied by the glossopharyngeal nerve.

Chapter 21

Nervous System Embryology

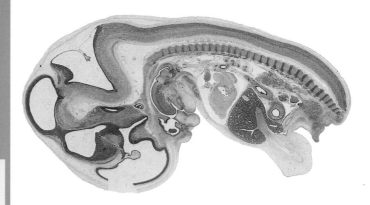

LEARNING OBJECTIVES

- ▶ Analyze the etiopathogenesis, clinical features, diagnosis, and complications of Chiari malformations.
- ▶ Describe the development of cranial nerve nuclei. Correlate these with their functions.
- ▶ Describe the pathway for the corneal reflex.
- ▶ Describe the development of motor and sensory components of cranial nerves.
- ▶ Analyze the etiopathogenesis, clinical features, and diagnosis of lissencephaly.
- ▶ Analyze the etiopathogenesis, clinical features, diagnosis, and complications of neural tube defects.
- ▶ Determine the distribution and fate of neural crest cells during development.
- ▶ Describe the development, structure, and functions of central and peripheral glia.
- ▶ Analyze the etiopathogenesis, clinical features, and diagnosis of glossopharyngeal neuralgia.
- ▶ Analyze the etiopathogenesis, clinical features, diagnosis, and complications of congenital aqueductal stenosis.
- ▶ Define the primary and secondary brain vesicles and trace their derivatives in human.
- ▶ Describe the pathway for the taste.
- ▶ Analyze the etiopathogenesis, clinical features, and diagnosis of holoprosencephaly.
- ▶ Analyze the etiopathogenesis, clinical features, and diagnosis of tethered cord syndrome.
- ▶ Describe the histogenesis of the developing neural tube.
- ▶ Analyze the etiopathogenesis, clinical features, and diagnosis of Dandy-Walker malformation.

21.1 Questions

Easy	Medium	Hard

Consider the following case for questions 1 to 2:

A 6-year-old girl is brought to the physician because of headache and neck pain. A CT scan shows herniation of cerebellar tonsils through the foramen magnum, and a small posterior cranial fossa. No other structural abnormalities are seen.

1. Which of the following best describes this finding?

A. Chiari type I malformation

B. Arnold-Chiari malformation

C. Dandy-Walker malformation

D. Holoprosencephaly

E. Lissencephaly

2. Which of the following is the underlying cause for her defects?

A. Defective somitogenesis

B. Lack of distension of the embryonic ventricular system

C. Defective neural tube closure

D. Defective neural crest cell migration

E. Defective neuroblast migration

3. A 3-day-old male neonate presents with significant difficulty with sucking and swallowing. Physical findings are significant for absent facial and jaw movements. Eye and tongue movements appear normal for the age. Which of the following would explain this combination of deficits?

A. Defect in the motor nucleus of the facial nerve

B. Defect in the motor nucleus of the trigeminal nerve

C. Defect in the general somatic efferent cell columns

D. Defect in the general visceral efferent cell columns

E. Defect in the special visceral efferent cell columns

4. A 60-year-old woman is undergoing follow-up neurological examination during her recovery from a stroke. When a wisp of cotton is touched to her left cornea, she blinks. Which of the following is the source of cell bodies involved in the primary afferent limb of this reflex?

A. Ectoderm

B. Neuroectoderm

C. Neural crest

D. A and B

E. A and C

5. A 6-month-old baby presents with microcephaly, hypotonia, profound mental retardation, and seizures. An MRI of the brain reveals grossly abnormal outline, few shallow sulci and shallow Sylvian fissures, and gross cortical thickening. Which of the following fetal defects is consistent with these findings?

A. Failure of regression of Rathke's pouch

B. Failure of closure of the rostral neuropore

C. Failure of closure of the caudal neuropore

D. Failure of migration of the neural crest cells

E. Failure of migration of neuroblasts

6. A 23-year-old woman presents with a dimple and a tuft of hair over the lower lumbar region of the vertebral column. She was asymptomatic and had shown up for her regular checkup. There were no sensorimotor deficits noted during a detailed neurological examination. A plain radiograph revealed missing neural arches involving several lumbar vertebrae. Which of the following is a true statement regarding her?

A. An MRI is most likely to detect incomplete dura and arachnoid mater covering the spinal cord.

B. An MRI is most likely to detect cystic dilatation of several segments of the spinal cord.

C. Antenatal diagnosis of this condition could have been possible by noting decreased α fetoprotein levels in maternal serum.

D. Prevention of this condition might have been possible by maternal consumption of folic acid.

E. Defective gastrulation is the primary cause for this defect in her.

7. A 26-year-old first-time mother suffers from a viral illness during the third week of her pregnancy. The virus has a known inclination toward cells that form chromaffin cells of the adrenal medulla. Which of the following might also be defective in the fetus?

A. Scar formation during wound healing following injury to the brain

B. Myelination of spinal cord tracts

C. Sensation from skin of the upper limb

D. Modulation of neuronal activities by buffering K^+ concentration in the extracellular space of the brain

E. Phagocytosis of microorganisms invading the brain

8. A 48-year-old man presents with a 2-year history of severe, transient, and stabbing pain that initiates in the right side of his throat. It gradually radiates to the base of his tongue, right ear, and occasionally beneath the angle of his right jaw. The paroxysmal attacks are frequently precipitated by swallowing cold drinks. Which of the specific segments of the central nervous system does the affected structure in the individual connect to?

A. Telencephalon

B. Diencephalon

C. Mesencephalon

D. Metencephalon

E. Myelencephalon

Consider the following case for questions 9 to 10:

A 3-day-old girl presents with enlarging head size, bulging fontanelles, and gaping cranial sutures. Postnatal magnetic resonance imaging is suggestive of congenital aqueductal stenosis.

9. Which of the following is the most unlikely finding in her?

A. Headache

B. Sunset eye sign

C. Dilated lateral ventricles

D. Dilated third ventricle

E. Dilated fourth ventricle

10. Which of the following embryonic segments contributes to the development of the obstructed structure in her?

A. Diencephalon

B. Mesencephalon

C. Metencephalon

D. Myelencephalon

E. Telencephalon

11. A 39-year-old woman suffers a stroke involving the posterior inferior cerebellar artery that causes specific damage to the brainstem special somatic afferent column. Sensation from which of the following structures will be compromised?

A. Facial skin

B. Taste buds

C. Cochlea

D. Smooth muscle of the esophagus

E. Striated muscle of the face

12. A 48-year-old woman presents with loss of taste sensation from the pharyngeal part of her tongue. Which of the following is the embryonic source for cell bodies of the involved primary afferent neurons?

A. Ectoderm

B. Neuroectoderm

C. Neural crest

D. A and B

C. A and C

13. A 28-week fetal ultrasound in a 20-year-old pregnant mother showed absent interhemispheric fissure and corpus callosum, fused thalami, and fused cerebral hemispheres with one cerebral ventricle. The neonate, delivered preterm at 32 weeks, was born with cyclopia and macroglossia. Which of the following is a true statement regarding this anomaly?

A. Oligohydramnios, detected by antenatal ultrasound, is a common association.

B. Maternal alcohol consumption is a frequent cause.

C. Trisomy 21 is a common association.

D. A and B

E. B and C

F. A and C

14. A second trimester fetal ultrasound in a 28-year-old woman shows a midline cystic mass overlying the occipital bone that contains echoes from herniated brain tissue. Laboratory findings for her were within normal limits other than elevated serum α-fetoprotein. Which of the following fetal defects is consistent with these findings?

A. Failure of regression of Rathke's pouch

B. Failure of closure of the rostral neuropore

C. Failure of closure of caudal neuropore

D. Failure of migration of neural crest cells

E. Failure of migration of neuroblasts

15. An 18-year-old girl presents with overflow incontinence. On examination, she has decreased power around the ankle with absent reflex. Her sensation of pain and touch was lost in the lateral side of the foot with saddle type of perianal anesthesia. Lumbosacral bony defect was evident in an X-ray of her spine. An MRI identified extension of the conus medullaris to the disk between L3 and L4 vertebrae, and a thickened filum terminale. Which of the following is the most probable embryological basis for her problems?

A. Defective migration of neural crest cells

B. Defective histogenesis of the developing neural tube

C. Mechanical traction of the spinal cord due to restricted mobility

D. Slower growth of the spinal cord relative to vertebral column

E. Accelerated growth of thoracic spinal segments

16. A second-trimester fetal ultrasound in a 42-year-old woman suggests a developmental defect affecting the neuroectoderm of the diencephalon segment of the neural tube. Which of the following organs might be at risk in the newborn if the course of the remaining pregnancy stays otherwise uneventful?

A. Cerebral cortex

B. Cerebellar cortex

C. Adenohypophysis

D. Neurohypophysis

E. Medulla oblongata

17. A 48-year-old woman, being treated with colchicine (a drug that arrests mitosis) for chronic gout, finds out that she is 4 weeks pregnant. Cells within which of the following layers of the neural tube in the developing embryo would mostly be affected?

A. Marginal layer

B. Mantle layer

C. Ventricular layer

D. Marginal and mantle layers

E. Marginal, mantle, and ventricular layers

18. A 23-year-old pregnant woman shows up for a routine second-trimester checkup. Fetal ultrasonography reveals a neural mass protruding through arch defects in lower lumbar vertebrae. At what week of gestation did this defect most likely occur?

A. 1 to 3

B. 4 to 8

C. 9 to 11

D. 12 to 15

E. 16 to 19

Consider the following case for questions 19 to 20:

A 33-year-old woman, who is 24 weeks pregnant, reports for a routine antenatal checkup. Her physical examination is unremarkable. Fetal ultrasound reveals a triangular defect posterior to the cerebellum. The defect seems to be occupied by CSF, and the posterior fossa is markedly enlarged. The cerebellum appears markedly compressed and hypoplastic, and the vermis cannot be displayed.

19. Which of the following is the most probable diagnosis for the fetus?

A. Arachnoid cyst

B. Blake's pouch cyst

C. Chiari type I malformation

D. Arnold-Chiari malformation

E. Dandy-Walker malformation

20. Which of the following is the embryological basis for the fetal disorder?

A. Underdevelopment of the occipital somites

B. Primary atresia of foramina of Luschka

C. Primary agenesis of cerebellar vermis

D. Communication of the 4th ventricle with an abnormally persistent retrocerebellar cyst

E. Leakage of CSF from an incompletely closed neural tube

21.2 Answers and Explanations

Easy	Medium	Hard

1. Correct: Chiari type I malformation (A)

Chiari malformations are a group of congenital hindbrain abnormalities affecting the structural relationships between the cerebellum, brainstem, the upper cervical cord, and the skull base.

In type I, cerebellar tonsils are displaced into the upper cervical canal through the foramen magnum. Displacement of the medulla, fourth ventricle, and cerebellar vermis through the foramen magnum occur in type II (**B**, Arnold-Chiari malformation).

Dandy-Walker malformation (**C**) is characterized by agenesis or hypoplasia of the cerebellar vermis, cystic dilatation of the fourth ventricle, and enlargement of the posterior fossa. Holoprosencephaly (**D**) occurs when the prosencephalon fails to cleave down the midline such that the telencephalon contains a single ventricle. Lissencephaly (**E**) is a heterogeneous group of disorders of cortical formation characterized by a smooth brain, with absent or hypoplastic sulci.

2. Correct: Defective somitogenesis (A)

In type I Chiari malformation, an underdeveloped occipital bone, possibly due to underdevelopment of the occipital somite originating from the paraxial mesoderm, induces overcrowding in the posterior cranial fossa, which contains the normally developed hindbrain.

The cause of the Chiari II malformation in children born with a myelomeningocele can be explained by the lack of distention of the embryonic ventricular system (**B**). Defective neural tube closure (**C**) precludes the accumulation of fluid and pressure within the ventricles. This distention is critical to normal brain development. Decompression of the brain vesicles causes overcrowding in the posterior fossa and changes in the fetal skull.

Failure of migration of neural crest cells (**D**, neurocristopathies) or neuroblasts (**E**, causing agyria, pachygyria, heterotopia, etc.) does not contribute to Chiari malformations.

3. Correct: Defect in the special visceral efferent cell columns (E)

The neonate presents with absent facial (muscles innervated by motor nucleus of the facial nerve) and jaw (muscles innervated by motor nucleus of the trigeminal nerve) movements, and difficulty in swallowing (muscles innervated by the nucleus ambiguus). These nuclei belong to the special visceral efferent (branchiomotor) cell columns.

Defects in motor nucleus of the facial (**A**) nerve will not cause absent jaw movements or difficulty in swallowing. Defects in the motor nucleus of the trigeminal (**B**) nerve will not cause absent facial movements or difficulty in swallowing. The general somatic efferent column (**C**) includes oculomotor, trochlear, abducens, and hypoglossal nuclei. Normal eye and tongue movements preclude their involvement. The general visceral efferent column (**D**) innervates glands and smooth muscles. This includes the Edinger-Westphal, superior and inferior salivatory, and dorsal vagal nuclei. No indications for their involvement are present in the case.

4. Correct: A and C (E)

The corneal reflex is initiated by the free nerve endings in the cornea and involves the trigeminal nerve and ganglion, the spinal trigeminal tract and nucleus, interneurons in the reticular formation, motor neurons in the facial nucleus and nerve, and the orbicularis oculi. The cell body of the primary afferent neuron lies in the trigeminal (semilunar) ganglia, which develop from both the neural crest (**C**) and the trigeminal placode (localized regions of the columnar epithelium that develop from ectoderm, **A**). No known direct contribution from the neuroectoderm (**B, D**) exists.

5. Correct: Failure of migration of neuroblasts (E)

The neonate is suffering from lissencephaly (absence of cortical gyri) and possibly from neuronal heterotopia (normal neurons in abnormal locations), both of which are caused by neuroblast migration defects.

Rathke's pouch is an ectodermal outpouching of stomodeum which forms the adenohypophysis of the pituitary gland. The lumen of the pouch narrows to form a Rathke's cleft that normally regresses. Persistence of this cleft is believed to cause Rathke's cleft cyst and/or craniopharyngioma (**A**).

Failure of closure of the rostral (**B**) or caudal (**C**) neuropore causes neural tube defects; failure of migration of neural crest cells (**D**) are termed neurocristopathies. None of these defects contribute toward lissencephaly.

6. Correct: Prevention of this condition might have been possible by maternal consumption of folic acid. (D)

She is suffering from spina bifida occulta, the most common and least severe of neural tube defects (NTDs). This occurs due to failure of closure of one or several vertebral arches posteriorly; the meninges and spinal cord are normal. A dimple or small lipoma may overlie the defect. Most cases are asymptomatic and discovered incidentally. Folic acid supplements at the time of conception and in the first 12 weeks of pregnancy reduce the incidence of NTDs in the fetus by approximately 70%.

Incomplete cover of dura and arachnoid mater (**A**, meningocele) or cystic dilatation of several segments of the spinal cord (**B**, syringomyelia) is highly unlikely to be asymptomatic.

Antenatal diagnosis of NTDs is possible by finding elevated levels of α-fetoprotein levels in maternal serum or amniotic fluid (**C**).

Gastrulation (**E**) is the process of forming three definitive germ layers in the embryo. Spina bifida is the result of failure of closure of the posterior neuropore, which indicates defective neurulation. Less severe forms, such as spina bifida occulta, are the result of failure of secondary neurulation (debatable in humans).

7. Correct: Sensation from skin of the upper limb (C)

The virus targets neural crest cells (truncal), since chromaffin cells of the adrenal medulla form from these. Truncal neural crest cells also form dorsal root ganglia (cell bodies of somatic sensory nerves). Disruption of these, therefore, might lead to somatosensory loss.

Scar formation during wound healing following injury to the brain (**A**) and K$^+$ spatial buffering (**D**) are important functions of astrocytes, which develop from neuroepithelium (neuroectoderm). Myelination of the central nervous system (**B**) is a function

179

of oligodendrocytes. These cells also develop from neuroepithelium (neuroectoderm). Phagocytosis of microorganisms invading the brain (**E**) is the function of microglia. These cells develop from mesenchymal progenitors within the bone marrow.

8.   Correct: Myelencephalon (E)

The patient is suffering from glossopharyngeal neuralgia (GN). Clusters of unilateral attacks of sharp, stabbing, and shooting pain localized in the throat radiating to the ear or vice versa are characteristic of GN. The distribution of pain is diagnostic: it usually starts in the pharynx, tonsil, and tongue base, and then rapidly involves the eustachian tube and inner ear or spreads to the mandibular angle. Swallowing is the most common trigger factor, and cold liquids mainly induce the pain. Glossopharyngeal nerve (CN IX) is attached to the medulla oblongata, which is derived from myelencephalon.

CN I and II are attached to the forebrain [derived from telencephalon (**A**) and diencephalon (**B**), respectively]. CN III and IV attach to the midbrain (derived from mesencephalon, **C**). CN V is attached to the pons (derived from metencephalon, **D**). CN VI–VIII attach to the pontomedullary junction. CN IX–XII attach to the medulla.

9.   Correct: Dilated fourth ventricle (E)

Congenital aqueductal stenosis presents with obstructive hydrocephalus.

Because the obstruction lies at the level of the aqueduct of Sylvius, the fourth ventricle is often of normal size. The lateral (**C**) and third (**D**) ventricles are often dilated because of the obstruction. The usual symptoms and signs of raised intracranial pressure and hydrocephalus are headache (**A**), vomiting, decreased conscious state, and sunset eye sign (**B**, up-gaze paresis with the eyes appearing driven downward).

10.   Correct: Mesencephalon (B)

The obstruction lies at the level of the aqueduct of Sylvius, which is the cavity of the midbrain. Developmental defect in the mesencephalon, therefore, would cause the defect.

Diencephalon (**A**) and telencephalon (**E**) give rise to forebrain structures. Metencephalon (**C**) and myelencephalon (**D**) give rise to hindbrain structures.

11.   Correct: Cochlea (C)

The special somatic afferent column in the brainstem includes the vestibulocochlear nuclei. Therefore, hearing and balance sensation from the inner ear will be affected.

Sensation from skin (**A**) and striated muscle (**E**, proprioception) of the face relay to the general somatic afferent column (trigeminal sensory nuclei). Sensation from taste buds (**B**, special visceral afferent) and smooth muscles of the esophagus (**D**,

general visceral afferent) relay back to the nucleus tractus solitarii.

12.   Correct: Ectoderm (A)

The glossopharyngeal nerve supplies the pharyngeal part (posterior third) of the tongue. Cell bodies for the primary afferent neurons lie in the inferior glossopharyngeal (petrosal) ganglia, which develop from the second epibranchial placode. These placodes are localized regions of columnar epithelium that develop from ectoderm. No known direct contribution from the neuroectoderm (**B, D**) or neural crest (**C, E**) exists.

Note that the cell bodies for 2nd-order sensory neurons are located in the nucleus of the solitary tract, and those for 3rd-order neurons are located in the ventral posteromedial (VPM) nucleus of the thalamus. The VPM projects to the ipsilateral gustatory cortex.

13.   Correct: Maternal alcohol consumption is a frequent cause. (B)

The neonate is suffering from holoprosencephaly (alobar). The fundamental problem is a failure of the developing prosencephalon to divide into left and right halves (which normally occurs at the end of the 5th week of gestation). This results in variable loss of midline structures of the brain and face as well as fusion of lateral ventricles and the 3rd ventricle. Environmental factors such as maternal diabetes mellitus, alcohol use, and retinoic acid have been implicated in the pathogenesis, as has mutation of several genes including *Sonic Hedgehog*. On antenatal ultrasound there may be evidence of polyhydramnios (not oligohydramnios, **A, D**, and **F**), a secondary feature due to impaired fetal swallowing. Trisomy 13 (most common) and trisomy 18 have been frequently associated with holoprosencephaly, but not trisomy 21 (**C, E**, and **F**).

14.   Correct: Failure of closure of the rostral neuropore (B)

The fetus is suffering from an occipital encephalocele. This is a neural tube defect caused by defective closure of the rostral neuropore, where brain tissue encased in meninges herniates out through a defect in the cranium.

Rathke's pouch is an ectodermal outpouching of stomodeum which forms the adenohypophysis of the pituitary gland. The lumen of the pouch narrows to form a Rathke's cleft, which normally regresses. Persistence of this cleft is believed to cause Rathke's cleft cyst and/or craniopharyngioma (**A**).

Failure of closure of caudal neuropore (**C**) causes spinal dysraphism (meningocele, meningomyelocele, etc.) commonly involving lumbosacral segments.

Failure of migration of neural crest cells (**D**, neurocristopathies) or neuroblasts (**E**, causing agyria, pachygyria, heterotopia, etc.) does not contribute to encephalocele.

15. Correct: Mechanical traction of the spinal cord due to restricted mobility (C)

The girl is suffering from tethered cord syndrome, in which the thickened filum tethers the cord to the sacrum. Diagnosis is made by low-lying conus (below the L2 vertebral level) and a thick filum, when accompanied by neurogenic bladder with sensorimotor deficits of the lower limb. At week 8 of gestation, the spinal cord extends the length of the spinal canal. For the remainder of gestation, the bony spinal elements outgrow the spinal cord (**D**). This results in ascension of the conus to the normal position (lower border of L1 in adults and L3 in infants). Tethering prevents this rostral ascension. Partial traction on the cord can result in progressive ischemia, leading to lumbosacral neuronal dysfunction, which is manifest in neurological, musculoskeletal, and urological abnormalities.

Defective migration of neural crest cells (**A**), defective histogenesis of neural tube (**B**), or accelerated growth of thoracic spinal segments (**E**) does not contribute to the syndrome.

16. Correct: Neurohypophysis (D)

Neurohypophysis, or posterior pituitary, develops from the infundibulum, which is a downward extension of neural ectoderm from the floor of the diencephalon.

Cerebral cortex (**A**) develops from telencephalon; cerebellar cortex (**B**) develops from metencephalon; adenohypophysis (**C**), or anterior pituitary, develops from Rathke's pouch (upward extension of oral ectoderm from the roof of stomodeum); and medulla oblongata (**E**) develops from myelencephalon.

17. Correct: Ventricular layer (C)

Colchicine, a microtubule growth inhibitor, affects mitosis and other microtubule-dependent functions of cells. With the beginning of cellular differentiation in the neural tube, the layer of cells closest to the lumen of the neural tube remains epithelial and is called the ventricular zone. This zone, which still contains mitotic cells, ultimately becomes the ependyma.

Farther from the ventricular zone is the intermediate (formerly called mantle) zone, which contains the cell bodies of the differentiating postmitotic neuroblasts (**B**, future gray matter). As the neuroblasts continue to produce axonal and dendritic processes, these processes form a peripheral marginal zone (**A**, future white matter).

18. Correct: 4 to 8 (B)

The embryonic period (weeks 4–8) is most vulnerable to teratogens and structural defects. The fetus is suffering from myelomeningocele consequent to defective closure of the neural tube. The rostral and caudal neuropores normally close late in the 4th week.

The germinal period (**A**, weeks 1–3) is characterized by a high rate of spontaneous abortions, chromosomal abnormalities being the leading cause. Weeks 9 through 19 (**C–E**) are not considered as vulnerable to teratogens as the embryonic period. These are times when most organ systems grow and mature, rather than form.

19. Correct: Dandy-Walker malformation (E)

The fetus is suffering from Dandy-Walker malformation, which is classically presented with hypoplastic or absent cerebellar vermis consequent to an enlarged posterior fossa, a cystic dilatation of the 4th ventricle, and a dilated cisterna magna.

An arachnoid cyst (**A**) is a collection of CSF encased within a pia-arachnoid layer and not associated with abnormalities of the cerebellum or brainstem; severe hypoplasia of the cerebellum and its vermis help rule out the diagnosis; also, cystic structure in the posterior fossa is in actuality the fourth ventricle.

Late in the first trimester, a small appendage of the fourth ventricle, the Blake's pouch, protrudes into the cisterna magna, caudally to the cerebellum. It regresses, usually by 12 weeks of gestation, when it fenestrates to form the foramen of Magendie. Persistent Blake's pouch cysts (**B**) occur due to failed perforation. As the foramina of Luschka open later than the foramen of Magendie during the embryologic development, this lack of perforation of the foramen of Magendie causes enlargement of the 4th ventricle, that results in an isolated superior displacement of the cerebellar vermis (but not its agenesis or hypoplasia). Blake's pouch cyst is the mildest and Dandy-Walker syndrome is the most severe of a continuum of anatomic anomalies involving the fourth ventricle, Blake's pouch complex.

In Chiari type I malformation (**C**), cerebellar tonsils are herniate into the upper cervical canal through the foramen magnum. Displacement of the medulla, fourth ventricle, and cerebellar vermis through the foramen magnum occur in type II (**D**, Arnold-Chiari malformation). Chiari malformations present with a small posterior fossa.

20. Correct: Communication of the 4th ventricle with an abnormally persistent retrocerebellar cyst (D)

In Dandy-Walker malformation, the 4th ventricle communicates with a retrocerebellar cyst that may cause enlargement of the posterior fossa and elevation of the tentorium. Upward displacement of a cerebellar vermis is associated with a dilated 4th ventricle and a dilated cisterna magna, resulting in secondary hypoplasia (atresia) of the vermis.

Underdeveloped occipital somites (**A**) lead to an underdeveloped occipital bone, which induces overcrowding in the posterior cranial fossa (as seen in type I Chiari malformation).

Atresia of foramina of Magendie and Luschka (**B**) might contribute to the findings in patients with

Dandy-Walker malformation. The severity of symptoms depends on the atresia, but this is not the embryological basis for the disorder (explained in the previous question with Blake's pouch cyst).

Vermal agenesis is secondary (not primary, **C**) to an enlarged posterior fossa and a dilated 4th ventricle.

Leakage of CSF from an incompletely closed neural tube (**E**) occurs in neural tube defects, which may be associated with Dandy-Walker malformations. This, however, is not the cause for such malformation.

Chapter 22

Digestive System Embryology

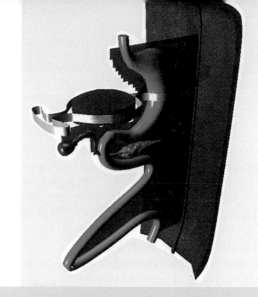

LEARNING OBJECTIVES

- ► Correlate the underlying developmental mechanisms in esophageal atresia (and VACTERL syndrome) with their clinical presentation, outcomes for the fetus/newborn, and pre/peri/postnatal diagnosis.
- ► Describe the mechanism and sequence of events in formation of the components of the gastrointestinal tract, liver, pancreas, and gall bladder.
- ► Correlate the underlying developmental mechanisms in gastroschisis with its clinical presentation, outcomes for the fetus/newborn, and pre/peri/postnatal diagnosis.
- ► Describe the developmental fate of the dorsal and ventral mesenteries associated with the primitive gut tube.
- ► Correlate the underlying developmental mechanisms in annular pancreas with its clinical presentation, outcomes for the fetus/newborn, and pre/peri/postnatal diagnosis.
- ► Correlate the underlying developmental mechanisms in vitelline cysts or fistulas with their clinical presentation, outcomes for the fetus/newborn, and pre/peri/postnatal diagnosis.
- ► Correlate embryological with anatomical definitions of foregut, midgut, and hindgut.
- ► Correlate the underlying developmental mechanisms in extrahepatic biliary atresia with its clinical presentation, outcomes for the fetus/newborn, and pre/peri/postnatal diagnosis.
- ► Correlate the underlying developmental mechanisms in nonrotation of the gut with its clinical presentation, outcomes for the fetus/newborn, and pre/peri/postnatal diagnosis.
- ► Correlate the underlying developmental mechanisms in achalasia with its clinical presentation, outcomes for the fetus/newborn, and pre/peri/postnatal diagnosis.
- ► Correlate the underlying developmental mechanisms in neonatal hypoglycemia with its clinical presentation, outcomes for the fetus/newborn, and pre/peri/postnatal diagnosis.
- ► Correlate the underlying developmental mechanisms in Hirschsprung's disease with its clinical presentation, outcomes for the fetus/newborn, and pre/peri/postnatal diagnosis.
- ► Correlate the underlying developmental mechanisms in omphalocele with its clinical presentation, outcomes for the fetus/newborn, and pre/peri/postnatal diagnosis.
- ► Correlate the underlying developmental mechanisms in Meckel's diverticulum with its clinical presentation, outcomes for the fetus/newborn, and pre/peri/postnatal diagnosis.
- ► Correlate the underlying developmental mechanisms in pancreas divisum with its clinical presentation, outcomes for the fetus/newborn, and pre/peri/postnatal diagnosis.
- ► Describe rotation of gut during development, including midgut herniation and physiological reduction of the hernia.
- ► Correlate the underlying developmental mechanisms in hypertrophic pyloric stenosis with its clinical presentation, outcomes for the fetus/newborn, and pre/peri/postnatal diagnosis.
- ► Correlate the underlying developmental mechanisms in duodenal atresia with its clinical presentation, outcomes for the fetus/newborn, and pre/peri/postnatal diagnosis.
- ► Correlate the underlying developmental mechanisms in imperforate anus with its clinical presentation, outcomes for the fetus/newborn, and pre/peri/postnatal diagnosis.
- ► Correlate the underlying developmental mechanisms in recto vesical, recto urethral, and recto vaginal fistulas with their clinical presentation, outcomes for the fetus/newborn, and pre/peri/postnatal diagnosis.

22.1 Questions

Easy	Medium	Hard

1. A newborn boy presents with excessive drooling. The baby chokes and turns blue with any attempt at feeding. A physical examination reveals moderate scoliosis, radial dysplasia, and syndactyly. Which of the following is a true statement regarding this disorder?

A. The pregnancy might have been complicated by oligohydramnios.

B. The neonate may also suffer from ventricular septal defect.

C. A nasogastric tube should easily insert into the stomach, and gastric drainage should immediately be performed.

D. The symptoms are primarily due to defective lateral folding of the embryo.

E. The symptoms are primarily due to defective migration of neural crest cells.

2. A newborn presenting with fecal incontinence was scheduled for sphincteroplasty. Given that the external anal sphincter was not fully functional in the child, which of the following germ layers might have suffered from a differentiation defect?

A. Endoderm

B. Surface ectoderm

C. Neuroectoderm

D. Neural crest cells

E. Mesoderm

3. A third-trimester ultrasound in a 20-year-old pregnant woman revealed a defect in the anterior abdominal wall of the fetus. Abdominal organs, including parts of the small and large bowels, herniated through the defect, which was located about an inch to the right of the umbilicus. No membrane covering the organs was identified. Which of the following might be an associated finding with this pregnancy?

A. Chromosomal abnormality of the fetus

B. Ventricular septal defect in the fetus

C. Scoliosis of the fetus

D. Elevated serum β-hCG many times above normal for the gestational age

E. Elevated α-fetoprotein level in the amniotic fluid

4. To understand malrotation involving the gastrointestinal tract, a resident reviews its early development. He understands that initially the tract, for the most part, was suspended from the ventral and dorsal body walls by the respective mesenteries. Which of the following is a remnant of the embryonic ventral mesentery?

A. Peritoneal fold that connects the sigmoid colon to the body wall

B. Peritoneal fold that connects the jejunum to the body wall

C. Peritoneal fold that connects the stomach to the transverse colon

D. Peritoneal fold that connects the stomach to the liver

E. Peritoneal fold that connects the stomach to the spleen

5. A 1-day-old preterm newborn girl was noted to have abdominal distension and bilious vomiting following an uneventful vaginal delivery. An abdominal CT scan revealed pancreatic tissue surrounding the second part of the duodenum. Which of the following might be an associated radiological finding in her?

A. Ileal diverticulum

B. Blindly ending esophageal stump

C. Absence of fundic gas shadow

D. Double-bubble sign

E. Abrupt narrowing at the gastroesophageal junction

6. A 2-week-old male infant was seen in the clinic with a history of persistent umbilical discharge since birth. A barium enema revealed a fistulous connection from the small bowel to the umbilicus. Which of the following might be the cause of the child's symptom?

A. Failure of the neural crest cells to migrate in the wall of midgut

B. Failure of the midgut to recanalize

C. Failure of the omphalomesenteric duct to involute

D. Failure of the allantoic diverticulum to involute

E. Failure of the urorectal septum to develop

7. A 6-year-old girl presents with a mass affecting a segment of her gastrointestinal tract that develops from the proximal hindgut. If the tumor cells metastasized via veins, which of the following would initially lodge these?

A. Ileal vein

B. Right colic vein

C. Superior mesenteric vein

D. Splenic vein

E. Inferior vena cava

8. A 4-week-old girl presents with increasing jaundice over the last week. Her parents report that 2 weeks ago, she began to have yellowing of her eyes with subsequent yellowing of her skin, and the jaundice appears to be worsening. Her stools have been pale in color for the past 10 days along with darker urine. Laboratory examinations reveal moderately increased total and direct bilirubin, and alkaline phosphatase. Which of the following is true of the infant?

A. Absence/agenesis of the liver

B. Absence/agenesis of the gall bladder

C. Absence/agenesis of the common bile duct

D. Absence/agenesis of the pancreas

E. Absence/agenesis of the spleen

9. A 48-year-old man presents with 3 days of left-sided abdominal pain, low-grade fever, and nausea. A CT scan of the abdomen revealed acute appendicitis superimposed on congenital intestinal malrotation leading to complete left-sided large gut and right-sided small gut. Which of the following is responsible for the embryological malformation in him?

A. Nonrotation of the primary intestinal loop

B. Reverse rotation of the primary intestinal loop

C. Failure of the primary intestinal loop to return into the abdominal cavity following physiologic herniation

D. Failure of the primary intestinal loop to detach from the yolk sac

E. Failure of the primary intestinal loop to maintain its blood supply from the superior mesenteric artery

10. A 6-month-old female infant presents with frequent regurgitation of food, recurrent chest infection, and failure to thrive. An upper GI contrast study revealed a dilated proximal esophagus with abrupt narrowing at the gastroesophageal junction. Which of the following tissue sources might be responsible for the underlying defect in the infant?

A. Surface ectoderm

B. Neuroectoderm

C. Neural crest cells

D. Endoderm

E. Mesoderm

11. A term male infant was born after an uneventful pregnancy to a 28-year-old diabetic woman. Immediately after birth, the neonate appeared jittery. Laboratory tests revealed blood glucose concentration below 30 mg/dL, and a diagnosis of neonatal hypoglycemia was made. Which of the following might be the source of the structure responsible for the newborn's symptoms?

A. Ectoderm

B. Endoderm

C. Mesoderm

D. Neuroectoderm

E. Neural crest cells

12. A 3-day-old male has not passed stool following several feeding sessions. Over the next few hours, he vomits (bilious), urinates, develops mild abdominal distension, but still has not had his first stool. Auscultation reveals normal peristaltic sounds in the upper abdomen and almost absent sounds in the lower abdomen. A per-rectal exam came back normal with meconium-covered gloved fingers. Which of the following might be the most probable cause of his symptoms?

A. Failure of rupture of the anal membrane

B. Failure of obliteration of the omphalomesenteric duct

C. Failure of migration of neural crest cells

D. Failure of the urorectal septum to develop

E. Failure of retraction of the primary intestinal loop following physiologic umbilical hernia

13. A 30-year-old pregnant woman presents for a routine third-trimester checkup. Her serum α-fetoprotein level is raised, and an ultrasound reveals a defect in the anterior abdominal wall of the fetus. An MRI demonstrates a fetal midline defect involving the umbilical cord, which contains intestinal loops covered in a membranous sac. Which of the following might the fetus be suffering from?

A. Congenital umbilical hernia

B. Exstrophy of the bladder

C. Cloacal exstrophy

D. Gastroschisis

E. Omphalocele

14. A gastroenterology resident was explaining to his intern how the enteric nervous system includes several neural circuits that control motor functions, local blood flow, and mucosal transport and secretions and modulates immune and endocrine functions. Which of the following is the source of such neurons?

A. Neural ectoderm

B. Neural crest cells

C. Visceral layer of the lateral plate mesoderm

D. Parietal layer of the lateral plate mesoderm

E. Endoderm

15. An 18-month-old boy is brought to the clinic with the chief complaint of passing large amounts of dark red blood from his rectum, and black jelly-like stools of two days duration. The child does not appear to be in acute distress at rest, has not vomited, and continues to feed regularly. A physical exam is significant for pale conjunctiva and lips. A Tc-99m pertechnetate scintigraphy scan (readily taken up by parietal cells) demonstrates immediate tracer localization in the stomach and in the right lower abdominal quadrant. Which of the following might be the cause of the child's symptoms?

A. Failure of the neural crest cells to migrate in the wall of midgut

B. Failure of the midgut to recanalize

C. Failure of the omphalomesenteric duct to involute

D. Failure of the allantoic diverticulum to involute

E. Failure of the urorectal septum to develop

16. A 75-year-old man with a clinical history of recurrent pancreatitis was hospitalized for epigastric pain and vomiting. Laboratory reports came back with elevated levels of serum amylase and serum lipase. MRCP revealed pancreas divisum. Which of the following is a probable underlying cause for his symptoms?

A. Failure of fusion of ventral and dorsal pancreatic buds

B. Failure of fusion of ventral and dorsal pancreatic ducts

C. Malrotation of the ventral pancreatic bud

D. Malrotation of the dorsal pancreatic bud

E. Drainage of most of the pancreas through the dorsal pancreatic duct, which opens into the major duodenal papilla

F. Drainage of most of the pancreas through the ventral pancreatic duct, which opens into the major duodenal papilla

17. A rotational defect causes the cranial limb of the primary intestinal (midgut) loop to undergo ischemic necrosis during physiologic herniation. Which of the organs might be affected in the growing fetus?

A. Stomach

B. Gallbladder

C. Jejunum

D. Cecum

E. Appendix

18. A 3-week-old infant presents with projectile nonbilious vomiting. Which of the following might be an additional finding in his case?

A. A characteristic double-bubble sign in X-ray

B. A prominent tracheoesophageal fistula

C. A pronounced circular layer of smooth muscle in the stomach wall

D. A prominent ileal diverticulum

E. Ectopic cordis

19. A 2-day-old male neonate presents with bilious vomiting since birth. A physical examination revealed features of Down's syndrome. A nasogastric tube is passed, and 40 to 50 mL bilious fluid is aspirated. An X-ray abdomen erect film showed a double-bubble sign. Which of the following is a probable diagnosis for the neonate?

A. Ankyloglossia

B. Esophageal atresia

C. Achalasia

D. Congenital hypertrophic pyloric stenosis

E. Duodenal atresia

20. A newborn girl presents on her first day of life for evaluation of a perineal mass. The child had normal external female genitalia and a sacral dimple, but the resident and the attending were unable to locate the anal opening. She did not pass meconium on the first day of life. On her second day, flecks of meconium were noted in her diapers. On further inspection, a small opening was noted in the posterior aspect of the vaginal vestibule. Which of the following might be the underlying cause of her symptoms?

A. Failure of rupture of the cloacal membrane

B. Defective development of the urorectal septum

C. Failure of migration of neural crest cells to the gut wall

D. Failure of rupture of the cloacal membrane and defective development of the urorectal septum

E. Failure of rupture of the cloacal membrane and failure of migration of neural crest cells to the gut wall

22.2 Answers and Explanations

Easy	Medium	Hard

1. Correct: The neonate may also suffer from ventricular septal defect. (B)

The neonate, soon after birth, regurgitates saliva and chokes and turns blue (cyanotic) with attempted feeding. This strongly suggests esophageal atresia with tracheoesophageal fistula. Accompanying vertebral and skeletal defects establish the diagnosis of VACTERL syndrome, which is frequently (~25%) associated. VACTERL stands for vertebral defects (scoliosis, fused, missing or extra vertebrae), anal atresia, cardiac defects (most commonly ventricular septal defect), tracheoesophageal fistula, renal anomalies (renal agenesis, polycystic kidneys), and limb abnormalities (radial dysplasia, syndactyly, polydactyly).

Esophageal atresia results in the inability to drink the amniotic fluid for the fetus, thus the pregnancy is complicated by polyhydramnios (not oligohydramnios, **A**).

Chest X-ray following a failed attempt to insert a nasogastric tube (**C**) confirms the diagnosis of esophageal atresia.

Dorsal deviation of the tracheoesophageal septum or failed recanalization of the gut tube results in esophageal atresia. Neither defective lateral folding of the embryo (**D**) nor defective migration of neural crest cells (**E**) causes the defect.

2. Correct: Mesoderm (E)

In the gastrointestinal tract, the lamina propria, muscularis mucosae, submucosa, inner circular and outer longitudinal (tenia coli) smooth muscle of the muscularis externa, the internal and external anal sphincters, and serosa/adventitia are derived from mesoderm.

The simple columnar absorptive cells lining hindgut derivatives and the upper anal canal, goblet cells, and enteroendocrine cells comprising the intestinal glands are derived from endoderm (**A**). The epithelia lining the lower anal canal are derived from ectoderm (**B**). Extrinsic innervation of the gastrointestinal tract develops from neuroectoderm (**C**). Neural crest cells (**D**) contribute to the formation of the enteric nervous system.

3. Correct: Elevated α-fetoprotein level in the amniotic fluid (E)

The fetus is affected by gastroschisis, in which intestinal loops herniate into the amniotic cavity through a lateral defect, usually to the right of the umbilicus. The contents are not covered by the amniotic membrane and are therefore exposed directly to the corrosive effect of the amniotic fluid. A second- or third-trimester ultrasound and an elevated α-fetoprotein (in maternal serum and/or amniotic fluid) are prenatal diagnostic indicators.

In contrast to omphalocele, gastroschisis is usually unrelated to chromosomal abnormalities (**A**) or other severe defects (**B**, **C**). Disproportionately elevated serum β-hCG (**D**) is not associated with either of these conditions.

4. Correct: Peritoneal fold that connects the stomach to the liver (D)

The ventral mesentery connecting the stomach (lesser curvature) to the ventral body wall is referred to as the ventral mesogastrium. The liver grows in it and divides it into lesser omentum (connects the liver to the stomach) and falciform ligament (connects the liver to the ventral body wall). Peritoneal folds that connect the sigmoid colon to the body wall (**A**, sigmoid mesocolon), jejunum to the body wall (**B**, the mesentery), stomach to the transverse colon (**C**, greater omentum), and stomach to the spleen (**E**, gastrosplenic ligament) are derived from the dorsal mesentery.

5. Correct: Double-bubble sign (D)

The neonate has annular pancreas, which occurs when pancreatic tissue surrounds and constricts the second part of the duodenum. The patient usually presents with features of duodenal obstruction (abdominal pain, bilious vomiting, nonperistaltic segment distal to and hyperperistaltic segment proximal to obstruction, double-bubble sign, electrolyte imbalance, etc.). The double-bubble sign is seen in infants and represents dilatation of the proximal duodenum and stomach. This is commonly seen with midgut obstruction.

While ileal diverticulum (**A**) might cause similar symptoms, it does not explain the CT scan finding. Also, the most common presentation in the infant with ileal diverticulum is painless hematochezia, not intestinal obstruction.

Blindly ending esophageal stump (**B**) is indicative of esophageal atresia. Absence of fundic gas shadow (**C**) is a sign of obstruction proximal to the stomach. Abrupt narrowing at the gastroesophageal junction (**E**) hints toward achalasia. Bilious vomiting should not be a presenting feature in any of these.

6. Correct: Failure of the omphalomesenteric duct to involute (C)

The omphalomesenteric or vitelline duct is the connection between the embryonic midgut and the yolk sac. This duct provides nutrition to the developing embryo until the placenta is established. By the 8th week of gestation, the duct separates from the intestines. If the duct is patent through its entire course from the small bowel to the umbilicus, fecal umbilical drainage occurs. The streaming of the contrast from the umbilicus during the barium enema confirms an enterocutaneous fistula.

Failure of migration of neural crest cells to the gut wall (**A**) will lead to motility disorders, which might present in the form of intestinal obstruction, but not bleeding. Failure of the midgut to recanalize (**B**) will present as gut atresia leading to intestinal obstruction. Again, there should not be any bleeding associated.

Patent urachus results when there is a persistence of an allantois remnant (**D**) which normally undergoes atresia during embryological development. It can lead to an abdominal wall defect similar in appearance on ultrasound to an omphalocele. Failure of the urorectal septum to develop normally (**E**) in a male infant would result in recto vesical or recto urethral fistula. Meconium-stained urine dribbles during micturition (recto vesical) or continuously (recto urethral) with urinary fistulas.

7. Correct: Splenic vein (D)

The proximal hindgut is drained by the inferior mesenteric vein, which drains into the splenic vein. The splenic vein then joins the superior mesenteric vein (**C**) to form the hepatic portal vein. Ileal (**A**, ileum) and right colic (**B**, ascending colon) veins drain portions of the midgut. The most distal part of the hindgut (lower rectum) drains into the inferior vena cava (**E**), through the internal pudendal and middle rectal veins.

8. Correct: Absence/agenesis of the common bile duct (C)

Elevated conjugated (direct) bilirubin and alkaline phosphatase, dark urine, and pale stool suggest obstructive jaundice. From the list, only agenesis of the common bile duct can cause a posthepatic (obstructive) jaundice where conjugated bilirubin would fail to reach the intestine. The infant is suffering from extrahepatic biliary atresia, the most common form of infantile pathological jaundice, which occurs due to failure of recanalization of the extrahepatic bile ducts. Typical symptoms include variable degrees of jaundice, dark urine, and light stools (develop over the first few weeks of life).

Agenesis of the liver (**A**) is incompatible with life, and if anything, will produce unconjugated hyperbilirubinemia. Agenesis of the gall bladder (**B**), pancreas (**D**), or spleen (**E**) will not produce obstructive jaundice because there is no obstruction in bile flow to the intestine.

9. Correct: Nonrotation of the primary intestinal loop (A)

During the 6th week, the primary intestinal loop grows rapidly to protrude into the umbilical cord (physiologic herniation). During the 10th week, it returns into the abdominal cavity. The jejunum is the first and the cecal bud is the last to re-enter the abdomen. While these processes are occurring, the midgut loop rotates 270° counterclockwise around the superior mesenteric artery. A nonrotated (misnomer) gut results from partial rotation of the midgut by only 90° counterclockwise. The small intestine ends up entirely to the right and the large intestine entirely to the left side of the abdominal cavity.

Reversed rotated (**B**) gut, where the midgut loop rotates clockwise 90° and the large intestine enters the abdominal cavity first, places the transverse colon behind the duodenum and the superior mesenteric artery.

Failure of the primary intestinal loop to return into the abdominal cavity following physiologic herniation (**C**) results in primary omphalocele, in which abdominal viscera (covered by amnion) herniate through the umbilicus.

Failure of the primary intestinal loop to detach from the yolk sac (**D**) might result in omphalomesenteric remnants in the form of Meckel's diverticulum, vitelline cysts, or fistulas.

Failure of the primary intestinal loop to maintain its blood supply from the superior mesenteric artery (**E**) will result in gut ischemia, which is a surgical emergency.

10. Correct: Neural crest cells (C)

The clinical presentation of the infant is suggestive of achalasia, which is an esophageal motility disorder due to defective migration of neural crest cells. Persons with achalasia lack inhibitory ganglion cells (derived from neural crest) in the lower esophageal sphincter, which results in an impaired relaxation of the sphincter in response to swallowing. A barium swallow facilitates the diagnosis, where the esophagus is seen enormously dilated proximal to and unusually narrow distal to the pathologic segment ("bird's-beak"). The other germ layers (**A, B, D,** and **E**) do not contribute to the ganglion cells of the enteric nervous system.

11. Correct: Endoderm (B)

Neonatal hypoglycemia is caused by hyperplasia of pancreatic islets, which occurs when fetal islets are exposed to high blood glucose levels (facilitated diffusion across the placenta), as in infants of diabetic mothers. The acinar cells, islet cells, and epithelium lining the ducts of the pancreas are derived from endoderm. While the surrounding connective tissue and vascular components of the pancreas are derived from visceral mesoderm (C), none of the other germ layers (A, D, and E) contribute to pancreatic development.

12. Correct: Failure of migration of neural crest cells (C)

The neonate seems to be suffering from Hirschsprung's disease. The disorder (also known as congenital megacolon), mostly affecting the rectosigmoid portion of the colon, is characterized by absence of myenteric and submucosal nerve plexuses in the gut wall, resulting in functional obstruction. Defective migration of neural crest cells (source of these neural elements within the enteric nervous system) is the possible cause for the disorder.

Failure of rupture of the anal membrane (A) is seen in imperforate anus. A normal per-rectal exam rules out its possibility.

Failure of obliteration of the omphalomesenteric duct (B, Meckel's diverticulum), although unlikely, might cause neonatal intestinal obstruction and present with bilious vomiting and abdominal distension. Painless hematochezia, however, is a much more common presentation in such cases.

Failure of the urorectal septum to develop normally (D) in males would result in recto vesical or recto urethral fistula. Meconium-stained urine dribbles during micturition (recto vesical) or continuously (recto-urethral) with urinary fistulas.

Failure of the primary intestinal loop to return into the abdominal cavity following physiologic herniation (E) results in primary omphalocele, in which abdominal viscera (covered by amnion) herniate through the umbilicus.

13. Correct: Omphalocele (E)

The fetus is affected by omphalocele, in which abdominal viscera (covered by amnion) herniate through the umbilicus. Primary omphalocele is due to failure of viscera to return to the body cavity following physiologic herniation. Secondary omphalocele is herniation of the abdominal viscera due to a defect in midline fusion of the body wall. This defect is usually associated with chromosomal abnormalities and other system involvement.

Umbilical herniation (A) is due to weakening of the muscles/fascia around the umbilicus, and protrudes tissue/organs through that area. Skin will be covering the herniation. Also, this usually has a gradual presentation after birth.

Bladder exstrophy (B) involves protrusion of the urinary bladder through a defect in the anterior abdominal wall. Nonvisualization of the bladder, lower abdominal bulge, and low insertion of the umbilical cord are chief prenatal ultrasound indicators of the condition.

Cloacal exstrophy (C) presents as a complex abdominal wall defect, with its main components as omphalocele, bladder exstrophy, and imperforate anus. Primary ultrasound criteria for diagnosing cloacal exstrophy prenatally are nonvisualization of the bladder, a large midline infraumbilical anterior wall defect or cystic anterior wall structure (persistent cloacal membrane), omphalocele, and lumbosacral anomalies.

In gastroschisis (D), intestinal loops herniate into the amniotic cavity through a lateral defect, usually to the right of the umbilicus. The contents are not covered by the amniotic membrane and are therefore exposed directly to the corrosive effect of the amniotic fluid.

14. Correct: Neural crest cells (B)

Neural crest cells contribute to the formation of the enteric nervous system. Extrinsic innervation of the gastrointestinal tract develops from neuroectoderm (A). The epithelial lining and the glandular parenchyma of the gastrointestinal tract develop from endoderm (E). Mesentery, connective tissue, smooth muscles, blood vessels, and the visceral peritoneum associated with gastrointestinal organs develop from the visceral mesoderm (C). Parietal peritoneum develops from the parietal mesoderm (D).

15. Correct: Failure of the omphalomesenteric duct to involute (C)

The infant seems to have a peptic ulcer affecting a Meckel's diverticulum (an omphalomesenteric remnant caused by failure of the vitelline duct to involute by the eighth week of gestation, located in the distal ileum, usually within 100 cm of the ileocecal valve). Heterotopic gastric mucosa (by far the most common tissue found in the diverticulum) may form a chronic ulcer and may damage the adjacent ileal mucosa via increased acid secretion. Such peptic ulceration can lead to pain, bleeding, and/or perforation. Painless melena or hematochezia (bright red blood from the rectum) are classic presentations. Consequently, severe anemia affects many of these children. A technetium-99m pertechnetate scintiscan (Meckel's scan), administered intravenously, identifies ectopic gastric mucosa, as it is readily taken up by parietal cells. In a positive scan, the patient develops immediate tracer localization in the stomach and in the right lower quadrant.

Failure of migration of neural crest cells to the gut wall (A) will lead to motility disorders, which might present in the form of intestinal obstruction, but not bleeding.

189

Failure of the midgut to recanalize (**B**) will present as gut atresia leading to intestinal obstruction. Again, there should not be any bleeding associated.

Patent urachus results when there is a persistence of an allantois remnant (**D**), which normally undergoes atresia during embryologic development. It can lead to an abdominal wall defect similar in appearance on ultrasound to an omphalocele. A failure of the urorectal septum to develop (**E**) would result in recto vesical, recto urethral, or recto vaginal fistulas. Meconium-stained urine dribbles during micturition (recto vesical) or continuously (recto urethral) with urinary fistulas. Meconium-stained vaginal secretion suggests recto vaginal fistula.

16.   Correct: Failure of fusion of ventral and dorsal pancreatic ducts (B)

Pancreas divisum occurs when the dorsal pancreatic duct drains the major portion of the pancreas and opens into the duodenum through minor papillae, resulting in an increased incidence of pancreatitis. It occurs due to failure of fusion of the ventral and dorsal ducts with persistence of both.

Failure of fusion (**A**) or malrotation (**C, D**) of pancreatic buds might contribute toward annular pancreas, not pancreas divisum.

The dorsal pancreatic duct drains most of the pancreas and opens into the major duodenal papilla (**E**) in normal population, not pancreas divisum. The ventral pancreatic duct in pancreas divisum opens into the major duodenal papilla but does not drain most of the pancreas (**F**). It drains only a portion of the head and uncinate process.

17.   Correct: Jejunum (C)

The midgut forms the primary intestinal loop that consists of a cranial and a caudal limb. The cranial limb forms the jejunum and upper part of the ileum. The caudal limb forms the cecal bud, from which the cecum (**D**) and appendix (**E**) develop. The stomach (**A**) and gallbladder (**B**) are foregut derivatives.

18.   Correct: A pronounced circular layer of smooth muscle in the stomach wall (C)

The clinical scenario is typical for infantile hypertrophic pyloric stenosis. This commonly occurs due to defective migration of neural crest cells and results in an impaired relaxation of the pyloric sphincter (formed by the circular layer of muscularis externa of the stomach wall). The infant (usually during age 3–4 weeks) presents with projectile, nonbilious vomiting ~ 15 to 20 minutes following feeding. A barium meal demonstrates a dilated stomach proximal to the hypertrophic sphincter.

Double-bubble sign in X-ray (**A**) is indicative of intestinal obstruction (duodenal atresia, annular pancreas, etc.). The vomitus would normally contain bile.

Tracheoesophageal fistula (**B**) usually presents at birth when the infant regurgitates saliva (drools), chokes, and turns blue (cyanotic) with attempted feeding.

An ileal diverticulum (**D**) in the pediatric population commonly presents with painless hematochezia. If it presents as an intestinal obstruction, the vomitus (if at all) will contain bile.

Ectopia cordis (**E**) is caused by defective fusion of the anterior thoracic wall and has no apparent association with infantile hypertrophic pyloric stenosis.

19.   Correct: Duodenal atresia (E)

Duodenal atresia, due to failure of lumen recanalization, presents with features of intestinal obstruction. It is typically characterized by onset of bilious vomiting within hours of birth. It also features the double-bubble sign (gas in stomach and duodenum) on postnatal abdominal X-ray of the neonate.

Ankyloglossia (**A**) or tongue-tie is the result of a short lingual frenulum causing difficulty in speech articulation due to limitation in tongue movement. This is not associated with vomiting.

Esophageal atresia (**B**) results in regurgitation of food and saliva immediately at birth. Neither will the neonate have bilious vomiting, nor will a nasogastric tube pass beyond the esophagus.

The neonate in achalasia (**C**) presents with progressive difficulty swallowing, regurgitation of swallowed foods and liquids, heartburn, difficulty burping, and sensation of a lump in the throat. A barium swallow demonstrates a "bird's-beak," where the esophagus is enormously dilated proximal to and unusually narrow distal to the pathologic segment.

Infantile hypertrophic pyloric stenosis (**D**) presents with projectile, nonbilious vomiting shortly following feeding. The usual age of presentation is 3 to 4 weeks. A barium meal demonstrates a dilated stomach proximal to the hypertrophic sphincter.

20.   Correct: Failure of rupture of the cloacal membrane and defective development of the urorectal septum (D)

The newborn is suffering from imperforate anus with recto vaginal fistula. The cloaca is partitioned by the urorectal septum into the posterior anorectal canal and anterior urogenital sinus. The cloacal membrane is partitioned by the urorectal septum into the posterior anal membrane and anterior urogenital membrane. Rupture of these membranes will establish continuity of these canals with the exterior (forming urethral, vaginal, and anal orifices). Failure of rupture of anal membrane (**A**) results in imperforate anus. The neonate has a dimple in place of the normal anal orifice and presents with the inability to pass meconium. Failure of the urorectal septum to develop normally (**B**) results in recto vesical, recto urethral, or recto vaginal fistulas. Meconium-stained diaper and gap in the posterior vaginal wall indicate recto vaginal fistula.

Failure of migration of neural crest cells to the gut wall (**C, E**)) will lead to motility disorders, which might present in the form of intestinal obstruction.

Chapter 23

Cardiovascular System Embryology

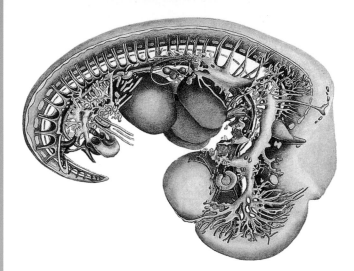

LEARNING OBJECTIVES

▶ Describe the etiopathogenesis, hemodynamic changes, clinical features, and diagnosis of Ebstein's anomaly.

▶ Describe the role of neural crest cells in development of the heart.

▶ Describe the etiopathogenesis, hemodynamic changes, clinical features, and diagnosis of ventricular septal defect.

▶ Describe the development of aortic arches. Define major arteries derived from these.

▶ Describe the etiopathogenesis, hemodynamic changes, clinical features, and diagnosis of patent ductus arteriosus.

▶ Define the precursors within the primary and secondary heart fields during formation of the primitive heart tube.

▶ Describe the contribution of sinus venosus, pulmonary veins, and primitive atria in development of the right and left atria in the adult heart.

▶ Describe the etiopathogenesis, hemodynamic changes, clinical features, and diagnosis of patent truncus arteriosus.

▶ Describe the etiopathogenesis, hemodynamic changes, clinical features, and diagnosis of double-outlet right ventricle.

▶ Describe the etiopathogenesis, hemodynamic changes, clinical features, and diagnosis of atrial septal defect.

▶ Describe the etiopathogenesis, hemodynamic changes, clinical features, and diagnosis of tetralogy of Fallot.

▶ Analyze the changes within the venous (inflow) system during the development of heart.

▶ Describe the etiopathogenesis, hemodynamic changes, clinical features, and diagnosis of transposition of the great arteries.

▶ Describe the etiopathogenesis, hemodynamic changes, clinical features, and diagnosis of coarctation of the aorta.

▶ Describe the development and septation of the outflow tracts in the primitive heart.

▶ Describe the role of cardiac mesenchyme in partitioning of the heart and development of the heart valves.

▶ Differentiate between fetal and adult circulation.

▶ Describe the etiopathogenesis, hemodynamic changes, clinical features, and diagnosis of tricuspid atresia (hypoplastic right ventricle).

23.1 Questions

Easy	Medium	Hard

1. A 33-year-old woman delivers a full-term infant. After 3 days and several feeding sessions, the baby has still not passed a stool. Over the next 8 hours, the baby wets his diaper, has a bulge in the abdomen, but still has not had his first stool. Auscultation reveals normal peristaltic sounds in the upper abdomen and almost absent sounds in the lower abdomen. A per-rectal exam came back normal with meconium-covered gloved fingers. Which of the following additional disorders might the baby be suffering from?

A. Atrial septal defect, ostium primum type

B. Atrial septal defect, ostium secundum type

C. Ventricular septal defect, muscular type

D. Ventricular septal defect, membranous type

E. Ebstein's anomaly

2. A 6-week-old infant presents with poor feeding, decreased weight gain, tachypnea, tachycardia, sweating (especially with feeding), and lethargy. Physical examination reveals a holosystolic murmur along the left sternal border that widely radiates throughout the precordium. An echocardiogram demonstrates a large ventricular septal defect affecting the membranous part of the septum. Which of the following structures might have suffered from a developmental defect?

A. Septum primum

B. Septum secundum

C. Endocardial cushions

D. Bulbus cordis

E. Truncus arteriosus

3. A 6-day-old neonate presents with diffuse neurodeficit. A color Doppler revealed an insufficient blood flow through the circle of Willis. Which of the following arterial arches might have suffered from developmental defects during embryogenesis?

A. Aortic arches 1 and 2

B. Aortic arches 2 and 3

C. Aortic arches 3 and 4

D. Aortic arches 3 and 6

E. Aortic arches 4 and 6

4. A male neonate born at 30 weeks gestation and weighing 2.1 lbs. develops respiratory distress immediately after birth. He did not have any bluish discoloration of skin, but physical examination revealed a continuous "machinery" murmur loudest at the left upper sternal border. Which of the following is the probable abnormality in the infant?

A. Failure of septation of truncus arteriosus

B. Failure of the shunt between the pulmonary artery and the descending aorta to close

C. Atresia of the tricuspid valve with accompanying atrial septal defect

D. Severe pulmonary stenosis with accompanying ventricular septal defect

E. An aorta that arises from the right ventricle and a pulmonary artery that arises from the left ventricle

5. A 28-year-old pregnant woman is very disappointed that she can't hear fetal heart sounds at least until 10 weeks' gestation (with Doppler ultrasound). If an ideal (hypothetical) device was available, what is the earliest gestational week when she could have heard these?

A. 2 weeks

B. 3 weeks

C. 4 weeks

D. 6 weeks

E. 8 weeks

6. A 12-year-old girl presented to the clinic with complaints of dyspnea-on-exertion for the past 2 months. She also complained of intermittent chest pains and palpitations. An echocardiogram revealed a giant left atrial myxoma affecting the smooth part of the atrium and causing severe mitral insufficiency. Which of the following embryonic structures is the source for the affected region of the heart?

A. Right horn of the sinus venosus

B. Left horn of the sinus venosus

C. Bulbus cordis

D. Primitive atrium

E. Primitive pulmonary vein

7. A male neonate born at 32 weeks' gestation was tachypneic and diaphoretic. Physical examination revealed moderate cyanosis and a pansystolic murmur best heard at the left sternal border. Which of the following is a probable cause for his symptoms?

A. Patent ductus arteriosus

B. Patent ductus venosus

C. Patent truncus arteriosus

D. Ventricular septal defect

E. Atrial septal defect

8. A full-term male neonate presents with dyspnea and a systolic murmur at birth. An echocardiogram revealed a double-outlet right ventricle with a subpulmonary ventricular septal defect. Which of the following additional findings is expected in the neonate?

A. Anemia

B. Cyanosis

C. Jaundice

D. Pulmonary embolism

E. Cerebral embolism

9. A 2-month-old infant presents with a systolic ejection murmur heard loudest at the upper left sternal border. Echocardiogram reveals an ostium primum atrial septal defect. Which of the following processes might have been defective in him?

A. Fusion of septum primum with septum secundum

B. Fusion of septum primum with endocardial cushions

C. Fusion of septum secundum with endocardial cushions

D. Apoptosis within the septum primum

E. Apoptosis within the septum secundum

10. A 2-day-old neonate needed intubation for progressive tachypnea. An umbilical artery catheterization was planned to sample arterial blood gas and monitor arterial pressure. Which of the following is an absolute contraindication to the procedure that the surgeon must exclude before planning on such catheterization?

A. Patent ductus arteriosus

B. Patent ductus venosus

C. Aortic arch aneurysm

D. Circle of Willis aneurysm

E. Internal iliac artery aneurysm

11. A 3-week-old infant presents with severe cyanosis, polycythemia, hypoxia, and a systolic ejection murmur heard best over the pulmonic area and the left sternal border. An echocardiogram revealed ventricular septal defect, an overriding aortic arch straddling the defect, and right ventricular hypertrophy. Which of the following additional findings, responsible for the severe cyanosis, is expected in the infant?

A. Septum primum atrial septal defect

B. Septum secundum atrial septal defect

C. Patent ductus arteriosus

D. Pulmonary stenosis

E. Left ventricular hypertrophy

12. A 2-day-old neonate presents with a blockage in the channel responsible for most of the venous drainage of the heart. An unruptured aneurysm during development was suspected to be the underlying cause. Which of the following is the most probable location where the aneurysm was lodged?

A. Left horn of sinus venosus

B. Right horn of sinus venosus

C. Bulbus cordis

D. Conus cordis

E. Truncus arteriosus

13. A 36-year-old mother gives birth to a male neonate at 40 weeks' gestation. He develops cyanosis within hours of birth, which progresses considerably in the next 24 hours. The physical examination, other than the cyanosis, is unremarkable. Which of the following is the most likely developmental defect in the neonate?

A. Ventricular septal defect

B. Atrial septal defect

C. Ventricular septal defect, an overriding aortic arch, and pulmonary stenosis

D. Failure of spiral partitioning of the conus cordis and the truncus arteriosus

E. Failure of the shunt between the pulmonary artery and the descending aorta to close

14. A 1-day-old male neonate presents with tachypnea, tachycardia, and increased work of breathing. While pulses in all his extremities were recorded to be normal at birth, the attending nurse was unable to locate his femoral pulses after a couple hours. A systolic murmur was best heard at the left interscapular area with radiation to the left axilla. Which of the following might be an additional finding in the neonate?

A. Cyanosis

B. Differential cyanosis (pink upper extremities with blue lower extremities)

C. Reversed differential cyanosis (pink lower extremities with blue upper extremities)

D. Systolic blood pressure discrepancies between the upper and lower extremities > 20 mm Hg

E. Strong arteria dorsalis pedis pulsation

15. A 26-year-old mother had a viral infection during her first trimester that caused widespread damage to the developing vasculature in the embryo. Which of the following structures would still be functional if the embryonic brachial arch arteries were prime targets for the virus?

A. Ascending aorta

B. Arch of the aorta

C. Internal carotid artery

D. Pulmonary artery

E. Ductus arteriosus

16. A pediatric resident is eager to study septation of the fetal heart. At what earliest week of gestation should she schedule a fetal echocardiography to visualize the completely formed septa?

A. End of 2 weeks

B. End of 3 weeks

C. End of 4 weeks

D. End of 5 weeks

E. End of 8 weeks

17. A researcher is in the process of developing an antibody that is capable of binding to proteins exclusively located within the primary source for cardiogenic tissue in a 3-week-old embryo. Which of the following tissues is the target for the antibody?

A. Paraxial mesoderm

B. Intermediate mesoderm

C. Lateral plate mesoderm, splanchnic layer

D. Lateral plate mesoderm, somatic layer

E. Endoderm

18. A developmental defect causes malformation of the conotruncal cushions in the fetus. You are concerned that it may lead to transposition of the great vessels. Which of the following additional defects would you want to consider during the fetal echocardiogram?

A. Atrial septal defect of the ostium primum type

B. Atrial septal defect of the ostium secundum type

C. Muscular ventricular septal defect

D. Tricuspid stenosis

E. Aortic stenosis

19. A pediatric resident in training has been advised to closely monitor circulatory changes that occur through the neonatal period and infancy. Which of the following structures can she appreciate in a 3-month-old infant with normal growth?

A. Ductus venosus

B. Ductus arteriosus

C. Foramen ovale

D. Fossa ovalis

E. Left umbilical vein

20. An 18-hour-old male neonate presents with minimal cyanosis and signs of heart failure. Physical examination reveals a holosystolic murmur at the left lower sternal border. A fetal echocardiogram demonstrates atresia of the tricuspid valve and an enlarged right atrium. Which of the following would be an essential additional finding in his echocardiogram?

A. Pulmonary stenosis

B. Ventricular septal defect

C. Enlarged right ventricle

D. Hypoplastic left ventricle

E. Hypoplastic left atrium

23.1 Answers and Explanations

Easy	Medium	Hard

1. Correct: Ventricular septal defect, membranous type (D)

Not passing stool for the first 3 days raises the suspicion of a lower GI motility disorder or an imperforate anus. A normal per-rectal exam rules out the possibilities of imperforate anus or anal atresia. The clinical feature is consistent with Hirschsprung's disease, which results from lack of ganglia in the distal colon due to a defect in migration of neural crest cells.

Neural crest cells in the fetal heart contribute to the conotruncal cushions that lead to septum formation in the truncus arteriosus and conus cordis, formation of semilunar valves, and formation of the membranous part of the ventricular septum. Defective migration of neural crest cells could result in a variety of defects that include pulmonary stenosis, aortic stenosis, persistent truncus arteriosus, tetralogy of Fallot, transposition of great vessels, and membranous type of ventricular septal defects (VSD).

The atrial septum (**A, B**), and the muscular part of the ventricular septum (**C**) have no contributions from the neural crest.

Ebstein's anomaly (**E**) results from a defective tricuspid valve and an accompanying atrial septal defect. Atrioventricular (tricuspid and mitral) valves are formed from endocardial cushions that have no contribution from the neural crest.

2. Correct: Endocardial cushions (C)

Normal closure of the membranous portion of the ventricular septum occurs through multiple concurrent embryologic mechanisms: (1) downward growth of the bulbar and truncal ridges forming the outlet septum, (2) growth of the endocardial cushions forming the inlet septum, and (3) growth of the muscular ventricular septum.

Septum primum (**A**) and secundum (**B**) are essential for forming the atrial septum. The bulbus cordis (**D**) develops into outflow tracts for the ventricles. Truncus arteriosus (**E**) develops into the aorta and the pulmonary trunk.

3. Correct: Aortic arches 3 and 4 (C)

The circle of Willis (circulus arteriosus) is formed by two interconnecting arterial sources—the internal carotid arteries and the vertebrobasilar system (which is formed by two vertebral arteries and the basilar artery). The internal carotid arteries are formed from the 3rd aortic arches. The vertebral arteries are branches off the subclavian arteries. The right subclavian artery and the arch of the aorta are formed from the right and left 4th aortic arches, respectively. Although left subclavian arteries are formed from the 7th left intersegmental arteries and not directly from the 3rd- or 4th-arch arteries, none of the other listed arches contribute to the circle of Willis.

Remnants of aortic arches 1 (**A**) in the neonate/adult are the maxillary arteries. Remnants of aortic arches 2 (**A, B**) in the neonate/adult are the stapedial and hyoidal arteries. Remnants of aortic arches 6 (**D, E**) in the neonate/adult are the right and left pulmonary arteries, and ductus arteriosus on the left.

4. Correct: Failure of the shunt between the pulmonary artery and the descending aorta to close (B)

Given the infant was acyanotic, it rules out the possibility of any right-to-left shunt being present in him. Failure of the shunt between the pulmonary artery and the descending aorta to close (patent ductus arteriosus → left-to-right shunt) would give rise to an acyanotic child with continuous machinery murmur.

Failure of septation of truncus arteriosus (**A**, persistent truncus arteriosus), atresia of the tricuspid valve with accompanying atrial septal defect (**C**), severe pulmonary stenosis with accompanying ventricular septal defect (**D**, as seen in tetralogy of Fallot), an aorta that arises from the right ventricle and a pulmonary artery that arises from the left ventricle (**E**, transposition of great vessels)—all present with right-to-left shunts and consequent cyanosis.

5. Correct: 4 weeks (C)

The heart begins to form late in the 3rd week (**B**) and starts to beat at the 4th week. During the 5th week cardiac septation occurs and the heart is almost fully formed by the 6th week (**D**). The 2nd week (**A**) is too early, while the 8th week (**E**) is too late for the heart to start functioning.

Fetal heart sounds are detectable by hand held Doppler (after 10 weeks' gestation) or by fetoscope (after 18–20 weeks' gestation). The normal heart rate is 110 to 160 beats per minute.

6. Correct: Primitive pulmonary vein (E)

The primitive pulmonary vein and its branches are incorporated into the left atrium, forming the smooth-walled part of the adult left atrium.

The right horn of the sinus venosus (**A**) develops into the smooth part of the right atrium, while the left horn (**B**) develops into the coronary sinus and the oblique vein of the left atrium. The bulbus cordis (**C**) develops into outflow tracts for the ventricles. The primitive atrium (**D**) develops into the trabeculated parts of atria.

7. Correct: Patent truncus arteriosus (C)

Pathophysiology of truncus arteriosus is typified by cyanosis where outflow from both ventricles is directed into the common arterial trunk. Neonates typically present with poor feeding, diaphoresis, tachypnea, and cyanosis.

Failure of the shunt between the pulmonary artery and the descending aorta to close (patent ductus arteriosus, **A**) would give rise to an acyanotic neonate with a continuous machinery murmur.

The ductus venosus (**B**) connects the umbilical vein to the inferior vena cava during fetal life and subsequently closes rapidly after birth. The patient with a persistent ductus venosus would usually present with hepatic encephalopathy and fatty degeneration of the liver at adulthood and is unlikely to have cyanosis.

Atrial (**E**) and ventricular (**D**) septal defects present with left-to-right shunts, which do not make the newborn cyanotic.

8. Correct: Cyanosis (B)

Double-outlet right ventricle (DORV, both the pulmonary trunk and the aorta arising out of the right ventricle) with subpulmonary ventricular septal defect (VSD) is also known as the Taussig-Bing anomaly. With this type of DORV, oxygen-rich blood flows from the left ventricle, through the VSD, and into the pulmonary artery. Oxygen-poor blood from the right ventricle flows mainly into the aorta. Cyanosis is often present at birth, and varies from mild to severe. Infants suffer from repeated chest infections and congestive heart failure.

Anemia (**A**), jaundice (**C**), pulmonary emboli (**D**), and systemic emboli (**E**) are not usual presenting features.

9. Correct: Fusion of septum primum with endocardial cushions (B)

During fetal development, the rudimentary atrium is divided by the septum primum, except for an anterior and inferior space that forms the ostium primum. The ostium primum is sealed by fusion of the septum primum with the endocardial cushions around 5 weeks' gestation. Failure to do so results in an ostium primum atrial septal defect.

Failure of apoptosis within the septum primum (**D**), that is, failure to develop the ostium secundum, is incompatible with life, since the connection between the right and the left atria is obliterated. On the other hand, excessive resorption of the septum primum might result in an ostium secundum atrial septal defect, where the normal septum secundum could prove insufficient to cover the large ostium secundum.

Fusion of septum primum with septum secundum (**A**) never really occurs, and the gap between these forms the foramen ovale. When the upper part of the septum primum gradually disappears, the remaining part becomes the valve of the oval foramen. After birth, when lung circulation begins and pressure in the left atrium increases, the valve of the oval foramen is pressed against the septum secundum, obliterating the oval foramen and separating the right and left atria. A defect in this process would result in an ostium secundum (persistent foramen ovale) type of atrial septal defect.

Fusion of septum secundum with endocardial cushions (**C**) or apoptosis within the septum secundum (**E**) never occurs during normal development.

10. Correct: Internal iliac artery aneurysm (E)

The umbilical arteries develop from and are direct continuation of the internal iliac arteries. In the adult, the distal part degenerates and forms the medial umbilical ligament, while the proximal part persists as the internal iliac and the superior vesical arteries. Umbilical artery catheterization is a common procedure in the neonatal intensive care unit and has become the standard of care for arterial access in neonates. Such catheterization would increase the chances of rupture of an aneurysm in the internal iliac artery, from which the umbilical artery arises. Other major contraindications to umbilical artery catheterization include omphalocele, peritonitis, necrotizing enterocolitis, and vascular compromise to the kidneys.

The ductus arteriosus (**A**) is a shunt between the pulmonary artery and the descending thoracic aorta; it is in the thorax and is not related to the umbilical arteries.

The ductus venosus (**B**) connects the umbilical vein to the inferior vena cava during fetal life and subsequently closes rapidly after birth. It derives from the left umbilical vein and is not related to the umbilical artery.

The arch of the aorta (**C**), derived from the left 4th aortic arch, is in the thorax and is not related to the umbilical artery.

The circle of Willis (**D**), formed by two interconnecting arterial sources (the internal carotid arteries and the vertebrobasilar system), supplies the brain and is not related to the umbilical artery.

11. Correct: Pulmonary stenosis (D)

Tetralogy of Fallot consists of a ventricular septal defect, an overriding aortic arch straddling the defect, pulmonary stenosis, and right ventricular hypertrophy. Pulmonary stenosis usually results in reduced blood flow to the lungs and an increase in pressure to the right ventricle. This pressure gradient leads to the right-to-left shunting of oxygen-poor blood across the septal defect and out into the systemic circulation, determines the degree of cyanosis, and results in symptoms of cyanosis, polycythemia, and hypoxia.

Atrial septal defects (**A, B**), patent ductus arteriosus (**C**), and left ventricular hypertrophy (**E**) neither contribute to cyanosis nor are associated with tetralogy of Fallot.

12. Correct: Left horn of sinus venosus (A)

The majority of veins draining the heart empty into the coronary sinus, which delivers deoxygenated blood to the right atrium. The coronary sinus and the oblique vein of the left atrium derive from the left horn of the sinus venosus.

The right sinus horn (**B**) is absorbed to form the smooth part of the right atrium. The bulbus cordis (**C**), and the conus cordis (**D**, also considered as the middle third of the bulbus cordis or conus arteriosus), develops into the outflow parts of the ventricles (infundibulum of the right and aortic vestibule of the left ventricles). The truncus arteriosus (**E**), also considered as the distal third of the bulbus cordis, develops into the pulmonary trunk and the aorta.

13. Correct: Failure of spiral partitioning of the conus cordis and the truncus arteriosus (D)

Failure of spiral partitioning of the conus cordis and the truncus arteriosus results in transposition of the great arteries (TGA), in which the aorta and the pulmonary artery arise from the morphologic right and left ventricles, respectively. This arrangement results in deficient oxygen supply to the tissues and is incompatible with prolonged survival unless mixing of oxygenated and deoxygenated blood occurs at some anatomic level, such as ventricular septal defect (VSD), atrial septal defect (ASD), or patent ductus arteriosus (PDA). Prominent and progressive cyanosis, within the first 24 hours of life, is the usual finding in neonates with TGA with intact atrial and ventricular septum. Other than cyanosis, the physical examination is often unremarkable (an important differentiating feature from tetralogy of Fallot).

VSD, an overriding aortic arch, and pulmonary stenosis (**C**) are three integral components of tetralogy of Fallot and would present with identical clinical features. However, the VSD and the pulmonary stenosis would result in a harsh systolic ejection murmur, which can be heard best over the pulmonary area and the left sternal border.

VSDs (**A**), ASDs (**B**), and failure of the shunt between the pulmonary artery and the descending aorta to close (**E**, PDA) result in left-to-right shunts and, consequently, acyanotic neonates.

14. Correct: Systolic blood pressure discrepancies between the upper and lower extremities > 20 mm Hg (D)

Coarctation of the aorta may be defined as a constricted aortic segment that comprises localized medial thickening. The classic location involves the thoracic aorta distal to the origin of the left subclavian artery. Dilatation of the descending aorta immediately distal to the coarctation segment (post-stenotic dilatation) is usually present. Neonates present with tachypnea, tachycardia, and increased work of breathing. These patients may have appeared well at birth, and abrupt deterioration coincides with closure of the ductus arteriosus. Keys to the diagnosis include blood pressure discrepancies between the upper and lower extremities and reduced or absent lower extremity pulsation. The murmur associated with coarctation of the aorta is usually a systolic murmur best heard posteriorly in the left interscapular area, usually with some degree of radiation to the left axilla, apex, and anterior precordium.

Cyanosis (**A**) is not associated with coarctation of the aorta, unless there is an associated defect that creates a right-to-left shunt. No such symptoms and signs were hinted at in the question.

Differential cyanosis (**B**)—pink upper extremities with cyanotic lower extremities—may occur when right-to-left shunt across a patent ductus arteriosus provides flow to the lower body. Reversed differential cyanosis (**C**)—upper body cyanosis with normal lower-body oxygen saturation—may occur with transposition of the great arteries (TGA) with patent ductus arteriosus (PDA) and elevated pulmonary vascular resistance or in TGA with PDA and preductal aortic coarctation. In both cases, saturated blood enters the pulmonary artery from the left ventricle and is then shunted through the PDA to supply the lower part of the body. **B** and **C** can be ruled out in our patient by absence of a continuous "machinery" murmur consequent to PDA, which can be heard loudest at the left upper sternal border.

Coarctation of the aorta presents with absent or reduced arterial pulsation in femoral, popliteal, dorsalis pedis (**E**), or any other lower extremity vessel.

15. Correct: Ascending aorta (A)

The ascending aorta develops from the truncus arteriosus of the primitive heart and not from the arch arteries. The arch of the aorta (**B**) develops from the left 4th-arch artery. Internal carotid arteries (**C**) develop from 3rd-arch arteries. Pulmonary arteries (**D**) develop from the 6th-arch arteries. Ductus arteriosus (**E**), a communication between the descending thoracic aorta and the pulmonary artery, develops from the left 6th arterial arch.

16. Correct: End of 5 weeks (D)

The heart begins to form late in the 3rd week (**B**) and starts to beat by the 4th week. During the late 4th week (**C**) cardiac septation begins and is almost fully complete by the end of the 5th week. The end of the 2nd week (**A**) is too early, while septation occurs well ahead of the 8th week (**E**).

17. Correct: Lateral plate mesoderm, splanchnic layer (C)

The heart develops from two sources: splanchnic or visceral mesoderm (primary source) and neural crest cells (contribute to conotruncal cushions and their derivatives).

Paraxial mesoderm (**A**) develops into most of the axial skeleton, striated muscles, and dermis of the neck and dorsal trunk. Intermediate mesoderm (**B**) develops into genitourinary structures. Somatic mesoderm (**D**) develops into inner lining of body walls (ventral dermis of trunk, parietal layers of mesothelia, etc.) and limbs (bones and dermis). Endoderm (**E**) develops into the primitive gut tube.

18. Correct: Aortic stenosis (E)

The conotruncal cushions contribute to septate the outflow tracts of the ventricles (conus and truncus) and form the aorticopulmonary septum. Differential growth of tissue from these cushions also contributes to the formation of the semilunar (pulmonary and aortic) valves. Therefore, malformation of these cushions can lead to a variety of outflow tract septation or obstruction defects, including aortic stenosis.

Atrial septa (**A, B**) are formed by septum primum, secundum, and endocardial cushions. The muscular part of the ventricular septum (**C**) is formed by a growth from the primitive ventricular wall, while the membranous part has contributions from the conotruncal (bulbar ridges) and endocardial cushions. Atrioventricular (**D**) valves are formed from endocardial cushions.

19. Correct: Fossa ovalis (D)

Fossa ovalis is an oval depression on the atrial septum and is a remnant of foramen ovale and its valve.

The ductus venosus (**A**), a channel that shunts oxygenated blood from the umbilical veins to the inferior vena cava, closes soon after birth. Its adult remnant is the ligamentum venosum.

The ductus arteriosus (**B**), a communication between the descending thoracic aorta and the pulmonary artery, constricts within a day after birth. Its adult remnant is the ligamentum arteriosum.

The foramen ovale (**C**) serves as a physiologic conduit for right-to-left shunting between the atria. Functional closure of the foramen occurs with increase in left atrial pressure once the pulmonary circulation is established following birth. Anatomic closure of the foramen (fusion of the septum primum and septum secundum) usually occurs within 3 months of birth.

Umbilical vessels (**E**) obliterate at birth with clamping of the umbilical cord and separation of the placenta. The adult remnant of the left umbilical vein is the ligamentum teres hepatis.

20. Correct: Ventricular septal defect (B)

With absence of the tricuspid valve and no continuity between the right atrium and right ventricle, venous blood returning to the right atrium can exit only by an interatrial communication: an atrial septal defect (ASD), which is necessary for survival. Also, oxygenation of blood with tricuspid atresia would be possible only if there is a ventricular septal defect (VSD) or a patent ductus arteriosus (PDA). The type of murmur indicates presence of VSD in this case (PDA would have presented with a continuous murmur).

Degree of cyanosis in a patient with tricuspid atresia depends on the pulmonary blood flow. Minimal cyanosis is indicative of pulmonary plethora and rules out pulmonary oligemia and hence, pulmonary stenosis (**A**).

The right ventricle is small and hypoplastic (**C**, not enlarged), since blood from both venae cavae is forced across the patent foramen ovale into the left heart.

The left ventricle (**D**) and the atrium (**E**) are hypertrophied, because of the volume overload (receives all venous return from systemic and pulmonary circulation). The right atrium is characteristically enlarged and hypertrophied and is responsible for the signs of heart failure.

Chapter 24

Respiratory System Embryology

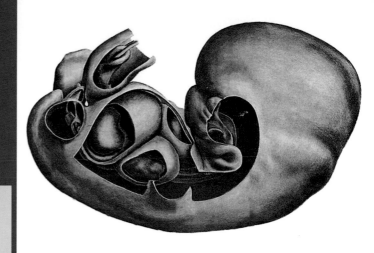

LEARNING OBJECTIVES

- ▶ Describe the development of the diaphragm.
- ▶ Analyze the pathogenesis, clinical features, and diagnosis of congenital diaphragmatic hernias.
- ▶ Describe the development of components of the blood-air barrier.
- ▶ Describe the etiopathogenesis, hemodynamic changes, clinical features, and diagnosis of acute lung injury.
- ▶ Analyze the pathogenesis, clinical features, and diagnosis of hyaline membrane disease.
- ▶ Describe the developmental changes with each of the stages during lung formation.
- ▶ Analyze the pathogenesis, clinical features, and diagnosis of tracheomalacia.
- ▶ Describe the development of the trachea.
- ▶ Describe the microstructure, location, and development of the olfactory epithelium.
- ▶ Analyze the pathogenesis, clinical features, and diagnosis of pulmonary sequestration.
- ▶ Describe the development of laryngeal cartilages.
- ▶ Correlate the underlying developmental mechanisms in tracheoesophageal fistulas (and VACTERL syndrome) with their clinical presentation, outcomes for the fetus/newborn, and pre/peri/postnatal diagnosis.

24.1 Questions

Easy	Medium	Hard

Consider the following case for questions 1 to 3:

A newborn male infant presents with severe cyanosis, tachypnea, and dyspnea. Despite 100% oxygen via mask, the baby becomes bradycardic and requires mechanical ventilation. Auscultation of the lungs reveals good breath sounds in the right chest, but no breath sounds in the left. The heart sounds seemed loudest in the right chest, and the abdomen appears scaphoid. A chest X-ray is done, which reveals intestinal loops in the left chest cavity.

1. Which of the following is a probable diagnosis for the neonate?

A. Tracheoesophageal fistula

B. Bochdalek's hernia

C. Kartagener's syndrome

D. Bronchogenic cysts

E. Pulmonary sequestration

2. Which of the following might be the developmental basis for the symptoms and signs in the neonate?

A. Defective formation of the tracheoesophageal septum

B. Defective fusion of septum transversum across the midline

C. Defective fusion of pleuroperitoneal membranes with septum transversum

D. Defective formation of dynein arms in cilia

E. Defective budding of embryonic foregut

3. Which of the following is the most important predictor of survival for the neonate?

A. Fetal age at presentation

B. Types of organs (small or large bowel) present in the chest cavity

C. Degree of pulmonary hypoplasia

D. Degree of cardiac hypertrophy

E. Anatomical location of the defect

4. A 26-year-old woman presents to the ER with a 2-day history of a flu-like illness characterized by dry cough and breathlessness. Physical examination was significant for a temperature of 102°F and a respiratory rate of 40 breaths per minute. Despite maximal supplemental oxygen therapy, arterial blood gas analysis showed type 2 respiratory failure. She tired rapidly, requiring tracheal intubation and invasive mechanical ventilation. Investigation revealed bilateral infiltrates on chest radiograph. From which of the following sources is the defective structure, responsible for her pulmonary edema, derived?

A. Ectoderm

B. Endoderm

C. Mesoderm

D. A and B

E. B and C

F. A and C

Consider the following case for questions 5 to 9:

A newborn male presents with tachypnea, progressive cyanosis, and expiratory grunting at birth. He was born at 28 weeks' gestation to a diabetic mother. Chest X-rays show diffuse bilateral atelectasis and air bronchograms. Despite advanced resuscitation efforts, the neonate expired 10 hours after birth. Postmortem histological examination of the lungs reveals acellular, proteinaceous material lining the alveolar septa.

5. Which of the following is the most likely diagnosis?

A. Cystic fibrosis

B. Bochdalek's hernia

C. Respiratory distress syndrome of the newborn

D. Pulmonary sequestration

E. Tracheoesophageal fistula

6. Which of the following cells secrete the substance that was deficient/defective in the neonate?

A. α cell, pancreatic islet

B. Parafollicular cell, thyroid

C. Zona fasciculata, adrenal

D. Basophil, pituitary

E. Type II pneumocyte, lung

7. During which of the following weeks does the substance that was deficient/defective in the neonate first appear in fetal circulation?

A. Week 12

B. Week 16

C. Week 20

D. Week 26

E. Week 32

8. Which of the following antenatal measures might have prevented the condition?

A. Maternal administration of antibiotics

B. Maternal administration of progesterone

C. Maternal administration of corticosteroids

D. Maternal administration of surfactant

D. A and B

E. B and C

F. C and D

9. Which of the following is a common complication of using hyperbaric oxygen therapy to treat the affected neonate?

A. Left ventricular hypertrophy

B. Pulmonary hypertension

C. Renal failure

D. Retinopathy

E. Type I diabetes mellitus

10. During a routine antenatal checkup of a 26-year-old expecting mother, the sonologist finds that the fetal respiratory bronchioles have formed but the epithelium is still too thick for gaseous exchange. During which of the following weeks was the checkup most likely scheduled?

A. Weeks 3 to 5

B. Weeks 5 to 16

C. Weeks 16 to 26

D. Weeks 26 to 32

E. Weeks 32 to 40

Consider the following case for questions 11 to 12:

A 6-month-old infant is brought to the clinic for a 6-week history of noisy breathing that has worsened following an upper respiratory infection. On examination, the infant is afebrile, has a coarse wheezing, and does not appear distressed. Her symptoms did not improve with a week of bronchodilator therapy.

11. Which of the following is the most probable diagnosis for her?

A. Laryngomalacia

B. Tracheomalacia

C. Bronchiolitis

D. Bronchial asthma

E. Bronchogenic carcinoma

12. Which of the following is the source of the defective structure in her?

A. Ectoderm

B. Endoderm

C. Paraxial mesoderm

D. Intermediate mesoderm

E. Lateral plate mesoderm

Consider the following case for questions 13 to 14:

A 16-year-old girl presents with anosmia following an upper respiratory tract infection. Mucosal scraping from her upper airway reveals dysfunctional ciliated cells in an otherwise normal pseudostratified columnar epithelium that lacks goblet cells.

13. Which of the following is the source for the defective cells in her?

A. Ectoderm

B. Endoderm

C. Visceral mesoderm

D. Parietal mesoderm

E. Neural crest

14. Which of the following is the source for the mucosal specimen?

A. Paranasal sinus

B. Nasopharynx

C. Roof of the nasal cavity

D. Floor of the nasal cavity

E. Nasal vestibule

Consider the following case for questions 15 to 16:

An 8-week-old infant presents with a 3-week history of mild cough. He is currently afebrile and has no history of any recent episodes of chest infection. Physical examination was significant for mild tachypnea and wheezing. A chest X-ray showed an area of opacity behind the cardiac silhouette in the lower area of the left hemithorax. A CT scan of the thorax with intravenous contrast revealed a mass, within a separate pleural investment, with necrosis in the lower lobe of the left lung. It also revealed two separate aortic branches directed toward the pulmonary opacity. He subsequently underwent surgery, and the anomalous tissue was removed by mass excision. Histologic findings of the mass included uniformly dilated bronchioles, alveolar ducts, and alveoli.

15. Which of the following is the possible diagnosis?

A. Bronchogenic cyst

B. Intralobar pulmonary sequestration

C. Extralobar pulmonary sequestration

D. Bronchiolitis

E. Bronchogenic carcinoma

16. In which of the following weeks of gestation did this anomaly most probably occur?

A. Weeks 3 to 6

B. Weeks 7 to 17

C. Weeks 18 to 26

D. Weeks 24 to 32

E. Weeks 34 to 40

201

Chapter 25

Endocrine System Embryology

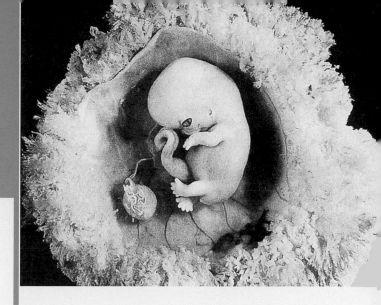

LEARNING OBJECTIVES

- ▶ Summarize the available precursors, sequence of events, and developmental mechanisms in the formation of the pituitary gland.
- ▶ Analyze the pathophysiology, clinical features, and diagnosis for remnants of Rathke's pouch (craniopharyngioma and Rathke's cleft cysts).
- ▶ Summarize the available precursors, sequence of events, and developmental mechanisms in the formation of the adrenal gland.
- ▶ Analyze the pathophysiology, clinical features, and diagnosis for pheochromocytoma.
- ▶ Summarize the available precursors, sequence of events, and developmental mechanisms in the formation of the thyroid gland.
- ▶ Analyze the pathophysiology, clinical features, and diagnosis for congenital hypothyroidism.
- ▶ Summarize the available precursors and illustrate the specialized developmental mechanisms in the formation of the thymus.
- ▶ Analyze the pathophysiology, clinical features, and diagnosis for DiGeorge's syndrome.
- ▶ Analyze the pathophysiology, clinical features, and diagnosis for thyroglossal cysts.
- ▶ Analyze the pathophysiology, clinical features, and diagnosis of congenital adrenal hyperplasia.

25.1 Questions

Easy	Medium	Hard

Consider the following case for questions 1 to 2:

A 39-year-old woman presents to the ER with a severe headache. She has had gradually worsening headaches for the past 3 months that were not relieved with over-the-counter medication. Her history reveals occasional blurring of vision, and amenorrhea for the past 5 months. Her physical examination reveals horizontal nystagmus. A brain MRI reveals a large cystic sellar mass.

1. Which of the following embryonic sources contributes for the mass that is responsible for the symptoms in the woman?

A. Surface ectoderm

B. Neuroectoderm

C. Neural crest cells

D. Endoderm

E. Mesoderm

2. Which of the following structures, irritated by the mass, might be the cause of such severe headache in the patient?

A. Falx cerebelli

B. Tentorium cerebelli

C. Dorsum sellae

D. Diaphragma sellae

E. Tuberculum sellae

3. A 1-year-old girl presents with hypotonia and decreased activity. She was the first child of a 24-year-old mother and was born at 42 gestational weeks. Her mother reports that she also suffers from lack of interest, poor appetite, sluggishness, oversleep, and constipation. Physical findings were significant for macroglossia and coarse facial features. Which of the following developmental processes might have been defective in the affected child?

A. Ectodermal evagination from the stomodeum

B. Endodermal invagination from foramen cecum

C. Ectodermal invagination from the oral cavity

D. Mesodermal distribution from occipital somites

E. Endodermal distribution within the third pharyngeal pouch

Consider the following case for questions 4 to 6:

A 6-year-old female child presents with facial flushing, palpitation, severe headache, and sweating. Most of her symptoms have occurred in paroxysms several times a week during the past 6 months. She also has lost significant weight over these months. Physical examination reveals moderate hypertension and tachycardia. The laboratory confirms an increase in plasma metanephrine.

4. Which of the following is the source for the pathologic cells in the child?

A. Ectoderm

B. Neuroectoderm

C. Endoderm

D. Neural crest

E. Mesoderm

5. Which of the following zones in the figure might lodge pathologic cells in the child?

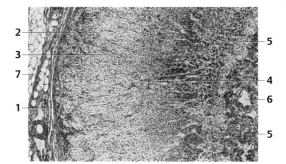

A. Zone 1

B. Zone 2

C. Zone 3

D. Zone 4

E. Zone 5

6. Which of the following arteries should be clamped during surgical removal of the pathologic organ?

A. Inferior phrenic

B. Celiac trunk

C. Lumbar arteries

C. Ovarian artery

D. Uterine artery

Consider the following case for questions 7 to 11:

A 3-week-old male infant presents with seizures and failure to thrive. On admission, he received packed red blood cells for anemia of unknown etiology and prophylactic antibiotics for possible sepsis. A chest X-ray revealed an enlarged heart. His echocardiogram confirmed persistence of truncus arteriosus and a large ventricular septal defect.

7. Which of the following germ layers might be the underlying cause of his defect?

A. Surface ectoderm

B. Neuroectoderm

C. Neural crest

D. Paraxial mesoderm

E. Endoderm

8. To make a diagnosis, fluorescence in situ hybridization (FISH) chromosomal analysis from the buccal mucosa was done. Which of the following is the expected finding?

A. Deletion of the short arm of chromosome 4

B. Deletion on the short arm of chromosome 5

C. Microdeletion on chromosome 15

D. Microdeletion on chromosome 17

E. Microdeletion on chromosome 22

9. Which of the following might be the underlying cause for sepsis in the infant?

A. Developmental defect involving the first pharyngeal pouch

B. Developmental defect involving the first pharyngeal pouch

C. Developmental defect involving the third pharyngeal pouch

D. Developmental defect involving the fourth pharyngeal pouch

E. Developmental defect involving both third and fourth pharyngeal pouches

10. Which of the following might be the underlying cause for seizures in the infant?

A. Developmental defect involving the first pharyngeal pouch

B. Developmental defect involving the second pharyngeal pouch

C. Developmental defect involving the third pharyngeal pouch

D. Developmental defect involving the fourth pharyngeal pouch

E. Developmental defect involving both third and fourth pharyngeal pouches

11. Which of the following might be an associated echocardiogram finding in the infant?

A. Atrial septal defect, ostium primum type

B. Atrial septal defect, ostium secundum type

C. Interrupted aortic arch

D. Ebstein's anomaly

E. Mitral stenosis

Consider the following case for questions 12 to 13:

A 4-year-old girl presents with visual disturbance and headache, which have progressed over a couple of months. Computed tomography (CT) and magnetic resonance imaging (MRI) of the brain revealed a suprasellar calcified cystic mass in the anterior part of the third cerebral ventricle.

12. Which of the following embryonic sources contributes for the mass that is primarily responsible for her symptoms?

A. Surface ectoderm

B. Neuroectoderm

C. Neural crest cells

D. Endoderm

E. Mesoderm

13. Which of the following vessels is the principal feeder for the cystic mass in the child?

A. Petrous segment of the internal carotid artery

B. Cavernous segment of the internal carotid artery

C. Supraclinoid segment of the internal carotid artery

D. Posterior cerebral artery

E. Vertebral artery

Consider the following case for questions 14 to 15:

A 9-year-old girl presents with an anterior midline neck mass that gradually appeared over 3 weeks. She has a history of an upper respiratory tract infection that occurred about a month ago and was successfully treated with antibiotics. A physical examination of the patient reveals a tender, smooth, hard, and well-demarcated mass that is localized above the thyroid gland. A computed tomography scan reveals a large, heterogeneous, enhancing soft tissue mass with a cystic component in the midline of the anterior neck space, extending from the base of the tongue to the superior extent of the thyroid gland. The mass is completely separated from the tongue muscles.

14. Which of the following is a true statement for her case?

A. These masses are usually symptomatic and necessitate prompt surgery.

B. These masses are always benign, and histopathology for an excised mass is unnecessary.

C. There is likely to be vertical movement of the mass on tongue protrusion.

D. She is likely to have elevated serum levels for thyroid hormones.

E. She is likely to have an elevated serum level for the thyroid-stimulating hormone.

15. Which of the following developmental processes might have been defective in her?

A. Ectodermal evagination from stomodeum

B. Endodermal invagination from foramen cecum

C. Ectodermal invagination from the oral cavity

D. Mesodermal distribution from occipital somites

E. Endodermal distribution within the third pharyngeal pouch

Consider the following case for questions 16 to 20:

A 2-week-old phenotypic female infant presents with lethargy, irritability, poor feeding, vomiting, and poor weight gain. On physical examination, the child had ambiguous genitalia with clitoral hypertrophy and labial hyperpigmentation. Laboratory investigations showed high levels of 17-hydroxyprogesterone.

16. Which of the following is the source for the pathological cells in the infant?

A. Ectoderm

B. Neuroectoderm

C. Endoderm

D. Neural crest

E. Mesoderm

17. To help with the diagnosis, a karyotype was ordered for the infant. Which of the following might be the genetic finding in her case?

A. 46, XX

B. 46, XY

C. 47, XXY

D. 47, XYY

E. 45, XO

18. To confirm the diagnosis, a serum hormonal assay was done for the infant. Which of the following is an expected finding in her case?

A. Increased glucocorticoid, decreased mineralocorticoid, increased adrenal androgen

B. Increased glucocorticoid, decreased mineralocorticoid, decreased adrenal androgen

C. Decreased glucocorticoid, decreased mineralocorticoid, increased adrenal androgen

D. Decreased glucocorticoid, decreased mineralocorticoid, decreased adrenal androgen

E. Increased glucocorticoid, increased mineralocorticoid, increased adrenal androgen

19. To establish a treatment plan, a measure of serum electrolyte levels for the infant is necessary. Which of the following is an expected finding in her case?

A. Increased sodium, increased potassium

B. Decreased sodium, decreased potassium

C. Increased sodium, decreased potassium

D. Decreased sodium, increased potassium

E. Decreased sodium, normal potassium

20. Which of the following zones might be involved with the electrolyte disturbances in the infant?

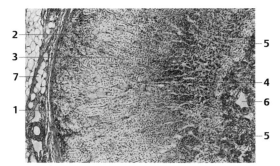

A. Zone 1

B. Zone 2

C. Zone 3

D. Zone 4

E. Zone 5

25.2 Answers and Explanations

| Easy | Medium | Hard |

1. Correct: Surface ectoderm (A)

The patient might be affected with Rathke's cleft cysts (RCCs). Rathke's pouch has an anterior and posterior wall in addition to a central embryonic cleft. The pars distalis and pars tuberalis of the anterior pituitary arise from the anterior wall, while the posterior wall develops into the pars intermedia. The central lumen becomes Rathke's cleft and normally regresses. However, this structure may persist and enlarge, resulting in the formation of a cyst. Extension of these cysts might lead to irritation of the adjacent meninges and cause headaches. Blurring of vision might be due to irritation of the optic chiasm by the cyst. Horizontal nystagmus might be due to pressure on the cavernous sinus with associated abducens nerve involvement. Hyperprolactinemia (due to compression of the pituitary stalk by RCCs that impairs dopamine transport to the anterior pituitary, or a commonly associated prolactin-secreting adenoma) presents with galactorrhea, amenorrhea, and hypogonadism.

Rathke's pouch is an epithelialized rostral invagination of the stomodeum (surface ectoderm).

2. Correct: Diaphragma sellae (D)

Diaphragma sellae is a fold of dura mater that covers the sella turcica and forms the roof of the hypophyseal fossa. An expanding pituitary mass is likely to irritate this structure and cause headaches.

Falx cerebelli (A) is a dural fold in the sagittal plane over the floor of the posterior cranial fossa. It partially separates the two cerebellar hemispheres.

Tentorium cerebelli (B) is a dural fold that is attached perpendicularly to falx cerebelli. It separates the cerebellum from the occipital lobe.

Tuberculum sellae (E) and dorsum sellae (C) are plates of bones (part of the sphenoid bone) that form the anterior and posterior boundaries of the hypophyseal fossa, respectively.

3. Correct: Endodermal invagination from foramen cecum (B)

The girl has classical signs and symptoms of congenital hypothyroidism and seems to have escaped an earlier diagnosis. A large number of these cases is due to thyroid dysgenesis (absent or hypoplastic thyroid gland). The thyroid gland develops as an endodermal outgrowth from foramen cecum, which is present in the floor of the primitive pharyngeal gut. It stays attached to the tongue via a thyroglossal duct till it reaches the adult final position.

The anterior lobe of the pituitary gland develops from an ectodermal evagination from the stomodeum (A). The parotid salivary gland develops from an ectodermal invagination from the oral cavity (C). Striated muscles of the tongue develop from occipital somites (D). Thymus and the inferior parathyroid glands develop from endoderm of the third pharyngeal pouch (E).

4. Correct: Neural crest (D)

The child is suffering from pheochromocytoma, which is a neoplasm of the chromaffin cells of the adrenal medulla. The paroxysms are related to sudden catecholamine discharge from the tumor. The sudden catecholamine excess causes hypertension, palpitations, tachycardia, chest pain, headache, anxiety, blanching, and excessive sweating. Weight loss is secondary to metabolic effects of excessive circulating catecholamines. These include an increase in basal metabolic rate, glycolysis, and glycogenolysis, leading to hyperglycemia and glycosuria. Pheochromocytoma is diagnosed by demonstrating abnormally high concentrations of catecholamines or their breakdown products in the plasma or urine. Increases in plasma metanephrine and normetanephrine concentrations are greater and more consistent than increases in plasma catecholamines or urinary metanephrines.

Chromaffin cells within the adrenal medulla derive from neural crest cells.

5. Correct: Zone 5 (E)

Adrenal medulla is represented by zone 5 in the image. Zones 1 (A), 2 (B), 3 (C), and 4 (D) represent the capsule, zona glomerulosa, zona fasciculata, and zona reticularis, respectively.

6. Correct: Inferior phrenic (A)

Adrenal glands are supplied from three arterial sources. Superior suprarenal is from the inferior phrenic, middle suprarenal is from the abdominal aorta, and inferior suprarenal is from the renal arteries.

7. Correct: Neural crest (C)

The infant is suffering from DiGeorge syndrome, which results in abnormal cephalic neural crest cell migration and defective development of the third and fourth pharyngeal pouches. Clinical characteristics include congenital heart defects, hypocalcemia, distinctive craniofacial features (micrognathia, hypertelorism, antimongoloid slant of the eyes, and ear malformations), renal anomalies, and thymic hypoplasia. Presentation usually results from cardiac failure or from hypocalcemia (seizures).

DiGeorge syndrome is developmentally related to neural crest migration anomalies. Their clinical features involve structures that develop from neural crest cells.

8. Correct: Microdeletion on chromosome 22 (E)

Microdeletion of chromosome 22q11.2 (Del22) is detectable in the majority of patients with DiGeorge syndrome. The diagnosis is confirmed via fluorescence in situ hybridization (FISH).

9. Correct: Developmental defect involving the third pharyngeal pouch (C)

The immunodeficiency in Del22 syndrome is due to poor formation of thymic tissue and impaired production of T cells. Thymus develops from the third pharyngeal pouch.

10. Correct: Developmental defect involving both third and fourth pharyngeal pouches (E)

Neonatal hypocalcemia is recognized in most of the children with Del22. Hypocalcemia may cause tremors, seizures, and arrhythmia. This symptom is related to hypoparathyroidism due to the absence or underdevelopment of parathyroid glands, which leads to low blood calcium levels. The superior (from the 4th) and inferior (from the 3rd) parathyroid glands develop from pharyngeal pouches.

11. Correct: Interrupted aortic arch (C)

Del22 is particularly common in patients with interrupted aortic arch, type B. In these cases, the infundibular septum is often hypoplastic or absent and is deviated posteriorly and to the left.

The atrial septum (**A, B**) has no contributions from the neural crest. Ebstein's anomaly (**D**) results from a defective tricuspid valve and an accompanying atrial septal defect. Atrioventricular (tricuspid and mitral, **E**) valves are formed from endocardial cushions that have no contribution from the neural crest.

12. Correct: Surface ectoderm (A)

The child may have been affected by craniopharyngioma. This is a benign, suprasellar, calcified, cystic mass that arises near the pituitary stalk, commonly extending into the suprasellar cistern. More than half of all patients present before the age of 20, usually with signs of raised intracranial pressure (headache, vomiting, papilledema, and hydrocephalus). Associated symptoms might include visual field abnormalities, cranial nerve involvement, and weight gain (related to hypothyroidism). Hypopituitarism can be documented in ~ 90%. The radiologic hallmark of a craniopharyngioma is the appearance of a suprasellar calcified cyst.

Craniopharyngiomas are derived from Rathke's pouch, which is an epithelialized rostral invagination of the stomodeum (surface ectoderm).

13. Correct: Supraclinoid segment of the internal carotid artery (C)

Adenohypophysis is principally supplied by the superior hypophyseal vessels, which are given off from the supraclinoid segment of the internal carotid artery (from its penetration of dura to its bifurcation into anterior and middle cerebral arteries).

The petrous segment of the internal carotid artery (**A**) ascends in the carotid canal. Branches off it are the caroticotympanic (enters tympanic cavity) and pterygoid (enters pterygoid canal) arteries.

The inferior hypophyseal arteries are off the cavernous segment of the internal carotid artery (**B**, passes through cavernous sinus). These principally supply the pars nervosa of the neurohypophysis.

The posterior cerebral (**D**) and vertebral (**E**) arteries do not provide branches to the anterior pituitary.

14. Correct: There is likely to be vertical movement of the mass on tongue protrusion. (C)

The girl is suffering, most probably, from an infected thyroglossal cyst consequent to an upper respiratory tract infection. These cysts present most frequently in the midline of the neck, either at or just below the level of the hyoid bone.

A pathognomonic sign on physical examination is vertical motion of the mass with swallowing and tongue protrusion, demonstrating the intimate relation to the hyoid bone. These generally are asymptomatic (**A**) unless secondarily infected, or affected by carcinomatous changes. Thyroid carcinomas can occur (papillary thyroid carcinoma commonly) in a small percentage of thyroglossal duct cysts (**B**), and all excised cysts and tracts should undergo careful histologic examination. These cysts rarely complicate thyroid function, so thyroid and thyroid-stimulating hormones are usually within normal limits (**D, E**).

15. Correct: Endodermal invagination from foramen cecum (B)

The primitive thyroid gland originates as an endodermal invagination from the foramen cecum, which is present in the floor of the pharyngeal gut during the 3rd week of gestation. The gland then descends in front of the pharynx as a bilobed diverticulum that is initially patent. It reaches its final position in the neck by the 7th week of the gestation. During migration it is connected to the tongue by a narrow tubular structure—the thyroglossal duct. The duct usually disappears by the 10th week of gestation. Persistence of any portion of this duct and secretion from its lining epithelium may give rise to the cystic lesion.

The anterior lobe of the pituitary gland develops from an ectodermal evagination from stomodeum (**A**). The parotid salivary gland develops from an ectodermal invagination from the oral cavity (**C**). Striated muscles of the tongue develop from occipital somites (**D**). Thymus and the inferior parathyroid glands develop from endoderm of the third pharyngeal pouch (**E**).

16. Correct: Mesoderm (E)

The infant is suffering from congenital adrenal hyperplasia (CAH), salt-wasting type. This typically manifests as an acute crisis in the second week of life. Symptoms are vague and include lethargy, irritability, poor feeding, vomiting, and poor weight gain. More than 90% of cases are due to deficiency of the enzyme 21β-hydroxylase, which is encoded by the gene *CYP21A2*. Impaired *CYP21A2* activity causes deficient production of both cortisol and aldosterone. The low serum cortisol stimulates adrenocorticotropic hormone (ACTH) production; adrenal hyperplasia occurs, and precursor steroids—in particular 17-hydroxyprogesterone—accumulate. The accumulated precursors cannot enter the cortisol synthesis pathway and thus spill over into the androgen synthesis pathway, forming androstenedione and dehydroepiandrosterone (DHEA). Prenatal exposure to excessive androgens results in masculinization of the female fetus, leading to ambiguous genitalia at birth. Increased pigmentation, especially of the labia majora and nipples, is common with excessive ACTH secretion.

Adrenal cortical cells are pathological in the infant, and these develop from intermediate mesoderm.

17. Correct: 46, XX (A)

Androgen excess is present in all patients with CAH and manifests with broad phenotypic variability, including severe virilization of the external genitalia in neonatal girls. However, the genotype of this infant is that of a normal female (46, XX).

18. Correct: Decreased glucocorticoid, decreased mineralocorticoid, increased adrenal androgen (C)

21-Hydroxylase deficiency disrupts glucocorticoid and mineralocorticoid synthesis, resulting in diminished negative feedback via the hypothalamus-pituitary axis. This leads to increased pituitary ACTH release, which drives increased synthesis of adrenal androgen precursors and subsequent androgen excess.

19. Correct: Decreased sodium, increased potassium (D)

The classic electrolyte abnormalities in salt-wasting congenital adrenal hyperplasia are hyponatremia and hyperkalemia. This is due to deficiency of aldosterone, which leads to natriuresis and consequent potassium retention in the patient.

20. Correct: Zone 2 (B)

As stated earlier, electrolyte abnormalities in this patient are due to aldosterone deficiency. Aldosterone is secreted by the zona glomerulosa cells (zone 2). The capsule (**A**, zone 1), zona fasciculata (**C**, zone 3), zona reticularis (**D**, zone 4), and adrenal medulla (**E**, zone 5) do not synthesize aldosterone.

Chapter 26

Genitourinary System Embryology

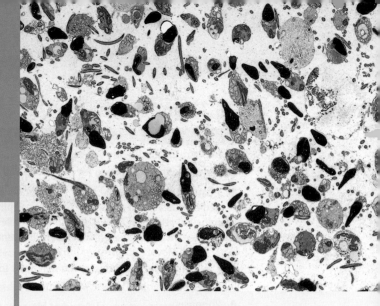

LEARNING OBJECTIVES

- ▶ Analyze the etiology, clinical features, and diagnosis of hypospadias.
- ▶ Analyze the etiology, clinical features, and diagnosis of androgen insensitivity syndrome.
- ▶ Analyze the etiology, clinical features, and diagnosis for Potter's sequence.
- ▶ Analyze the etiology, clinical features, and diagnosis for exstrophy–epispadias complex.
- ▶ Analyze the etiology, clinical features, and diagnosis of 5-α reductase deficiency.
- ▶ Describe the derivatives of the mesonephric duct in the adult human.
- ▶ Analyze the etiology, clinical features, and diagnosis of hydrocele.
- ▶ Analyze the etiology, clinical features, and diagnosis of müllerian agenesis.

Consider the following case for questions 16 to 17:

A 3-month-old boy presents with right-sided scrotal swelling. According to his parents, the bulge has not changed in size since birth and there has been no noticeable discomfort. Physical exam reveals a noncompressible, nonfluctuant, and nontender right scrotal mass that brilliantly transilluminates. No inguinal or abdominal masses are appreciated on palpation. An ultrasound reveals an anechoic mass along the spermatic cord, separated from the testis and the epididymis.

16. Which of the following is the diagnosis for the infant?

A. Inguinal hernia

B. Communicating hydrocele

C. Noncommunicating hydrocele

D. Varicocele

E. Spermatocele

17. Which of the following might be the underlying defect in the infant?

A. Complete patency of the processus vaginalis

B. Partial patency of the processus vaginalis

C. Congenital dilatation of the testicular veins

D. Congenital obstruction of the epididymal ducts

E. Congenital absence of vas deferens

Consider the following case for questions 18 to 20:

A 16-year-old girl presents with primary amenorrhea. A physical examination reveals age appropriate growth of external genitalia, axillary and pubic hair, and breasts. A pelvic ultrasound failed to locate the uterus or the uterine tube, but could identify normally placed bilateral ovaries.

18. Which of the following might be responsible for the primary amenorrhea in the patient?

A. 17-α hydroxylase deficiency

B. 5-α reductase deficiency

C. Monosomy of X chromosome

D. Müllerian agenesis

E. Mutation in the androgen receptor gene

19. Which of the following is the expected genotype for the patient?

A. 45, X

B. 46, XY

C. 46, XX

D. 47, XXY

E. 47, XYY

20. Which of the following might be an associated finding in this patient?

A. Decreased serum follicle-stimulating hormone levels

B. Decreased serum luteinizing hormone levels

C. Decreased serum estrogen levels

D. Increased serum estrogen levels

E. Renal abnormalities

26.2 Answers and Explanations

Easy	Medium	Hard

1. Correct: Hypospadias (B)

The neonate is suffering from hypospadias.

In hypospadias, the urethral meatus is located on the ventral surface of the penis. It is often associated with ventral curvature of the penis, a condition called chordee. Although newborns and young children seldom have symptoms related to hypospadias, older children and adults may complain of difficulty directing the urinary stream and stream spraying. Chordee can prevent sexual intercourse.

Phimosis (**A**) is a condition in which the contracted foreskin cannot be retracted over the glans. Chronic infection from poor local hygiene is its most common cause.

Epispadias (**C**) is a developmental anomaly in which the urethral meatus is on the dorsal side of the penis.

Exstrophy of the bladder (**D**) occurs with a complete ventral defect of the urogenital sinus and the overlying skeletal system. The posterior wall of the bladder is exteriorized due to nonclosure of the ventral body and bladder walls. Urine is seen to trickle from the upper lateral corners (ureteric orifices) of the mass.

Cloacal exstrophy (**E**) includes the triad of omphalocele, bladder exstrophy, and imperforate anus. It is a more severe defect—nonfusion of the ventral body wall is accompanied by an improper growth of the urorectal septum. Therefore, the entire cloaca is exteriorized, both urine and fecal matter are discharged through the protruding mass.

2. Correct: Failure of fusion of cloacal folds (C)

By the end of 6 weeks, the urorectal septum has separated the hindgut and urogenital sinus portions of the cloaca, such that the cloacal folds are divided into urethral folds anteriorly and anal folds posteriorly. The urethra is formed by the fusion of the urethral folds along the ventral surface of the penis, which extends to the corona on the distal shaft. The glandular urethra is formed by canalization of an ectodermal cord that has grown through the glans to communicate with the fused urethral folds. Hypospadias results when fusion of the urethral folds is incomplete.

Failure of obliteration of allantois (**A**) results in an urachal fistula in which urine dribbles through the umbilicus. Failure of formation of the ventral wall of the urogenital sinus (**B**) accompanied by failure of fusion of the ventral body wall (**E**) can lead to bladder exstrophy. In males, genital swellings (**D**) eventually fuse to form the scrotum, and the line of fusion forms the scrotal raphe.

3.　Correct: Cryptorchidism (D)

Hypospadias in the male is evidence of feminization. Because urethral development occurs under the influence of dihydrotestosterone (which is converted in peripheral tissue from testosterone by 5-α-reductase), the development of hypospadias can be related either to a reduction in 5-α-reductase activity, to a lack of testosterone production, or to failure of the local receptors to recognize the hormone. An undescended testis is a common association with hypospadias.

Discharge of fecal matter through the umbilicus (**A**) occurs due to nonobliteration of the vitelline duct. Discharge of urine through the umbilicus (**B**) occurs due to nonobliteration of the urachus (allantois). Rectourethral fistula (**C**) occurs due to defective formation of the urorectal septum. Penile enlargement (**E**) is a sign of androgen excess in males, not deficiency.

4.　Correct: Androgen insensitivity syndrome (C)

The patient is suffering from complete androgen insensitivity syndrome (CAIS). It is caused by mutations in the androgen receptor (AR) gene, abolishing the target cells' responses to testosterone (T) and dihydrotestosterone (DHT). The syndrome is characterized by bilateral testes [dependent on testis-determining factor or sex-determining region Y (SRY) protein encoded by the *SRY* gene], absent or hypoplastic wolffian ducts (dependent on T), female-appearing external genitalia and a blind vaginal pouch (secondary sexual characteristics primarily dependent on DHT), and absent müllerian derivatives (dependent on müllerian inhibiting factor). At puberty, female secondary sexual characteristics develop, but menarche does not ensue. Pubic and axillary hair is usually sparse or absent. Breast development is normal due to aromatization of excess testosterone into estrogen.

Congenital adrenal hyperplasia (**A**) is highly unlikely with normal serum cortisol, aldosterone, and electrolyte levels. One of its variants, 17-α hydroxylase deficiency, can have a very similar presentation but will have accompanying hypertension and hypokalemia.

Turner's syndrome (**B**) will fail to explain the presence of testes.

Klinefelter's syndrome (**D**) will fail to explain the absence of wolffian duct structures (epididymis, vas deferens, and seminal vesicles).

Müllerian agenesis (**E**) will fail to explain the absence of ovaries.

5.　Correct: Mutation in androgen receptor gene (E)

CAIS is caused by mutations in the androgen receptor (AR) gene, abolishing the target cells' responses to testosterone (T) and dihydrotestosterone (DHT).

A defect in 17α-hydroxylation (**A**) in the zona fasciculata of the adrenal and in the gonads results in impaired synthesis of 17–hydroxyprogesterone and 17-hydroxypregnenolone and, consequently, cortisol and sex steroids. The secretion of large amounts of corticosterone and deoxycorticosterone leads to hypertension, hypokalemia, and alkalosis. Affected 46, XY individuals present with female genitalia with a blind vaginal pouch or hypoplastic male genitalia. Müllerian structures are absent. Wolffian structures are hypoplastic.

5-α reductase deficiency (**B**) causes defective conversion of T to DHT. This results, in the most severely affected individuals, ambiguous external genitalia that are characterized by a small hypospadiac phallus bound down in chordee, a bifid scrotum, and a urogenital sinus that opens onto the perineum. A blind vaginal pouch is present, opening either into a urogenital sinus or directly into the urethra. Normal development of testes and wolffian duct structures (epididymis, vas deferens, and seminal vesicle), due to normal T levels, is characteristic.

Turner's syndrome (**C**, monosomy of X chromosome) leads to hypoplastic external and internal female genital organs (streak ovaries and uterus) responsible for poorly developed secondary sexual characteristics. An ultrasound will not reveal the presence of testes.

Klinefelter's syndrome (**D**, an extra X chromosome) is characterized by small undescended testes, relatively reduced penile length, gynecomastia, diminished facial and body hair, hypotonia, and disproportionately long legs. Absence of wolffian duct structures precludes its possibility.

6.　Correct: 46, XY (D)

Genotype in androgen insensitivity syndrome is that of a normal male, i.e., 46, XY.

As noted previously, 45, X (**A**, Turner's syndrome) and 47, XXY (**B**, Klinefelter's syndrome) do not present with features of this patient.

47, XYY (**C**, Jacob's syndrome) or 46, XX (**E**, normal female or müllerian agenesis) karyotypes are not associated with androgen insensitivity syndrome.

7. Correct: Increased serum luteinizing hormone (LH) levels (D)

At puberty, in patients with CAIS, androgen resistance results in augmented LH secretion with an increase in T secretion (**A**) and estradiol production (**C**) due to a lack of T feedback on the hypothalamus. Estradiol arises mainly from peripheral conversion (aromatization) of T and androstenedione as well as from direct secretion by the testes. FSH levels are normal (**E**) because of estradiol feedback. Enzymatic conversion of T to DHT is not impaired (**B**) in this syndrome.

8. Correct: Oligohydramnios (C)

The newborn had suffered from Potter's sequence (syndrome). It predominantly affects male babies and is accompanied by severe oligohydramnios due to polycystic kidneys, bilateral renal agenesis, or obstructive uropathy during the middle gestational weeks. Renal failure is the main defect in Potter's sequence and the primary cause of death-in-utero. Other characteristic features include premature birth, breech presentation, atypical facial appearance, and limb malformations. Severe respiratory insufficiency due to pulmonary hypoplasia leads to a fatal outcome in most newborns.

Fetal urine is critical for the proper development of the lungs by aiding in the expansion of the airways by means of hydrodynamic pressure and by also supplying a critical amino acid (proline) for lung development. It also serves to cushion the fetus from being compressed by the mother's uterus as it grows. Oligohydramnios is the cause of the typical facial appearance of the fetus and fatal pulmonary hypoplasia in the fetus.

Breech presentation (**B**) is a consequence of oligohydramnios and not a cause for the defects. Advanced maternal age (**A**), defective migration of neural crest cells (**E**), or polyhydramnios (**D**) is not associated with Potter's sequence.

9. Correct: Mesonephric duct (B)

Mesonephric ducts persist in the male and, under the stimulatory influence of testosterone, differentiate into internal genital ducts (epididymis, ductus deferens, and ejaculatory ducts). The ureteric bud, which is a diverticulum off the mesonephric duct, induces the metanephric blastema (definitive kidney). Bilateral renal agenesis is mostly due to faulty induction by the ureteric bud.

Embryologically, the allantois (**A**, diverticulum of the yolk sac) connects the urogenital sinus with the umbilicus. Normally, the allantois is obliterated and is represented by a fibrous cord (urachus) extending from the dome of the bladder to the umbilicus. The paramesonephric duct (**C**) forms the internal genital tracts (uterine tubes, uterus, and vagina) in females. The primitive urogenital sinus (**D**), developed from endoderm, gives rise to the urinary bladder, urethra, and the paraurethral glands. The urorectal septum (**E**) divides the endodermal cloaca into an anterior urogenital sinus and a posterior anorectal canal of the hindgut.

10. Correct: A and B (D)

The newborn has presented at birth with a genitourinary defect consistent with the classic bladder exstrophy variant of the exstrophy–epispadias complex (EEC). Bladder exstrophy is characterized by an infraumbilical abdominal wall defect, incomplete closure of the bladder with mucosa continuous with the abdominal wall, epispadias, and alterations in the pelvic bones and muscles. It is part of the EEC, with cloacal exstrophy on the severe and isolated epispadias on the mild ends of the spectrum.

The mass is an exposed and everted urinary bladder (**B**); the dorsally opened plate that ran from the bladder neck down to the open glans is the epispadiac urethra (**A**). A normally developed anus precludes the diagnosis of cloacal exstrophy (**C, E,** and **F**), which results in exteriorization of the entire cloaca due to an accompanying defect in separation of urogenital sinus (anterior) from the anorectal canal (posterior).

11. Correct: Defective midline migration of mesenchymal tissue (B)

In EEC, overgrowth of the cloacal membrane prevents medial migration of the mesenchymal tissue. This prevents fusion of midline structures below the umbilicus. Depending on the extent of the abdominal wall defect, the cloacal membrane ruptures prematurely, resulting in the spectrum of the exstrophy–epispadias complex. Classic bladder exstrophy results if rupture occurs after the separation of the genitourinary and gastrointestinal tracts.

Cloacal exstrophy occurs if rupture occurs before separation of the genitourinary and gastrointestinal tracts by the urorectal septum (**C, D,** and **E**). Defective migration of neural crest cells (**A, D**) is not related to EEC.

12. Correct: 5-α reductase deficiency (B)

The patient is suffering from 5-α reductase enzyme deficiency. The defect lies in conversion of testosterone (T) to dihydrotestosterone (DHT) in androgen-sensitive tissues including the prostate, seminal vesicle, and external genitalia. This results in normal development of the testes and wolffian duct structures (epididymis, vas deferens, and seminal vesicle) due to normal levels of T, but ambiguous external genitalia (secondary sexual characteristics primarily dependent on DHT).

A defect in 17α-hydroxylation (**A**) in the zona fasciculata of the adrenal and in the gonads results in impaired synthesis of 17–hydroxyprogesterone and 17-hydroxypregnenolone and, consequently, cortisol and sex steroids. The secretion of large amounts of corticosterone and deoxycorticosterone leads to hypertension, hypokalemia, and alkalosis. Affected 46, XY individuals present with female genitalia with a blind vaginal pouch or hypoplastic male genitalia. Müllerian structures are absent. Wolffian structures (epididymis, vas deferens, and seminal vesicle) are hypoplastic or absent.

Turner's syndrome (**C**, 45, X) leads to hypoplastic external and internal female genital organs (streak ovaries and uterus) responsible for poorly developed secondary sexual characteristics.

Klinefelter syndrome (**D**, 47, XXY) is characterized by small undescended testes, relatively reduced penile length, gynecomastia, diminished facial and body hair, hypotonia, and disproportionately long legs.

Androgen insensitivity syndrome (**E**) results from mutation in the androgen receptor gene. This abolishes the target cells' response to testosterone and dihydrotestosterone. The syndrome is characterized by bilateral testes [*SRY* (sex-determining region of Y) dependent], absent or hypoplastic wolffian ducts (T dependent), female-appearing external genitalia, and a blind vaginal pouch.

13. Correct: Increased serum testosterone-to-dihydrotestosterone ratio (C)

Elevated serum T-to-DHT ratio is the hallmark of 5-α-reductase deficiency. Typically, T levels are normal to mildly elevated (**A**, **D**, and **E**) and DHT levels are low to undetectable (**B** and **D**).

14. Correct: Major urinary calyces (B)

Mesonephric ducts persist in the male and, under the stimulatory influence of testosterone, differentiate into internal genital ducts (epididymis, ductus deferens, and ejaculatory ducts). The ureteric bud, which is a diverticulum off the mesonephric duct, induces the metanephric blastema (definitive kidney).

The ureteric bud gives rise to the collecting and the papillary ducts, minor and the major calyces, renal pelvis, and the ureter.

Distal convoluted tubules (**A**) derive from the metanephric blastema. The urinary bladder (**C**) and the urethra (**D**) derive from endoderm of the urogenital sinus. Navicular fossa of the urethra (**E**) develops from an ectodermal invagination.

15. Correct: Prostate gland (D)

The prostate gland is derived from an endodermal outgrowth from the prostatic urethra, which itself is a derivative from the urogenital sinus (endoderm). The rest of the listed structures of the male internal genital organs are derived from the mesonephric duct.

16. Correct: Noncommunicating hydrocele (C)

The infant is suffering from a noncommunicating hydrocele (hydrocele of the cord).

A hydrocele is a collection of peritoneal fluid between the parietal and visceral layers of the tunica vaginalis surrounding the testicle. This occurs when the processus vaginalis obliterates proximally and distally but remains patent in the middle.

Inguinal hernias (**A**) and communicating hydroceles (**B**) increase in size with increased intraabdominal pressure (activity, crying or straining). Also, both of these are compressible (that is, they decrease in size with pressure), and inguinal hernia does not transilluminate.

A varicocele (**D**) is an abnormal tortuosity and dilation of the pampiniform venous plexus and internal spermatic vein. This, also, will not transilluminate.

Spermatocele (**E**) is a retention cyst of a tubule of the rete testis or the head of the epididymis. The cyst is distended with a milky fluid that contains sperm. Located at the superior pole of the testis and caput epididymis, the spermatocele is soft and fluctuant and can be transilluminated. At sonographic examination, spermatoceles are well-defined epididymal hypoechoic lesions.

17. Correct: Partial patency of the processus vaginalis (B)

Noncommunicating hydrocele occurs due to partial patency of the processus vaginalis, when it obliterates proximally and distally but remains patent in the middle.

Complete patency of the processus vaginalis (**A**) will result in a communicating hydrocele and might lead to, if large enough, herniation of abdominal contents through it (indirect inguinal hernia). Dilatation of testicular veins (**C**) causes varicocele. Both congenital obstruction of epididymal ducts (**D**) and congenital absence of vas deferens (**E**) will result in spermatocele.

18. Correct: Müllerian agenesis (D)

Müllerian agenesis (Mayer-Rokitansky-Kuster-Hauser syndrome) results in congenital absence of structures developed from the paramesonephric (müllerian) duct (uterine tubes, uterus, and upper vagina). These individuals have normal ovarian development, normal endocrine function, and normal female sexual development.

A defect in 17α-hydroxylation (**A**) in the zona fasciculata of the adrenal and in the gonads results in impaired synthesis of 17-hydroxyprogesterone and 17-hydroxypregnenolone and, consequently, cortisol and sex steroids. The secretion of large amounts of corticosterone and deoxycorticosterone leads to hypertension, hypokalemia, and alkalosis. Affected

46, XY individuals present with female genitalia with a blind vaginal pouch or hypoplastic male genitalia. Müllerian structures are absent; wolffian structures are hypoplastic. Affected 46, XX females have normal development of the internal genital ducts and external genitalia.

5-α reductase deficiency (**B**) causes defective conversion of testosterone (T) to dihydrotestosterone (DHT). This results, in the most severely affected individuals, in ambiguous external genitalia that are characterized by a small hypospadiac phallus bound down in chordee, a bifid scrotum, and a urogenital sinus that opens onto the perineum. A blind vaginal pouch is present, opening either into a urogenital sinus or directly into the urethra. Normal development of testes and well-differentiated wolffian duct structures (epididymis, vas deferens, and seminal vesicle) are characteristic.

Turner's syndrome (**C**, monosomy of X chromosome) leads to hypoplastic external and internal female genital organs (streak ovaries and uterus) responsible for poorly developed secondary sexual characteristics.

Androgen insensitivity syndrome (**E**) results from mutation in the androgen receptor gene. This abolishes the target cells' response to testosterone and dihydrotestosterone. The syndrome is characterized by bilateral testes [*SRY* (sex-determining region of Y) dependent], absent or hypoplastic wolffian ducts (T dependent), female-appearing external genitalia and a blind vaginal pouch (DHT dependent), and absent müllerian derivatives (müllerian inhibiting factor dependent).

19.   Correct: 46, XX (C)

Individuals with müllerian agenesis have normal female (46, XX) karyotype. 45, X (**A**, Turner's syndrome), 46, XY (**B**, normal male or androgen insensitivity syndrome), 47, XXY (**D**, Klinefelter's syndrome), and 47, XYY (**E**, Jacob's syndrome) karyotypes are not associated with müllerian agenesis.

20.   Correct: Renal abnormalities (E)

Given the common developmental source for the paramesonephric ducts and the kidneys (intermediate mesoderm), renal abnormalities would be commonly expected in these patients. As a matter of fact, ~ 50% of patients with müllerian agenesis present with associated defects involving the urinary tract.

Individuals with müllerian agenesis typically have normal ovaries and ovarian function (**C, D**); thus, they develop normal secondary sexual attributes. Circulating levels of luteinizing hormone (**B**) and follicle-stimulating hormone (**A**) are normal, indicating appropriate ovarian function.

Chapter 27

Placenta and Fetal Circulation

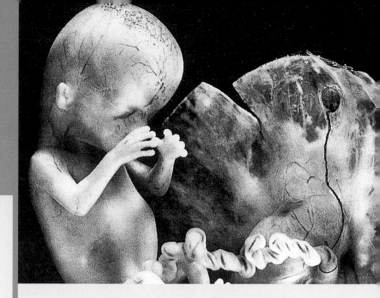

LEARNING OBJECTIVES

- ▶ Analyze the pathophysiology, clinical presentation, and diagnosis of spontaneous (and its types including threatened, incomplete or inevitable, complete, and missed) and septic abortion.

- ▶ Describe the development of placental structures during pregnancy.

- ▶ Differentiate between fetal and newborn circulation; predict changes in oxygenation as a result of birth.

- ▶ Analyze pathogenesis, clinical presentation, diagnosis, and complications of placenta previa.

- ▶ Contrast between oligohydramnios and polyhydramnios; describe possible causes and clinical outcomes for these.

- ▶ Analyze pathogenesis, clinical presentation, diagnosis, and complications of erythroblastosis fetalis.

- ▶ Analyze pathogenesis, clinical presentation, diagnosis, and complications of abruptio placentae.

- ▶ Identify primary embryonic venous channels entering the primitive heart tube and trace these to their adult derivatives.

- ▶ Define the uteroplacental and fetoplacental circulation during embryonic and fetal development.

- ▶ Describe the role of amniocentesis as a tool for assessing embryonic and fetal health.

- ▶ Describe various mechanisms of twinning in the human.

- ▶ Analyze the development of decidual structures essential for hemochorial placentation during embryonic and fetal growth.

- ▶ Describe the role of placental membrane (barrier) in establishment of selective transplacental transport.

27.1 Questions

Easy	Medium	Hard

Consider the following case for questions 1 to 2:

A 5-weeks-pregnant 32-year-old woman presents to your clinic with vaginal bleeding and abdominal cramping. Three days prior to admission, she had experienced crampy abdominal pain located in the hypogastric area with a pain scale of 7 out of 10. Physical examination reveals pale conjunctiva, slightly increased pulse rate, and normal blood pressure, temperature, and respiratory rate. Pelvic examination reveals tissue segments accompanying vaginal bleeding, placental fragments within the uterine cavity, and a dilated cervical os. The expelled tissue segments are examined for chorionic villi.

1. Which of the following is the diagnosis for the pregnant woman?

A. Threatened abortion

B. Incomplete abortion

C. Complete abortion

D. Missed abortion

E. Septic abortion

2. Which of the following findings should be consistent with the chorionic villi?

A. Cytotrophoblastic core surrounded by syncytiotrophoblast

B. Cytotrophoblastic and syncytiotrophoblastic shell

C. Extraembryonic somatic mesodermal core

D. Blood vessels in the core

E. A and D

F. B and D

G. B, C, and D

H. C and D

Consider the following case for questions 3 to 5:

A female neonate, born at 42 weeks' gestation, was admitted within the first few hours after birth with respiratory distress. Bilateral pneumothorax were diagnosed and treated with needle aspiration followed by chest tube placement. There was no significant improvement in the respiratory status, and ventilator support was initiated. She was eventually diagnosed with persistent pulmonary hypertension of the newborn, and the attending physician explained to her parents how their daughter failed the transition from fetal to adult circulation.

3. Within fetal circulation, which of the following structures carries blood with the lowest oxygen saturation?

A. Right atrium

B. Left atrium

C. Umbilical vein

D. Inferior vena cava, proximal segment

E. Inferior vena cava, distal segment

F. Descending aorta

4. Within fetal circulation, which of the following structures carries blood with the highest oxygen saturation?

A. Right atrium

B. Inferior vena cava, proximal segment

C. Inferior vena cava, distal segment

D. Ductus venosus

E. Ductus arteriosus

F. Descending aorta

5. During fetal life, oxygenated blood is shunted away from the less functional liver and lungs to more important organs such as the brain. Which of the following structure(s) is/are responsible for this important function?

A. Ductus venosus

B. Ductus arteriosus

C. Foramen ovale

D. A and B

E. B and C

F. A and C

G. A, B, and C

6. A 26-year-old pregnant woman experiences repeated episodes of bright red vaginal bleeding during the third trimester of her pregnancy. The bleeding, mostly painless, spontaneously subsides each time. An ultrasound shows that the placenta is located in the lower uterus, almost covering the internal os. Which of the following might be an associated finding in her case?

A. Uterine enlargement greater than expected for gestational age

B. Abnormally elevated human chorionic gonadotropin level

C. Previous pregnancy delivered by caesarean section

D. Accessory placental lobes

E. A retroplacental clot

7. Ultrasound examination of a 39-year-old pregnant woman, during her routine 2nd-trimester checkup, reveals fetal growth retardation consequent to severe oligohydramnios. Which of the following abnormalities might you expect in her unborn child?

A. Renal agenesis

B. Anencephaly

C. Diaphragmatic hernia

D. Esophageal atresia

E. Duodenal atresia

8. A first-time pregnant 26-year-old woman is found to be Rh negative, while her husband is Rh positive. Which of the following would be the most reasonable approach at this point?

A. Nothing is really required because it is uncertain if the fetus will be Rh positive.

B. Nothing is really required because IgG doesn't cross placental barrier.

C. Nothing is really required because this is her first pregnancy.

D. Injecting anti-D antibody into her during this pregnancy

E. Excess folic acid in her diet

9. A 21-year-old pregnant woman presents with sudden painless vaginal bleeding during the early third trimester. A diagnosis of placenta previa was made. Which of the following embryonic components contribute to the development of the placenta?

A. Embryoblast

B. Trophoblast

C. Hypoblast

D. Amnioblast

E. Notochord

10. A 36-year-old woman presents in her third trimester with vaginal bleeding, abdominal pain, uterine contractions, and fetal distress. An ultrasound reveals a retroplacental clot, suggesting a premature separation of the placenta. Which of the following might be an associated finding in her case?

A. Uterine enlargement greater than expected for gestational age

B. Abnormally elevated human chorionic gonadotropin level

C. Low-lying placenta partially covering the internal os

D. Hypertension

E. Accessory placental lobes

11. A female neonate was diagnosed with portal hypertension, due to abnormality in formation of the hepatic portal vein. Her mother recalls having suffered from a viral infection during the late third week of her pregnancy. Which of the following fetal blood vessels might have been affected by the virus?

A. Left umbilical vein

B. Right umbilical vein

C. Vitelline vein

D. Right anterior cardinal vein

E. Right posterior cardinal vein

Consider the following case for questions 12 to 13:

A male neonate, born to a 36-year-old mother, presents with an absent right thumb and a hypoplastic left thumb. History reveals that her mother was on an antidepressant that she had taken until late in the 4th week of the pregnancy. The OB/GYN resident explains to the mother how that might account for the underlying problem in her child.

12. While the placental barrier is essential to prevent transport of toxic substances, it eventually thins out to facilitate gas exchange. Which of the following is/are component(s) of the mature placental barrier?

A. Cytotrophoblast

B. Syncytiotrophoblast

C. Endothelial lining of fetal capillaries

D. Basement membrane of fetal capillaries

E. A and C

F. A, C, and D

G. B and C

H. B, C, and D

13. The intervillous space of the placenta is an important site within the uteroplacental circulation. Which of the following might be found in this space?

A. Maternal blood

B. Fetal blood

C. Amniotic fluid

D. Oxygen, carbon dioxide, and electrolytes

E. A and D

F. B and D

G. C and D

14. A second-time-pregnant 35-year-old woman comes to your clinic for a regular antenatal checkup. She reports that her first child was born with chromosomal abnormalities. You discuss the option of amniocentesis for her. Which of the following is true regarding the procedure?

A. It is routinely done during the 6th to 8th week of pregnancy.

B. Results of fetal karyotype can be obtained on the same day of the procedure.

C. Risk associated with the procedure is less than that of chorionic villus sampling.

D. Chances of diagnosing neural tube defects with amniocentesis is very low.

E. Ultrasound is contraindicated for being used simultaneously with amniocentesis.

15. A 25-year-old woman comes to the physician because of a positive result on her home pregnancy test. She has a history of twins in her family. A transvaginal ultrasound confirms that the embryo (formed from a single fertilized ovum) had split at day 5 during the blastocyst stage. This will, most likely, result in which of the following?

A. Genetically identical twins with shared chorion

B. Genetically identical twins with shared chorion and amnion

C. Genetically identical twins with two chorions and two amnions

D. Fraternal twins

E. A male and a female twin with similar phenotype

Consider the following case for questions 16 to 17:

A 26-year-old first-time pregnant woman comes to your clinic at 8 weeks, gestation with painless vaginal bleeding. The bleeding, which has appeared over the past couple of hours, is mild. There was no significant abnormality detected on her physical examination. A pelvic examination revealed a closed cervical os. An ultrasound failed to reveal a fetal pole within a sizeable gestational sac and a thin decidual reaction of less than 2 mm.

16. Which of the following is the diagnosis for the pregnant woman?

A. Threatened abortion

B. Incomplete abortion

C. Complete abortion

D. Missed abortion

E. Anembryonic pregnancy

17. As noted with the ultrasound, an abnormal decidual structure was found within the endometrial biopsy obtained from her. Which of the following is true regarding normal decidua?

A. The most important region of decidua for nourishment of the conceptus is decidua capsularis.

B. The most important region of decidua for nourishment of the conceptus is decidua parietalis.

C. Apposition of decidua basalis and decidua capsularis functionally obliterates the uterine cavity during the 4th month of pregnancy.

D. Apposition of decidua basalis and decidua parietalis functionally obliterates the uterine cavity during the 4th month of pregnancy.

E. Apposition of decidua parietalis and decidua capsularis functionally obliterates the uterine cavity during the 4th month of pregnancy.

18. A 26-year-old mother who has been pregnant for 12 weeks presents with vaginal bleeding. Physical examination reveals a uterine size that corresponds to a 20-week pregnancy. Her laboratories came back with an excessively high serum hCG (human chorionic gonadotropin) and a reduced level of serum AFP (α fetoprotein). Which of the following is the most likely diagnosis?

A. Ruptured ectopic pregnancy

B. Hydatidiform mole

C. Dizygotic twins

D. Placenta previa

E. Anencephaly

19. An embryologist notices a segment of tissue made up of large, multinucleated, and fused mass of cells related to a partially implanted blastocyst. Which of the following parts of the developing embryo will this tissue ultimately become?

A. Skin

B. Brain

C. Lining of stomach

D. Biceps brachii muscle

E. Placenta

20. A female neonate, born to a 21-year-old mother, presents with jaundice 4 hours after birth. Over the course of a few hours, the neonate developed heart failure, bipedal edema, and ascites. Her blood group antigen typed as D+, as opposed to a D-type for the mother. Which of the following might be a true statement for this pregnancy?

A. This is likely to be the firstborn child, and the neonate is suffering from a condition that is due to transplacental transport of maternal IgM antibodies.

B. This is likely to be the second-born child, and the neonate is suffering from a condition that is due to transplacental transport of maternal IgM antibodies

C. This is likely to be the firstborn child, and the neonate is suffering from a condition that is due to transplacental transport of maternal IgG antibodies

D. This is likely to be the second-born child, and the neonate is suffering from a condition that is due to transplacental transport of maternal IgG antibodies

E. The neonate is suffering from a condition that is due to transplacental transport of maternal IgE antibodies

27.2 Answers and Explanations

Easy	Medium	Hard

1. Correct: Incomplete abortion (B)

The patient is suffering from an incomplete abortion. It is defined as the passage of some, but not all, of the products of conception from the uterine cavity, prior to 20 weeks' gestation. Bleeding and cramping usually continue until all products of conception have been expelled.

In threatened abortion (**A**), the cervix remains closed, and slight vaginal bleeding (prior to 20 weeks gestation), with or without cramping, may be noted.

In a complete abortion (**C**), all products of conception have passed from the uterine cavity, prior to 20 weeks gestation, and the cervix is closed. Slight bleeding and mild cramping may continue for several weeks.

Missed abortion (**D**) is defined as a pregnancy that has been retained within the uterus after embryonic or fetal demise. Cramping or bleeding may be present, but often there are no symptoms. The cervix is closed, and the products of conception remain in situ.

Septic abortion (**E**) presents with infection of the uterus and the product of conception. Clinical findings include signs of infection (fever and leuko-

cytosis, for example), diffuse pelvic tenderness, and profuse and foul vaginal discharge in most cases.

2. Correct: B, C, and D (G)

Because the woman was 5 weeks pregnant, tertiary villi (formed during the later 3rd week) must have been formed in the developing embryo. These are characterized by fetal blood vessels (**D**) that develop in the mesodermal (extraembryonic) core (**C**), with the shell comprising both cytotrophoblast and syncytiotrophoblast (**B**). Primary villus, formed during the 2nd week, has a cytotrophoblastic core surrounded by syncytiotrophoblast (**A**). In the secondary villus, formed early during the 3rd week, a core of mesoderm penetrates the cytotrophoblast, but blood vessels are yet to form.

3. Correct: Inferior vena cava, distal segment (E)

Pulmonary circulation is attenuated in the fetus by high intrinsic vascular resistance in the pulmonary arterioles and bypass shunting around the lungs via the ductus arteriosus. The rapid transition from fetal to newborn circulation includes a precipitous drop in pulmonary vascular resistance concomitant with lung expansion, followed by increased pulmonary blood flow in the first minutes of life and a gradual closing of the ductus arteriosus over the next 48 hours. Any condition that disrupts this progression leads to persistent pulmonary hypertension of the newborn.

The distal segment of the inferior vena cava (IVC) carries poorly oxygenated blood returning from the lower fetal body. The right atrium (**A**) receives a mixture of deoxygenated [brought in by superior vena cava (SVC) and distal IVC] and highly oxygenated (brought in via umbilical vein, ductus venosus, and proximal IVC) blood. The left atrium (**B**) receives blood from the right atrium through the foramen ovale. Most of the blood crossing the foramen ovale corresponds to the stream of well-oxygenated blood in the IVC coming from the ductus venosus.

Well-oxygenated blood returns to the fetus from the placenta by way of the umbilical vein (**C**). The umbilical vein enters the liver, where it joins with the portal venous system. Most of this blood is shunted directly to the proximal IVC (**D**) through the ductus venosus.

Blood entering the right atrium from the SVC joins with the remaining blood in the IVC, which corresponds mainly to the less-oxygenated bloodstream from the distal IVC (fetal lower body). This blood primarily enters the right ventricle. From here, most blood is shunted through the ductus arteriosus, which joins the descending aorta (**F**). This blood is still more oxygenated than the distal segment of IVC, because it is a mixture of oxygenated (less) and deoxygenated (more) blood, obtained from the right atrium.

4.   Correct: Ductus venosus (D)

As noted earlier, well-oxygenated blood is shunted directly to the proximal IVC through the ductus venosus. The oxygen saturation of blood in the proximal IVC (**B**) is lower than that in the ductus venosus, because it has mixed with poorly oxygenated blood returning from the fetal lower body through the distal IVC (**C**). As noted earlier, blood entering the right ventricle from the right atrium (**A**) is less oxygenated. From here, most blood is shunted through the ductus arteriosus (**E**), which joins the descending aorta (**F**).

5.   Correct: A and C (F)

As noted earlier, well-oxygenated blood is shunted directly to the proximal IVC through the ductus venosus (**A**). The IVC blood enters the right atrium, and ~ 40% is diverted to the left atrium through the foramen ovale (**C**). Most of the blood crossing the foramen ovale corresponds to the stream of well-oxygenated blood in the IVC coming from the ductus venosus. In the left atrium, this blood mixes with a relatively small quantity of pulmonary venous blood, enters the left ventricle, and then proceeds to the vessels supplying the brain. Therefore, both ductus venosus and foramen ovale play important roles in shunting oxygenated blood to the brain, bypassing the liver and lungs.

Blood entering the right atrium from the SVC joins with the remaining (60%) blood in the IVC, which corresponds mainly to the less-oxygenated bloodstream from the distal IVC (fetal lower body). This blood enters the right ventricle. From here, most blood is shunted through the ductus arteriosus (**B, D, E,** and **G**), which joins the descending aorta.

6.   Correct: Previous pregnancy delivered by caesarean section (C)

The woman is suffering from placenta previa, in which the placenta implants in the lower uterine segment, adjacent to or overlying the internal cervical os. Placenta previa typically presents with painless vaginal bleeding, usually in the third trimester. There are several risk factors, including multiparity, increasing maternal age, history of prior caesarean section, and multiple gestation.

Uterine size (**A**) or human chorionic gonadotropin (**B**) greater than expected for gestational age is found in several diseases, including gestational trophoblastic disease, but not in placenta previa. Abnormal uterine bleeding, usually during the first trimester, is the most common presenting symptom of gestational trophoblastic disease.

Accessory placental lobes (**D**), termed succenturiate placenta, are potential sources of postpartum hemorrhage, not antepartum hemorrhage.

A retroplacental clot (**E**) is formed in placental abruption, which results from premature separation of the placenta prior to delivery. Lack of pain with vaginal bleeding distinguishes placenta previa from placental abruption.

7.   Correct: Renal agenesis (A)

Fetal urination is the primary amniotic fluid source by the second half of pregnancy. Oligohydramnios is an abnormally decreased amount of amniotic fluid. This may reflect a fetal abnormality that precludes normal urination (renal agenesis, for example), or it may represent a placental abnormality severe enough to impair perfusion.

Hydramnios is an abnormally increased amniotic fluid volume. Impaired swallowing, secondary to either a central nervous system abnormality (anencephaly, **B**) or gastrointestinal tract obstruction [esophageal (**D**) or duodenal (**E**) atresia], can result in an impressive degree of hydramnios. Diaphragmatic hernia (**C**) may be associated with hydramnios due to mediastinal shift and impaired swallowing.

8.   Correct: Injecting anti-D antibody to her during this pregnancy (D)

Rh 0 (D antigen) incompatibility may develop when an Rh-negative woman is impregnated by an Rh-positive man, and conceives an Rh-positive fetus. In such cases, with fetomaternal hemorrhage (inevitable during delivery, or invasive procedures), fetal RBCs stimulate maternal antibody production against the Rh antigens. No complications develop during the initial sensitizing pregnancy; however, in subsequent pregnancies, maternal antibodies (IgG) cross the placenta (**B**) and lyse fetal RBCs (erythroblastosis fetalis), causing anemia and its complications (generalized edema, heart failure, etc.).

Prevention involves giving the Rh-negative mother anti-D immunoglobulin during the initial pregnancy (**C**). When fetal red blood cells cross into the maternal circulation, anti-D antibody binds to them, masking the D antigen from the mother, and preventing her from forming antibodies against it. This will prevent her from being sensitized to possible Rh positive fetal antigens.

On the first prenatal visit, all pregnant women should be screened for ABO blood group and Rh 0 antigen. They should also undergo antibody screening (indirect Coombs' test). All Rh-negative first-time mothers should be administered 300 mg of anti-D immunoglobulin at 28 weeks of gestation, regardless of the fetal blood group (**A**). If the infant is Rh 0 positive, 300 mg of anti-D immunoglobulin is administered to the mother (provided maternal antibody screening is negative), within 72 hours after delivery. If the antibody screen is positive, the patient is aggressively managed as if she will be Rh-sensitized during the next pregnancy. Folic acid has no role in prevention of erythroblastosis fetalis (**E**).

9. Correct: Trophoblast (B)

Approximately 3 days after fertilization, the embryo has divided to form a 16-cell morula by the time it enters the uterine cavity. Cells organize into an inner cell mass (embryoblast), and surrounding cells compose the outer cell mass (trophoblast). The embryoblast (**A**) gives rise to the embryo proper, while the trophoblast contributes to the placenta.

Beginning in the 2nd week, the embryoblast differentiates into a dorsal epiblast and a ventral hypoblast (**C**). Hypoblast is important for early signaling to establish the cranial-caudal axis (from anterior visceral endoderm/prechordal plate, which is the head organizer), but will eventually be displaced by definitive endoderm.

Early in the 2nd week, an amniotic cavity develops within the cells of the epiblast. Amnioblasts (**D**) proliferate from the edges of the epiblast and secrete amniotic fluid.

The notochord (**E**), a median cellular cord of mesoderm extending from the primitive node to the prechordal plate, acts as an embryonic organizer. The nucleus pulposus of the intervertebral disk is its adult remnant.

10. Correct: Hypertension (D)

The woman is suffering from abruptio placentae, in which premature separation of the normally implanted placenta occurs after 20 weeks of gestation but prior to delivery. Maternal hypertension and smoking have been strongly associated with the occurrence of placental abruption.

Uterine enlargement (**A**) or human chorionic gonadotropin (**B**) greater than expected for gestational age is found in several diseases, including gestational trophoblastic disease, but not in placental abruption. Also, uterine bleeding during the first trimester is the most common presenting symptom for gestational trophoblastic disease.

A low-lying placenta covering the internal os (**C**) is diagnostic of placenta previa. Lack of pain with the presence of bleeding is what distinguishes placenta previa from placental abruption.

Accessory placental lobes (**E**), termed succenturiate placenta, are potential sources of postpartum, but not antepartum, hemorrhage.

11. Correct: Vitelline vein (C)

The vitelline veins, carrying blood from the yolk sac into the sinus venosus, form the following structures in the adult: hepatic sinusoids, portal venous system (hepatic portal, superior mesenteric, and splenic veins), and part (hepatic) of the IVC.

The left umbilical vein (**A**), in the adult, forms the ligamentum teres hepatis. The right umbilical vein (**B**) degenerates during fetal development. The right anterior cardinal vein (**D**), in the adult, forms the right internal jugular vein and part of the superior vena cava. The right posterior cardinal vein (**E**) forms part of the inferior vena cava in the adult.

12. Correct: B, C, and D (H)

The placental barrier, at earlier stages, is composed of the syncytiotrophoblast, cytotrophoblast, and fetal capillary endothelium and the basement membrane.

At later stages, the barrier thins out with cytotrophoblast degeneration (**A**, **E**, and **F**), and is composed of syncytiotrophoblast (**B**) and fetal capillary endothelium (**C**) and basement membrane (**D**).

13. Correct: A and D (E)

The uteroplacental circulation starts with the maternal blood flow (**A**) into the intervillous space through spiral uterine arteries. The intervillous space, site of gas and metabolic exchange (**D**) lined by syncytiotrophoblast, contains maternal blood, which is separated from the fetal blood (**B**, **F**) by the placental barrier. The fetoplacental circulation enable the umbilical arteries to carry deoxygenated and nutrient-depleted fetal blood to the villus core fetal vessels. After the exchange of oxygen and nutrients, the umbilical vein carries fresh oxygenated and nutrient-rich blood circulating back to the fetal systemic circulation. Amniotic fluid (**C**, **G**) does not flow through the intervillous spaces.

14. Correct: Risk associated with the procedure is less than that of chorionic villus sampling. (C)

Amniocentesis is a primary screening procedure to detect fetal abnormalities. Performed under sonographic guidance, fluid is sampled from the amniotic cavity. Risks associated with the procedure are considered to be very low, compared with other common procedures (chorionic villus sampling, for example). Amniocentesis is performed usually during the 2nd trimester (15–20 weeks), and sometimes the 3rd trimester, but not the 1st trimester (**A**). There is usually a wait for about a week to obtain results for fetal karyotyping (**B**). Early in the 2nd trimester, amniocentesis provides a useful tool (diagnosis of choice) in AFP (α fetoprotein) evaluation for neural tube defect assessment (**D**). In amniocentesis, a needle is inserted transcutaneously through the maternal abdominal wall into the amniotic cavity under ultrasound guidance (**E**), and fluid is removed.

15. Correct: Genetically identical twins with shared chorion (A)

Monozygotic twins are the result of division of a single fertilized ovum that subsequently divides into two separate individuals. Normally, they share the same physical and genetic features. The outcome of the monozygotic twinning process depends on when division occurs:

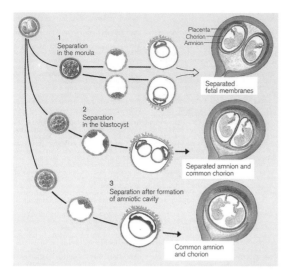

At 0 to 4 days postfertilization (morula stage), an early conceptus may divide into two. Division at this early stage creates two chorions and two amnions (**C**, dichorionic, diamnionic).

Division between 4 and 8 days (blastocyst stage) leads to formation of a blastocyst with two separate embryoblasts. Each embryoblast will form its own amnion within a shared chorion (**A**, monochorionic, diamnionic).

Between 8 and 12 days, the amnion and amniotic cavity form above the germinal disk. Embryonic division leads to two embryos with a shared amnion and shared chorion (**B**, monochorionic, monoamnionic).

Monozygotic twins are always of the same sex (**E**).

Dizygotic twins (fraternal twins, **D**) are produced from separately fertilized ova. They bear only the resemblance of brothers or sisters.

16. Correct: Anembryonic pregnancy (E)

Anembryonic pregnancy (blighted ovum) is an ultrasound diagnosis. It is a pregnancy in which the embryo fails to develop or is resorbed after loss of viability. Mild pain or bleeding may be present; however, the cervix is closed, and the nonviable pregnancy is retained in the uterus.

In threatened abortion (**A**), the cervix remains closed, and slight vaginal bleeding with or without cramping may be noted. A live intrauterine gestation is noted with an ultrasound.

Incomplete abortion (**B**) is defined as the passage of some, but not all, of the products of conception from the uterine cavity. Bleeding and cramping usually continue until all products of conception have been expelled, and the cervical os is dilated. Ultrasound findings of presence of prominent vascular supply and feeding vessel associated with normal uterine gestation help make the diagnosis.

In complete abortion (**C**), all of the products of conception have passed from the uterine cavity and the cervix is closed. The history of our patient is not suggestive of this. Ultrasound shows an empty uterus with no fetal components or products of conception.

Missed abortion (**D**) is defined as a pregnancy that has been retained within the uterus after embryonic or fetal demise. Cramping or bleeding may be present, but often there are no symptoms. The cervix is closed, and the products of conception remain in situ. A CRL (crown-rump length) of ≥7 mm without a heartbeat on ultrasound confirms the diagnosis.

17. Correct: Apposition of decidua parietalis and decidua capsularis functionally obliterates the uterine cavity during the 4th month of pregnancy. (E)

The concept is explained using the image:

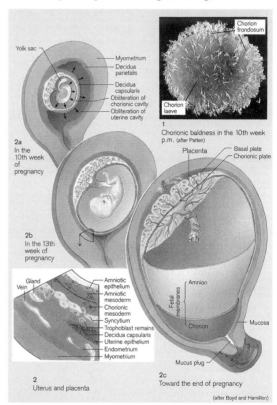

Decidua directly beneath blastocyst implantation is modified by trophoblast invasion and becomes the decidua basalis. This is most important for embryonic and fetal nourishment (**A, B**).

The decidua capsularis (**C**) overlies the enlarging blastocyst and initially separates the conceptus from the rest of the uterine cavity. Internally, it contacts the avascular chorion laeve. The remainder of the uterus is lined by decidua parietalis (**D**).

During early pregnancy, there is a space between the decidua capsularis and parietalis because the gestational sac does not fill the entire uterine cavity. By 14 to 16 weeks' gestation, the expanding sac has enlarged to fill the uterine cavity completely. The resulting apposition of the decidua capsularis and parietalis creates the decidua vera, and the uterine cavity is functionally obliterated.

18. Correct: Hydatidiform mole (B)

The woman has a hydatidiform mole, which represents an abnormal placenta characterized by marked proliferation of trophoblast. A complete mole is marked by absence of an embryo. Diagnostic clinical signs include 1st-trimester vaginal bleeding, uterine enlargement greater than expected for gestational age, and abnormally elevated hCG levels.

Ruptured ectopic pregnancy (**A**) commonly presents during the 1st trimester with abdominal pain and signs of internal bleeding (shock). Uterine enlargement greater than expected for gestational age does not occur.

Placenta previa (**D**) typically presents with painless vaginal bleeding, usually in the third trimester.

Twinning (**C**) and anencephaly (**E**) present with elevated levels of α fetoprotein.

19. Correct: Placenta (E)

Within an implanting blastocyst, cells organize into an inner cell mass (embryoblast) and surrounding cells that compose the outer cell mass (trophoblast). The embryoblast gives rise to the embryo proper, while the trophoblast contributes to the placenta. The trophoblast differentiates into cytotrophoblast and syncytiotrophoblast early during the 2nd week. The cells of cytotrophoblast are mitotically active and continuously contribute to the syncytiotropho-blast. The syncytiotrophoblast (large, multinucleated, and fused cells referred to in the question) is responsible for invading the uterine endometrium during implantation.

Skin (**A**, surface ectoderm), brain (**B**, neuroectoderm), lining of stomach (**C**, endoderm), and skeletal muscle (**D**, mesoderm) are formed from the inner cell mass.

20. Correct: This is likely to be the second-born child, and the neonate is suffering from a condition that is due to transplacental transport of maternal IgG antibodies. (D)

Erythroblastosis fetalis is hemolytic anemia in the fetus caused by transplacental transmission of maternal IgG antibodies to the fetus. It classically results from D (Rh 0) antigen incompatibility, which may develop when a D− woman is impregnated by a D+ man and conceives a D+ fetus. In such cases, with fetomaternal hemorrhage (inevitable during delivery, or invasive procedures), fetal RBCs stimulate maternal antibody production against the Rh antigens. No complications develop during the initial sensitizing pregnancy (**A, C**); however, in subsequent pregnancies, maternal antibodies (IgG) cross the placenta and lyse fetal RBCs, causing anemia and its complications (generalized edema, heart failure, etc.).

IgM (**A, B**) and IgE (**E**) do not cross the placental barrier.

Chapter 28

Comprehensive Review Exam

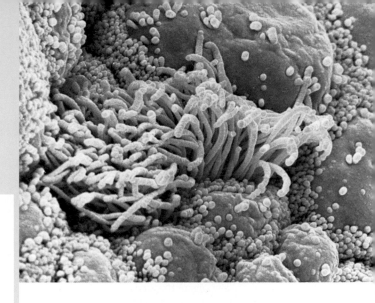

LEARNING OBJECTIVES

- ▶ Analyze the etiology, clinical features, and diagnosis of inguinal hernias.
- ▶ Illustrate the structure of the layers of the epidermis; correlate these with their functions.
- ▶ Outline the etiopathogenesis, hemodynamic changes, clinical features, and diagnosis of patent ductus arteriosus.
- ▶ Predict the etiopathogenesis and outcomes for splenic rupture.
- ▶ Illustrate the microstructure of the spleen.
- ▶ Evaluate the functions of the histological zones of the spleen.
- ▶ Analyze the etiology, clinical features, and diagnosis of Turner's syndrome.
- ▶ Illustrate the microstructure of the major salivary glands and correlate these with their functions.
- ▶ Trace the secretomotor pathways for the major salivary glands.
- ▶ Characterize the general features of development of the aortic arches.
- ▶ Trace the major arteries derived from the aortic arches.
- ▶ Outline the etiopathogenesis, hemodynamic changes, clinical features, and diagnosis of double aortic arch.
- ▶ Illustrate the microstructure of the small intestine.
- ▶ Contrast between the microstructures of duodenum, jejunum, and ileum.
- ▶ Analyze the etiology, clinical features, and diagnosis for exstrophy–epispadias complex.
- ▶ Illustrate the microstructure of the liver.
- ▶ Correlate the ultrastructure of hepatic components with their functions.
- ▶ Trace the stages of meiotic division during oocyte maturation.
- ▶ Describe how sinus venosus, pulmonary veins, and primitive atria contribute to the development of atria.
- ▶ Outline the etiopathogenesis, hemodynamic changes, clinical features, and diagnosis of Ebstein's anomaly.
- ▶ Illustrate the microstructure of seminal glands and correlate it with its functions.
- ▶ Illustrate gut rotation, including midgut herniation and physiological reduction of the hernia.
- ▶ Analyze embryological and anatomical definitions of foregut, midgut, and hindgut.

- ▶ Analyze etiopathogenesis, clinical features, and diagnosis of primary adrenal insufficiency.
- ▶ Trace the development of the adrenal gland.
- ▶ Illustrate the microstructure of the adrenal gland and correlate it with its functions.
- ▶ Illustrate the development of female external genitalia.
- ▶ Illustrate the microstructure of distal convoluted tubules and correlate it with their functions.
- ▶ Outline the etiopathogenesis, hemodynamic changes, clinical features, and diagnosis of aortic valve atresia (hypoplastic left heart syndrome).
- ▶ Analyze the etiopathogenesis, clinical features, and diagnosis for pulmonary emphysema.
- ▶ Illustrate the microstructure of conducting and gas-exchange portions of the respiratory tract and correlate these with their functions.
- ▶ Analyze the defects associated with horseshoe kidney.
- ▶ Analyze the etiopathogenesis, clinical features, and diagnosis of cystic fibrosis.
- ▶ Illustrate the microstructure of the pituitary gland and correlate it with its functions.
- ▶ Correlate the role of cardiac mesenchyme in partitioning of the heart with the development of the heart valves.
- ▶ Outline the etiopathogenesis, hemodynamic changes, clinical features, and diagnosis of patent foramen ovale.
- ▶ Illustrate the microscopic structure of central and peripheral glia (astrocytes, oligodendrocytes, microglia, ependyma, Schwann cells, and satellite cells).
- ▶ Correlate the ultrastructure of central and peripheral glia to their development and functions.
- ▶ Illustrate the microstructures of conducting fibers of the heart and correlate these with their functions.
- ▶ Demonstrate the developmental fate of the dorsal and ventral mesenteries associated with the primitive gut tube.

28.1 Questions

Easy	Medium	Hard

Consider the following case for questions 1 to 3:

A 2-month-old infant presents with a bulge in the right groin that mostly disappears when lying down. It becomes more noticeable when the infant cries or strains during defecation. Physical examination reveals a smooth, compressible, and nontender mass, most prominent above and lateral to the pubic crest, that does not transilluminate. Compression immediately above the mid-inguinal point does not reduce its size when the infant coughs.

1. Which of the following is the diagnosis for the infant?

A. Communicating hydrocele

B. Noncommunicating hydrocele

C. Indirect inguinal hernia

D. Direct inguinal hernia

E. Varicocele

2. Which of the following might be the underlying defect in the infant?

A. Complete patency of processus vaginalis

B. Partial patency of processus vaginalis

C. Congenital weakness of the posterior wall of the inguinal canal

D. Congenital dilatation of the testicular veins

E. Congenital obstruction of the epididymal ducts

3. Which of the following statement is true for the swelling in the infant?

A. The swelling is covered from outside inward by the external spermatic fascia, cremasteric fascia, and internal spermatic fascia.

B. At surgery, the inferior epigastric artery should be identified lateral to the neck of the swelling.

C. This swelling appears in the groin posterior to the inguinal ligament.

D. Aspiration from the swelling should reveal only amber-colored fluid.

E. Aspiration from the swelling should reveal only milky fluid containing sperm.

4. A 16-year-old boy presents with pruritus and scratching of his bilateral antecubital fossae of 3 weeks' duration. A physical examination reveals hyperpigmentation, lichenification, and scaling of the affected areas. He was diagnosed with an impaired epidermal barrier consequent to a mutation in the gene encoding filaggrin. Which of the following layers within the epidermis is the seat of pathology for him?

A. Layer that contains most macula adherens

B. Layer that contains cells devoid of nuclei

C. Layer that is usually absent in thin skin

D. Layer that contains cells that produce the major protein component of the cornified envelope

E. Layer that contains cells that are mitotically active

F. Layer that contains cells that form lamellar granules

5. A preterm infant, born at 24 weeks' gestation, was scheduled for ligation of a large hemodynamically significant ductus arteriosus after failure of two courses of indomethacin. Which of the following is a likely complication following the procedure?

A. Paralysis of the left vocal cord

B. Paralysis of the right vocal cord

C. Paralysis of the left hemidiaphragm

D. Paralysis of the right hemidiaphragm

E. Paralysis of the left infrahyoid muscles

6. A 27-year-old man presents with severe abdominal pain, tachycardia, hypotension, and dizziness 3 hours following a blunt abdominal trauma to his left lower rib cage. A physical examination revealed extreme tenderness around the left 10th rib. Which of the following is the likely histological finding for the organ that might have been damaged?

A. Bundles of serous acini interrupted by pale staining islands

B. Sinusoidal spaces with gaps between endothelial lining cells and discontinuous basal lamina

C. Simple columnar epithelial lining with villi, microvilli, and goblet cells

D. Simple columnar epithelial lining with variable invagination into the underlying connective tissue

E. Outer cortex predominantly packed with steroid-producing cells

Consider the following case for questions 7 to 10:

A 16-year-old girl presents with primary amenorrhea, obesity, and short stature. A physical examination reveals a webbed neck, hypertension (measured on the right arm), normal female external genitalia with sparse pubic hair, hypoplastic breasts, and decreased pulse volume in the lower extremities. Laboratory exams reveal impaired glucose tolerance, normal serum electrolytes, normal serum cortisol, and normal serum aldosterone levels. A pelvic ultrasound showed streaky uterus and ovaries.

7. Which of the following is the possible diagnosis for the patient?

A. Congenital adrenal hyperplasia

B. Turner's syndrome

C. Androgen insensitivity syndrome

D. Klinefelter's syndrome

E. Müllerian agenesis

8. Which of the following might be responsible for the primary amenorrhea in the patient?

A. 17-α hydroxylase deficiency

B. 5-α reductase deficiency

C. An additional X chromosome

D. Monosomy of the X chromosome

E. Mutation in the androgen receptor gene

9. Which of the following is the expected genotype for the patient?

A. 45, X

B. 47, XXY

C. 47, XYY

D. 46, XY

E. 46, XX

10. Which of the following might be an associated finding in the patient?

A. Increased serum thyroxine levels

B. Increased serum luteinizing hormone levels

C. Increased serum estrogen levels

D. Increased serum progesterone levels

E. Increased serum inhibin B levels

11. A 60-year-old man presents with pain and swelling within the right side of the oral cavity of 3 days' duration. Eating usually exacerbates the pain. Biopsies were obtained from all his major salivary glands, and one of these is shown in the figure. Which of the following is true for the biopsied specimen?

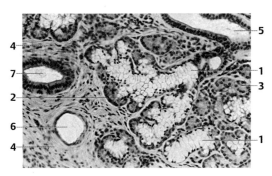

A. Its secretion is exclusively serous.

B. Its secretion is predominantly serous.

C. Its secretion is controlled by the nucleus solitarius in the brainstem.

D. Its secretion is controlled by the inferior salivatory nucleus in the brainstem.

E. Its secretion is controlled by the superior salivatory nucleus in the brainstem.

12. A 2-week-old girl presented to the ER with tachypnea, inspiratory stridor, retractions, and evidence of respiratory failure. She was placed on mechanical ventilation and required inotropic support to maintain perfusion and blood pressure. Clinical evaluation revealed a systolic murmur and echocardiography showed a vascular ring compressing the distal trachea. Which of the following is most likely responsible for her symptoms?

A. Abnormal obliteration of the right 4th aortic arch

B. Abnormal regression of the left 4th aortic arch

C. Abnormal obliteration of the left 4th aortic arch and left dorsal aorta

D. Persistence of the right dorsal aorta

E. Persistence of the left dorsal aorta

13. A 56-year-old man presents with acute abdominal pain, absolute constipation, and vomiting of 3 days' duration. Investigations revealed a large segment of strangulated intestine affected by volvulus. Biopsy from the surgically removed specimen from him is seen in the figure. Which of the following is a correct statement for the specimen?

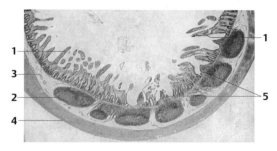

A. The ileocolic artery should have been clamped during its removal.

B. This intestinal segment derives from the embryonic foregut.

C. This intestinal segment is affected by the diverticulum consequent to a nonobliterated vitelline duct.

D. This intestinal segment is usually affected by cancer affecting the head of the pancreas.

E. This is a secondarily retroperitoneal segment of the intestine.

Consider the following case for questions 14 to 16:

A male preterm newborn presents with an infraumbilical midline mass with exposed mucous membrane. Urine is found to trickle from its upper right and left angles. A completely dorsally opened plate runs from the neck of the mass down to the open glans penis; left and right corpora cavernosa are clearly visible beneath and alongside the plate. On squeezing the abdomen, a speck of meconium was found to appear in the upper part of the exposed mucosa.

14. Which of the following is the diagnosis for the newborn?

A. Epispadias

B. Bladder exstrophy

C. Cloacal exstrophy

D. A and B

E. A and C

F. A, B, and C

15. Which of the following is the underlying cause for the defect?

A. Defective migration of neural crest cells

B. Defective midline migration of mesenchymal tissue

C. Defective formation of the urorectal septum

D. A and C

E. B and C

16. Which of the following is a likely associated finding in the newborn?

A. Diaphragmatic hernia

B. Hypertrophic pyloric sphincter

C. Meckel's diverticulum

D. Hirschsprung's disease

E. Imperforate anus

17. A 27-year-old primigravida presents at 28 weeks' gestation with abdominal cramps, spotting, and generalized pruritus. Investigations revealed an elevated serum direct bilirubin and elevated alkaline phosphatase. Which of the following zones in the figure may be affected in her?

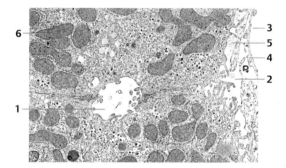

A. 1

B. 2

C. 3

D. 4

E. 5

18. A 26-year-old female shows up in the infertility clinic on June 28. She has been trying to conceive for about a year now. She reports that she has normal 28-day menstrual cycles and her LMP (last menstrual period) was on June 13. Which of the following stages of cell division would the oocyte that is most likely to be available to be fertilized by a spermatozoon be in on the day of her clinic visit (given the fact that she is not already pregnant)?

A. Leptotene stage of meiosis I

B. Diplotene stage of meiosis I

C. Metaphase of meiosis I

D. Metaphase of meiosis II

E. Prophase of meiosis II

19. A 6-week-old infant presents with severe cyanosis. Physical examination reveals a holosystolic murmur of tricuspid regurgitation at the lower left sternal border, an enlarged liver, and an elevated jugular venous pulse (JVP). An echocardiogram demonstrates apical displacement of the septal leaflet of tricuspid valve, and a hugely dilated heart chamber. Which of the following embryonic structures gives rise to the enlarged chamber?

A. Bulbus cordis

B. Ductus arteriosus

C. Truncus arteriosus

D. Right sinus horn

E. Left sinus horn

20. A 38-year-old man presents with infertility. He reports to have tried several over-the-counter medications and hormones for the previous 5 years without any result. Samples were obtained from various parts of his external and internal genital organs and one of these is shown in the figure. Which of the following is a true statement for the organ?

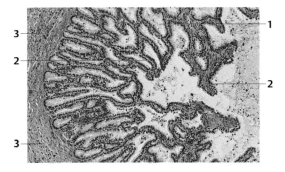

A. This organ traverses the inguinal canal.

B. This organ produces spermatozoa.

C. This organ is where spermatozoa mature and gain motility.

D. Secretion from this organ is the primary source of energy for spermatozoa to swim.

E. Secretion from this organ is rich in acid phosphatase.

21. A male neonate presents with ischemic necrosis of the caudal limb of the primary intestinal loop that undergoes physiologic herniation. Which of the following arteries might be affected in him?

A. Gastroduodenal artery

B. Jejunal artery

C. Ileocolic artery

D. Left colic artery

E. Superior rectal artery

Consider the following case for questions 22 to 24:

A 32-year-old woman presented with vague abdominal discomfort, fatigue, anorexia, and nausea for 6 months. She admitted to moderate weight loss over these months. A physical examination revealed obvious hyperpigmentation that involved her oral mucosa. Laboratory exams came back with a low cortisol level, which did not rise to expected levels when challenged with adrenocorticotrophic hormone.

22. Which of the following might be the embryonic source of the tissue responsible for her symptoms?

A. Oral ectoderm

B. Neuroectoderm

C. Neural crest

D. Intermediate mesoderm

E. Endoderm

23. Which of the following might be an associated finding in her?

A. Na+ ↑, K+ ↓, ACTH ↑

B. Na+ ↓, K+ ↑, ACTH ↑

C. Na+ ↓, K+ ↑, ACTH ↓

D. Na+ ↓, K+ ↓, ACTH ↓

E. Na+ ↑, K+ ↓, ACTH ↓

24. Which of the following might be an important normal histologic feature of a cell defective in her?

A. Hypersegmentation of the nuclei

B. Absence of lipid droplets

C. Abundance of smooth endoplasmic reticulum

D. Abundance of rough endoplasmic reticulum

E. Apical secretory granules

25. Which of the following structures will be affected due to a developmental defect of the genital tubercle?

A. Vagina

B. Urethra

C. Greater vestibular glands

D. Bulb of the vestibule

E. Labia majora

26. A renal biopsy obtained from a 60-year-old man presenting with hematuria is seen in the figure. Which of the following substances might have the most effect on the structure labeled 2?

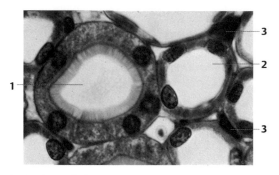

A. Angiotensin II
B. Aldosterone
C. Parathyroid hormone
D. Antidiuretic hormone
E. B and D

27. A 16-hour-old male neonate presents with progressive dyspnea and worsening cough. A physical examination reveals moderate cyanosis, and a fetal echo demonstrates atresia of the aortic valve. Which of the following would be an essential additional finding in his echocardiogram?

A. Patent ductus arteriosus
B. Ventricular septal defect
C. Hypertrophied left ventricle
D. Hypertrophied mitral valve
E. Hypoplastic right ventricle

28. A 56-year-old male presents with shortness of breath. He has smoked cigarettes for the past 35 years on an average of 1 pack per day. A physical examination reveals reduced breath sounds in the right side of his chest. Laboratory investigations came back with reduced serum α1-antitrypsin. A chest X-ray revealed hyperinflation of the right chest with flattening of the right hemidiaphragm. Which of the following represents the histology of the structure that is, most likely, affected in him?

A. Lined by ciliated simple cuboidal cells, absence of goblet cells, wall contains some smooth muscles but no cartilage.
B. Lined by ciliated low cuboidal cells, absence of goblet cells, wall contains some smooth muscles but no cartilage.
C. Lined by pseudostratified tall columnar cells, absence of goblet cells.
D. Lined by pseudostratified ciliated columnar cells, with presence of goblet cells, wall contains rings of hyaline cartilage.
E. Lined by pseudostratified ciliated columnar cells, presence of goblet cells, wall contains plates of hyaline cartilage and prominent smooth muscles.

29. A 5-year-old girl, being investigated for renal anomalies, was found to have low-lying kidneys. The lower poles of her kidneys were fused to form an isthmus opposite the L4 vertebra. Which of the following structures might have prevented ascent of her kidneys?

A. Duodenojejunal flexure
B. Superior mesenteric artery
C. Inferior mesenteric artery
D. Third part of the duodenum
E. Transverse colon

Consider the following case for questions 30 to 31:

A male newborn presents at age 24 hours with a distended abdomen and bilious vomiting. He has not passed meconium. He has passed scanty urine, which was normal in color. Digital rectal examination reveals normal meconium-stained gloved fingers. Blood testing reveals an increase in immunoreactive trypsin (IRT).

30. Which of the following might be an expected complication during his infancy, childhood, and/or adulthood?

A. Carbohydrate indigestion
B. Protein indigestion
C. Chronic renal failure
D. Infertility due to defective spermatogenesis
E. Recurrent respiratory infections

31. Which of the following might be the underlying pathogenesis for the neonate?

A. Defective migration of neural crest cells to the gut wall

B. Defective epithelial ion channel consequent to genetic mutation

C. Defective growth of the urorectal septum

D. Defective regression of the omphalomesenteric duct

E. Defective rupture of the cloacal membrane

Consider the following case for questions 32 to 35:

A 5-year-old girl presented with slowly progressive visual disturbance and headache, which lasted for a couple of months. Computed tomography (CT) and magnetic resonance imaging (MRI) of the brain revealed a suprasellar calcified cystic mass in the anterior part of the third cerebral ventricle. The mass was biopsied at surgery and is being examined for pathology.

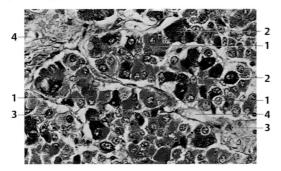

32. Which of the following is the probable source for the image?

A. Thalamus

B. Hypothalamus

C. Pineal gland

D. Adenohypophysis

E. Neurohypophysis

33. Which of the following vessel(s) need(s) to be clamped for surgical resection of the mass?

A. Petrous segment of the internal carotid artery

B. Cavernous segment of the internal carotid artery

C. Supraclinoid segment of the internal carotid artery

D. A and B

E. B and C

F. A and C

34. Which of the following is a likely product from the cells labeled 2?

A. Prolactin

B. Somatotropin

C. Follicle-stimulating hormone

D. Corticotropin-releasing hormone

E. Luteinizing hormone–releasing hormone

35. A histologist is trying to formulate immuno-fluorescent techniques to visualize cells within the displayed tissue in the image for questions 32 to 35. Developing antibodies targeted against which of the following substances will end up being a waste of resources?

A. ACTH (adrenocorticotrophic hormone)

B. ADH (antidiuretic hormone)

C. GH (growth hormone)

D. FSH (follicle-stimulating hormone)

E. TSH (thyroid-stimulating hormone)

36. A 3-day-old neonate presents with mild cyanosis that exacerbates during crying. Physical findings, other than the cyanosis, were normal. An echocardiogram revealed presence of persistent foramen ovale that created a sizable atrial septal defect. Which of the following structures in the neonate might have been defective during development?

A. Ostium primum

B. Septum secundum

C. Septum spurium

D. Endocardial cushions

E. Conotruncal cushions

37. A biopsy obtained from the lower brainstem of a 26-year-old man is examined under the microscope. Which of the following is true for the structure indicated by 1 in the figure?

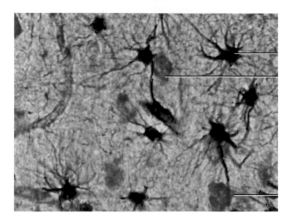

A. The chief source of the indicated structure is neuroectoderm.

B. The chief source of the indicated structure is neural crest.

C. It expresses neurofilament as the intermediate filament.

D. It expresses glial fibrillary acidic protein (GFAP) as the intermediate filament.

E. A and C

F. A and D

G. B and C

H. B and D

38. A cell from the heart wall stains strongly with PAS reagent. It seems larger than regular myocardial cells and has intercalated disks placed at variable intervals. Which of the following is/are the most likely location(s) from where it might have been obtained?

A. Right atrium next to SVC orifice, subendocardium

B. Atrial septum, triangle of Koch, subendocardium

C. Right and left ventricles, subendocardium

D. Epicardium

E. Parietal layer of serous pericardium

39. A routine third-trimester ultrasound in a 30-year-old pregnant woman revealed defective formation of the dorsal mesentery in the embryo. Which of the following might be affected in the newborn?

A. Falciform ligament

B. Ligamentum teres hepatis

C. Ligamentum venosum

D. Lesser omentum

E. Greater omentum

40. A developmental defect causes malformation of the endocardial cushions in the fetus. You are concerned that the fetus might develop an atrial septal defect. Which of the following additional defects would you want to consider during the fetal echocardiogram?

A. Transposition of great vessels (TGV)

B. Persistent truncus arteriosus (PTA)

C. Muscular ventricular septal defect

D. Tricuspid stenosis

E. Aortic stenosis

28.2 Answers and Explanations

Easy	Medium	Hard

1. Correct: Direct inguinal hernia (D)

The infant is suffering from a direct inguinal hernia. The sac of such hernia enters the inguinal canal through the inguinal triangle of Hesselbach. Although less common in infants, several cases have been reported in relevant literature.

A negative transillumination test precludes the swelling from being a hydrocele (**A, B**) or a varicocele (**E**). Also, a noncommunicating hydrocele (**B**) will not alter size or be compressible.

The facts that the swelling does not reduce on compression immediately above the mid-inguinal point (landmark for deep inguinal ring) and is most prominent above and lateral to the pubic crest (landmark for superficial inguinal ring) indicate that the hernia is partially traversing the inguinal canal and has not entered through the deep ring. Therefore, it is not an indirect inguinal hernia (**C**).

2. Correct: Congenital weakness of the posterior wall of the inguinal canal (C)

Direct inguinal hernias occur due to a defect in the posterior wall of the inguinal canal. Complete (**A**, communication hydrocele, indirect inguinal hernia) or partial (**B**, non-communicating hydrocele) patency of processus vaginalis, congenital dilatation of testicular veins (**D**, varicocele), or congenital obstruction of epididymal ducts (**E**, spermatocele, transillumination positive) does not contribute toward the formation of direct inguinal hernia.

3. Correct: At surgery, the inferior epigastric artery should be identified lateral to the neck of the swelling. (B)

The inferior epigastric artery, landmark to distinguish between direct and indirect inguinal hernias, lies lateral to the neck of a direct inguinal hernia.

Because the hernia did not enter the inguinal canal through the deep inguinal ring (gap in fascia transversalis), it will not be covered by the internal spermatic fascia (which is derived from fascia transversalis), which sheaths structures that pass through the deep ring (**A**).

Inguinal hernias appear in the groin anterior to the inguinal ligament, in contrast to femoral hernias, which appear in the femoral canal posterior to the ligament (**C**).

Amber-colored fluid (**D**) or milky fluid containing sperm (**E**) should be the only contents of the swelling in case of hydrocele or spermatocele, respectively. Intestinal coils are expected within a hernial sac.

4. Correct: Layer that contains cells that produce the major protein component of the cornified envelope (D)

The boy is suffering from atopic dermatitis (AD), a complex disorder clinically characterized by dry skin, defective epidermal barrier, susceptibility to cutaneous bacterial colonization, and infection. Recent studies establish strong associations of AD with filaggrin mutation. Filaggrin is synthesized as a high-molecular-weight precursor, profilaggrin, which contains multiple filaggrin molecules and is localized to keratohyalin granules. The granular layer cells are recognized by characteristic basophilic keratohyalin granules in the cytoplasm composed primarily of keratin filaments, filaggrin, and loricrin. Loricrin forms the major protein component of the cornified envelope. On its release from keratohyalin granules, it binds to desmosomal structures and is subsequently cross-linked to the plasma membrane by tissue transglutaminases to form the cornified cell envelope.

Stratum spinosum contains most macula adherens or desmosomes (**A**). Lamellar granules (**F**) are also formed in this layer of the epidermal cells. These secretory organelles deliver precursors of stratum corneum lipids into the intercellular space.

Stratum corneum contains keratinocytes that are devoid of nuclei (**B**), while stratum lucidum is absent in thin skin (**C**). Both stratum basalis and stratum spinosum contain mitotically active cells (**E**).

5. Correct: Paralysis of the left vocal cord (A)

Patent ductus arteriosus is a persistent communication between the descending thoracic aorta (most commonly distal to the origin of the left subclavian artery) and the pulmonary artery (junction of the main pulmonary artery and the origin of the left pulmonary artery). The left recurrent laryngeal nerve hooks around the ductus arteriosus to reach the larynx from the thorax, and it is maximally at risk during surgery on the structure. It supplies the left vocal cord, and unilateral palsy would result in hoarseness of voice.

Paralysis of the right vocal cord (**B**) would follow an injury to the right recurrent laryngeal nerve, which hooks around the right subclavian artery and is therefore not related to the ductus arteriosus.

Paralysis of the left (**C**) and right (**D**) hemidiaphragms would follow injuries to the left and right phrenic nerves, respectively, which also are not related to ductus arteriosus.

Infrahyoid muscles (**E**) are supplied by the ansa cervicalis (C1–C3, which is the sternohyoid, sternothyroid, and omohyoid) and C1 fibers carried via the hypoglossal nerve (thyrohyoid). These nerves are located in the neck and are not related to the ductus arteriosus.

6. Correct: Sinusoidal spaces with gaps between endothelial lining cells and discontinuous basal lamina (B)

The patient is suffering from splenic rupture consequent to a left 10th-rib fracture. The spleen (axis formed by left 10th rib) is most commonly injured in blunt trauma, with rupture usually due to trauma to the left lower rib cage. Bleeding into the peritoneal cavity causes abdominal pain and tenderness that may radiate to the left side of the neck or left shoulder (Kehr's sign). Patients present with features of shock.

Splenic sinusoids are specialized capillaries with wider lumen and gap between endothelial cells; the basal lamina is discontinuous; macrophages line the slits between endothelial cells. The arrangement permits an adequate filtration system for the red pulp of the spleen.

None of the other listed histological features are seen in the spleen, and the clinical features are not suggestive of ruptures of the pancreas (**A**), small gut (**C**), stomach (**D**), or adrenal (**E**).

7. Correct: Turner's syndrome (B)

The patient is suffering from Turner's syndrome. The syndrome is characterized by hypoplastic external and internal genital organs (streak ovaries and uterus) responsible for poorly developed secondary sexual characteristics. Almost all individuals with Turner's syndrome have short stature. These patients are at risk of congenital heart defects (coarctation of aorta in this case, diagnosed from hypertension in the right upper extremity and feeble pulse in the lower extremities), lymphedema, renal malformation, hearing loss, osteoporosis, obesity, and diabetes. Physical manifestations may include a webbed neck, widely spaced nipples, and cubitus valgus.

Congenital adrenal hyperplasia (**A**) is highly unlikely with normal serum cortisol, aldosterone, and electrolyte levels. Androgen insensitivity syndrome (**C**) presents with absent ovaries and uterus. Klinefelter's syndrome (**D**) presents with male external and internal genitalia with gynecomastia. Müllerian agenesis (**E**) will present with an absent uterus but normally developed ovaries.

Turner's syndrome is characterized by partial or complete absence of one X chromosome.

A defect in 17α-hydroxylation (**A**) in the zona fasciculata of the adrenal and in the gonads results in impaired synthesis of 17–hydroxyprogesterone and 17-hydroxypregnenolone and, consequently, cortisol and sex steroids. The secretion of large amounts of corticosterone and deoxycorticosterone leads to hypertension, hypokalemia, and alkalosis. Affected 46, XY individuals present with female genitalia with a blind vaginal pouch or hypoplastic male genitalia. Müllerian structures are absent. Wolffian structures are hypoplastic. Affected 46, XX females have normal development of the internal genital ducts and external genitalia.

5-α reductase deficiency (**B**) causes defective conversion of testosterone (T) to dihydrotestosterone (DHT). This results, in the most severely affected individuals, in ambiguous external genitalia that are characterized by a small hypospadiac phallus bound down in chordee, a bifid scrotum, and a urogenital sinus that opens onto the perineum. A blind vaginal pouch is present, opening either into a urogenital sinus or directly into the urethra. Normal development of testes and well-differentiated wolffian duct structures (epididymis, vas deferens, and seminal vesicle) are characteristic.

Klinefelter's syndrome (**C**, an extra X chromosome) is characterized by small undescended testes, relatively reduced penile length, gynecomastia, diminished facial and body hair, hypotonia, and disproportionately long legs.

Androgen insensitivity syndrome (**E**) results from mutation in the androgen receptor gene. This abolishes the target cells' response to T and DHT. The syndrome is characterized by bilateral testes [*SRY* (sex-determining region of Y) dependent], absent or hypoplastic wolffian ducts (T dependent), female-appearing external genitalia and a blind vaginal pouch (DHT dependent), and absent müllerian derivatives (müllerian inhibiting factor dependent). Breast development is normal due to aromatization of the excess testosterone into estrogen.

As noted earlier, Turner's syndrome is characterized by partial or complete absence of one X chromosome (45, X karyotype).

47, XXY (**B**, Klinefelter's syndrome), 47, XYY (**C**, Jacob's syndrome), 46, XY (**D**, normal male or androgen insensitivity syndrome), or 46, XX (**E**, normal female or müllerian agenesis) karyotypes are not associated with Turner's syndrome.

Turner's syndrome is characterized by gonadal dysgenesis that virtually precludes hypersecretion of any of the ovarian hormones (**C**, **D**, and **E**). High gonadotropin levels (**B**) are consequent to ovarian failure.

Approximately a third of individuals with Turner's syndrome have hypothyroidism (**A**), commonly caused by autoimmune (Hashimoto's) thyroiditis. Decreased levels of thyroxine support the diagnosis for the syndrome.

The image can be identified as the sublingual salivary gland from predominant tubules of mucus glands (structure 1), a few scattered serous acini (structure 3), and serous demilunes (structure 2). This is a predominantly mucous gland (**A, B**) that has preganglionic parasympathetic (secretory) fibers originating from the superior salivatory nucleus in the brainstem.

The parotid gland is exclusively serous (**A**) and is controlled by the inferior salivatory nucleus (**D**). The submandibular gland is predominantly serous (**B**). The nucleus solitarius (**C**) is a higher taste and cardiorespiratory center and does not control salivary secretion.

Double aortic arch is the most common form of symptomatic vascular ring, accounting for up to 40% of complete rings, and commonly occurs in isolation. It is due to persistence of the right dorsal aorta, which maintains its connection with the left dorsal aorta. The vascular ring compresses both the trachea and the esophagus. In this case, the child presented with clinical features of tracheal compression.

Abnormal obliteration of the right 4th aortic arch (**A**) causes the right 4th intersegmental artery (future right subclavian artery) to form an abnormal connection with the left dorsal aorta. The aberrant right subclavian artery crosses the midline posterior to the esophagus. It is asymptomatic for the most part, but cases with dysphagia have been reported.

Abnormal regression of the left 4th aortic arch (**B**, interrupted aortic arch) results in an interruption between the aortic arch and the descending aorta. There are different varieties of this defect (types A, B, and C); accompanying ventricular septal defect (VSD) and/or patent ductus arteriosus (PDA) ensures blood flow to the lower body. However, none of the types present with vascular rings.

Abnormal obliteration of the left 4th aortic arch and left dorsal aorta (**C**, right aortic arch) are accompanied by abnormal persistence of their right counterparts. Because the ductus arteriosus is now connected to the right aortic arch, occasionally the ligamentum arteriosum passes behind the esophagus and causes dysphagia. Again, a vascular ring is not formed and no tracheal compression occurs.

Persistence of the left dorsal aorta (**E**) is normal and it does not account for tracheal compression.

13. Correct: This intestinal segment is affected by the diverticulum consequent to a nonobliterated vitelline duct. (C)

The image can be identified as the ileum by the presence of villi (structure 1) and Peyer's patches (structure 2). Persistent vitelline duct can form Meckel's diverticulum, which affects distal ileum.

Ileum is supplied by the ileal branches of the superior mesenteric artery. Appendix removal needs clamping of the ileocolic artery (**A**). The appendix can be ruled out for this specimen because of the presence of villi. Ileum is derived from embryonic midgut (**B**).

Duodenum is usually affected by cancer of the pancreatic head (**D**). Secondary retroperitoneal intestinal segments (**E**) are duodenum and ascending and descending colons.

14. Correct: A, B, and C (F)

The newborn has presented at birth with a genitourinary defect consistent with the cloacal exstrophy variant of the exstrophy-epispadias complex (EEC). This is characterized by an infraumbilical abdominal wall defect, incomplete closure of the bladder with mucosa continuous with the abdominal wall, epispadias, alterations in the pelvic bones and muscles, and persistence of urogenital sinus.

Description of the mass matches with an exposed and everted urinary bladder (**B**). The dorsally opened plate that ran from the bladder neck down to the open glans is the epispadiac urethra (**A**). Presence of meconium indicates an incomplete separation of the urogenital sinus and consequent persistence of cloaca. This confirms the diagnosis of cloacal exstrophy (**C**), which results in exteriorization of the entire cloaca due to an accompanying defect in separation of the urogenital sinus (anterior) from the anorectal canal (posterior).

15. Correct: B and C (E)

Overgrowth of the cloacal membrane in EEC prevents medial migration of the mesenchymal tissue (**B**). This prevents fusion of midline structures below the umbilicus. Depending on the extent of the abdominal wall defect, the cloacal membrane ruptures prematurely, resulting in the spectrum of the exstrophy-epispadias complex. Classic bladder

exstrophy results if rupture occurs after the separation of the genitourinary and gastrointestinal tracts. Cloacal exstrophy occurs if rupture occurs before separation of the genitourinary and gastrointestinal tracts by the urorectal septum (**C**).

Defective migration of neural crest cells (**A, D**) is not related to EEC.

16. Correct: Imperforate anus (E)

Cloacal exstrophy includes the triad of omphalocele, bladder exstrophy, and imperforate anus. Ileal prolapse often accompanies cloacal exstrophy, but a classical Meckel's diverticulum (**C**) is not a common association. Other listed abnormalities (**A, B,** and **D**) are not frequently associated with cloacal exstrophy.

17. Correct: 1 (A)

The patient is suffering from intrahepatic cholestasis of pregnancy. Cholestasis can be diagnosed by generalized pruritus and elevated conjugated bilirubin and alkaline phosphatase. Biliary channels within the liver will be dilated. Structure 1 denotes biliary canaliculi that affect lateral domains of adjacent hepatocytes. These spaces collect bile synthesized by hepatocytes and are sealed off by tight junctions between them. Structure 2 (**B**) denotes space of Disse that lies between basolateral membrane of hepatocytes and sinusoidal endothelium. Bidirectional exchange of solutes between the sinusoidal blood and hepatocytes occurs here. Structure 3 (**C**) denotes lumen of hepatic sinusoid. This contains blood brought in by portal vein and hepatic artery, and is inaccessible for bile. Structures 4 (**D**) and 5 (**E**) denote an endothelial cell and a cross-sectioned reticular fiber, respectively.

18. Correct: Metaphase of meiosis II (D)

The female is on day 15 of the normal cycle, which implies ovulation has occurred. The oocytes remain arrested in the diplotene stage of the first meiotic prophase (**B**) until they are recruited to grow and mature (by FSH) to produce an ovum or they undergo apoptosis. The resumption of meiosis is mediated by the mid-cycle surge in LH, and meiosis I is completed at ovulation. Following ovulation, once again, the process is arrested (for the secondary oocyte that is supposed to be available to be fertilized by a sperm), this time in the second meiotic metaphase. Meiosis is completed only if fertilization occurs.

19. Correct: Right sinus horn (D)

Given the elevated JVP and enlarged liver, the infant has developed congestive cardiac failure (CCF), i.e., right heart failure. Also, a tricuspid regurgitation and cyanosis (accompanying atrial septal defect with reversal of shunt from right to left) in infancy heavily shifts the diagnosis toward Ebstein's anomaly. An echocardiogram confirms this diagnosis; apical displacement of the septal (most specific) and posterior tricuspid valve leaflets leads to atrialization of the right ventricle, hugely dilated right atrium, and eventual CCF. The smooth part of the right atrium develops from the sinus venosus and the right sinus horn.

Bulbus cordis (**A**) develops into outflow tracts of the ventricles—infundibulum for the right and aortic vestibule for the left ventricles.

Ductus arteriosus (**B**) is a communication between the descending thoracic aorta and the pulmonary artery. Ligamentum arteriosum is its remnant.

Truncus arteriosus (**C**) develops into the aorta and the pulmonary trunk.

Left sinus horn (**E**) develops into the coronary sinus and the oblique vein of the left atrium.

20.   Correct: Secretion from this organ is the primary source of energy for spermatozoa to swim. (D)

Highly folded mucosa with several levels of branching (structure 2, honeycomb pattern) is the characteristic feature for seminal glands (vesicles). It is often lined by simple or pseudostratified columnar epithelium. Its secretions are rich in fructose (provides energy for spermatozoa to swim) and also contain citrate, inositol, prostaglandins, and several proteins.

Ductus deferens (**A**) would present with a less complex mucosal branching pattern. It will also have several layers of prominent smooth muscles in its wall.

Seminiferous tubules of testis (**B**) would feature a complex germinal epithelium with spermatogenic cells at different levels of maturation.

Epididymis (**C**) presents with tall pseudostratified columnar epithelium with prominent stereocilia.

Tubuloalveolar glands embedded in the fibromuscular stroma of the prostate gland (**E**) are difficult to rule out. However, the extensive complex branching pattern of the mucosa weighs in for the seminal glands. Also, concretions could be confirmative, if found, in such extensive sections of the prostate.

21.   Correct: Ileocolic artery (C)

The midgut forms the primary intestinal loop, which consists of a cranial and a caudal limb. The cranial limb forms the jejunum and upper part of the ileum. The caudal limb forms the cecal bud, from which the cecum and appendix develop. The rest of the caudal limb forms the lower part of the ileum, ascending colon, and proximal two-thirds of the transverse colon. The ileocolic artery, through its ileal, cecal, appendicular, and colic branches, supplies the lower ileum, ileocecal junction, cecum, appendix, and ascending colon.

The gastroduodenal artery (**A**), off the common hepatic branch of the celiac artery, supplies foregut structures (stomach and proximal duodenum). The jejunal artery (**B**) supplies the jejunum, which is derived from the cranial limb of the primary intestinal loop. Left colic (**D**) and superior rectal (**E**) arteries supply structures derived from the hindgut.

22.   Correct: Intermediate mesoderm (D)

The patient is suffering from adrenal cortical failure (as in Addison's disease). Clinical features include fatigue, weakness, anorexia, nausea and vomiting, weight loss, abdominal pain, cutaneous and mucosal pigmentation, hypotension, and, occasionally, hypoglycemia.

Adrenal cortex develops from intermediate mesoderm (that also form the kidneys).

Oral ectoderm (**A**) gives rise to the anterior pituitary gland. In case of pituitary failure (i.e., secondary adrenal insufficiency), the ACTH challenge test would increase cortisol levels.

Neuroectoderm (**B**) gives rise to the central nervous system and the posterior pituitary gland. These are not primary offenders in Addison's disease.

Neural crest cells (**C**) form the chromaffin cells of adrenal medulla, among many other structures. These are not involved in Addison's disease.

Adrenal cortex does not derive from endoderm (**E**).

23.   Correct: Na+ ↓, K+ ↑, ACTH ↑ (B)

In primary adrenal insufficiency, aldosterone deficiency results in renal loss of Na⁺ and retention of K⁺, causing hyponatremia and hyperkalemia. With decreasing cortisol secretion, plasma levels of ACTH are increased because of decreased negative feedback inhibition of their secretion.

24.   Correct: Abundance of smooth endoplasmic reticulum (C)

Cells of the adrenal cortex have abundant smooth endoplasmic reticulum and lipid droplets (**B**) typical of steroid-producing cells. Abundance of rough endoplasmic reticulum (**D**) and apical secretory granules (**E**) are found in protein-synthesizing cells. Nuclear hypersegmentation (**A**) is not a noted feature in the adrenal cortical cells.

25.   Correct: Bulb of the vestibule (D)

The glans and corpora cavernosa of the clitoris, and bulbospongiosum of the vestibule are derived from the genital tubercle. The vagina (**A**) is derived from the paramesonephric duct; the urethra (**B**) and greater vestibular glands (**C**) are derived from the urogenital sinus; and labia majora (**E**) are derived from genital swellings (folds).

26.   Correct: Parathyroid hormone (C)

Structure 2 can be identified as distal tubule by presence of simple cuboidal lining cells and lack of brush border. Also note that the cell borders are barely visible. The site of parathyroid hormone regulation of Ca^{2+} reabsorption is the distal tubules.

Angiotensin II (**A**) acts on proximal convoluted tubules (structure 1). These tubules can be identified by the prominent brush border.

Aldosterone (**B**) and antidiuretic hormone (**D**) act primarily on principal cells of collecting ducts. These are difficult to distinguish from distal convoluted tubules given the similarity of epithelia. Two features that could help separate the two are that the collecting ducts usually have larger lumen in crosssection and have distinct borders separating the lining cells.

27. Correct: Patent ductus arteriosus (A)

Survival in case of aortic valve atresia (before surgical correction) is dependent on the presence of a functioning ductus arteriosus, because that is the only way to shunt blood to the systemic circulation. A patent foramen ovale is also usually present. It is the only mechanism to shunt oxygenated pulmonary venous blood from the left atrium to the right atrium and onto the systemic circulation via the patent ductus arteriosus.

A ventricular septal defect (**B**) may be an associated finding, but not an essential one.

Aortic atresia is usually associated with hypoplasia of the ascending aorta, of the left ventricle (**C**), and of the mitral valve (**D**), because the left chambers eventually become functionless, leading to the hypoplastic left heart syndrome.

The right ventricle (**E**) is hypertrophied, because it must pump blood to both the pulmonary and the systemic circulations, which are connected in parallel, rather than in series, by the ductus arteriosus. The right atrium, tricuspid valve, right ventricle, and the pulmonary trunk are larger than usual.

28. Correct: Lined by ciliated low cuboidal cells, absence of goblet cells, wall contains some smooth muscles but no cartilage. (B)

The patient is suffering from pulmonary emphysema, diagnosed from classical clinical and laboratory findings. This is a condition marked by irreversible enlargement of airspaces distal to terminal bronchioles, accompanied by destruction of their walls. The principal pathologic event in emphysema is thought to be a continuing destructive process resulting from an imbalance of local oxidant injury and elastolytic activity caused by a deficiency of protease inhibitors (α1-antitrypsin). Oxidants, whether endogenous (superoxide anion) or exogenous (e.g., cigarette smoke), can inhibit the normal protective function of protease inhibitors, allowing progressive tissue destruction.

Olfactory epithelium (**C**), trachea (**D**), or bronchi (**E**) are not involved in gas exchange and are not involved in pathologic changes in emphysema.

Histologic features of terminal bronchioles (**A**, last part of conducting airway) and respiratory bronchioles (**B**) are similar other than the facts that respiratory bronchioles are lined by a flatter epithelium and their walls have fewer smooth muscles.

29. Correct: Inferior mesenteric artery (C)

The normal ascent of the kidneys allows the organs to take their place in the abdomen below the adrenal glands. However, with a horseshoe kidney, ascent into the abdomen is restricted by the inferior mesenteric artery (IMA, given off at the level of the L3 vertebra from the abdominal aorta), which hooks over the isthmus. Therefore, horseshoe kidneys are low lying.

The ascending or the 4th part of the duodenum ascends as far as the upper border of the L2 vertebra and turns forward to form the duodenojejunal flexure (**A**). The superior mesenteric artery (**B**) is given off at the level of L1 vertebra from the abdominal aorta. Both of these structures lie above the level of IMA and would be next in line to obstruct ascent of a horseshoe kidney.

The horizontal or 3rd part of the duodenum (**D**) lies at the level of L3 vertebra but is not a midline structure.

Transverse colon (**E**) is located much anterior to the kidneys and could not possibly cause obstruction.

30. Correct: Recurrent respiratory infections (E)

The neonate is suffering from meconium ileus consequent to cystic fibrosis (CF). Meconium ileus is a severe intestinal obstruction resulting from inspissation of tenacious meconium in the terminal ileum and is virtually diagnostic of CF. Elevated serum immunoreactive trypsin (IRT) confirms the diagnosis.

The major morbidity and mortality associated with CF is attributable to respiratory compromise, characterized by copious hyperviscous and adherent pulmonary secretions that obstruct small and medium-sized airways. Chronic and recurrent respiratory infections are very common in this setting.

Tenacious exocrine secretions obstruct pancreatic ducts and impair production and flow of digestive enzymes to the duodenum. Although pancreatic amylase and trypsin are important for carbohydrate (**A**) and protein (**B**) digestion, respectively, other enzymes in gastric and intestinal juice can usually compensate for their loss.

Renal failure (**C**) is not a common reported complication of CF. Men typically exhibit complete involution of the vas deferens, and ~ 99% of males with CF are infertile. This is due to defective liquid secretion within the vas, while spermatogenesis is normal (**D**).

31. Correct: Defective epithelial ion channel consequent to genetic mutation (B)

The cause of CF is a defect in a single gene on chromosome 7 that encodes an epithelial chloride channel called the CF transmembrane conductance regulator (CFTR) protein. Abnormal ion transport functions underlie organ-specific pathologies in CF.

Defective migration of neural crest cells to the gut wall (**A**) might cause Hirschsprung's disease. While the clinical feature resembles that of CF, an elevated serum IRT shifts the diagnosis toward CF.

Defective growth of urorectal septum (**C**) in males would cause rectourethral or rectovesical fistulas. Fecal matter will be passed in the urine.

Defective regression of the omphalomesenteric (vitelline) duct (**D**) could cause a diverticulum (Meckel's) or a fistula (vitelline). Meckel's diverticulum usually presents with painless rectal bleeding, if at all, at that early age.

Imperforate anus (**E**) could resemble the clinical features, but a normal digital rectal exam precludes its possibility.

32. Correct: Adenohypophysis (D).

The patient might be affected by craniopharyngioma. These are benign, suprasellar, calcified, cystic masses that are derived from Rathke's pouch (an epithelialized rostral invagination of the stomodeum that develops into the adenohypophysis) and arise near the pituitary stalk, commonly extending into the suprasellar cistern. The radiologic hallmark of a craniopharyngioma is the appearance of a suprasellar calcified cyst.

The image can be identified as adenohypophysis (polymorphic cells) with basophils (2) dispersed among the acidophils (1). Structures 3 and 4 are chromophobes and capillaries, respectively.

The thalamus (**A**), hypothalamus (**B**), and neurohypophysis (**E**) will predominantly show neural tissue and less polymorphic cells.

The pineal gland (**C**) presents two types of cells: pinealocytes and glia. Pinealocytes have larger, lighter-staining nuclei, and glial cells have small, darker-staining nuclei. With age, calcified formations appear in the pineal gland (brain sand or corpora aranacea).

33. Correct: B and C (E)

Removal of a mass related to the pituitary gland will necessitate clamping of the superior and inferior hypophyseal vessels. Superior hypophyseal vessels are principally given off from the supraclinoid segment of the internal carotid artery (**C**, begins at penetration of dura and extends until its bifurcation into the anterior and middle cerebral arteries). Inferior hypophyseal arteries are off the cavernous segment of the artery (**B**, passes through the cavernous sinus). Although inferior hypophyseal arteries principally supply the posterior pituitary, they form an arterial ring surrounding the infundibulum and, therefore, need to be clamped.

The petrous segment of the artery (**A, D,** and **F**) ascends in the carotid canal. Branches off of it are the caroticotympanic (enters tympanic cavity) and pterygoid (enters pterygoid canal) arteries.

34. Correct: Follicle-stimulating hormone (C)

Cells labeled 2 are basophils. TSH, ACTH, FSH, and LH/ICSH are all secreted by basophils. Somatotropin (**B**) and prolactin (**A**) are secreted by acidophils. Corticotropin- (**D**) and luteinizing hormone (**E**) releasing hormones are secreted from the hypothalamus.

35. Correct: ADH (antidiuretic hormone) (B)

ADH is synthesized by hypothalamic neurons and stored in pars nervosa of the neurohypophysis. This could not be stained using a fluorescent antibody applied for adenohypophysis. ACTH (**A**), FSH (**D**), and TSH (**E**) are synthesized by basophils, while GH (**C**) is synthesized by acidophils of the adenohypophysis.

36. Correct: Septum secundum (B)

A gap between the septum secundum and the septum primum forms the foramen ovale. When the upper part of the septum primum gradually disappears, the remaining part becomes the valve of the oval foramen. After birth, when lung circulation begins and pressure in the left atrium increases, the valve of the oval foramen is pressed against the septum secundum, obliterating the oval foramen and separating the right and left atria. Persistent foramen ovale is due to inadequate development of the septum secundum. It can also, less frequently, be due to excessive resorption of the ostium secundum/septum primum. The trivial amount of left-to-right shunting through patent foramen ovale generally produces no symptoms. Patients with right-to-left shunting can experience transient or persistent periods of cyanosis. This can be exacerbated by acute increases in pulmonary vascular resistance, such as those that occur during breath holding, crying, or the Valsalva maneuver.

Ostium primum (**A**) is the gap between septum primum and endocardial cushions and is closed by their fusion. It has no role in the formation of foramen ovale.

Endocardial cushion (**D**) malformation might result in an ostium primum type of atrial septal defect, but not patent foramen ovale.

Right and left sinoatrial valves join above the opening of the coronary sinus, forming the septum spurium (**C**). This septum and the two sinoatrial valves obliterate and are not appreciated in the adult heart.

Conotruncal cushions (**E**) are not involved in the formation of the atrial septum.

37. Correct: A and D (F)

The cell labeled 1 is a protoplasmic astrocyte, which is a central glia. It can be identified by a large number of processes radiating from the perikaryon, resembling spiders. Glial cells, other than the microglia, are derived from neuroectoderm (**A**) and not from the neural crest (**B, G**, and **H**). Also, GFAP (**D**) is an important marker for astrocytes during their immunocytochemical staining. Neurofilament (**C, E**, and **G**) is expressed by neurons and not glial cells.

38. Correct: Right and left ventricles, subendocardium (C)

The cell described is a Purkinje cell (fiber), which is typically found within the subendocardial zone of ventricles.

Sinoatrial nodal cells (**A**) or atrioventricular nodal cells (**B**) are smaller than cardiac myocytes and lack intercalated disks. Epicardium (**D**, visceral layer of serous pericardium) and the parietal layer of serous pericardium (**E**) do not contain cardiac myocytes and constitute mesothelial lining of simple squamous cells and connective tissue cells. These cells do not possess intercalated disks.

39. Correct: Greater omentum (E)

Due to rotation of the stomach around an anteroposterior axis, the dorsal mesogastrium (mesentery) extends down (from the greater curvature of the stomach) over the transverse colon and covers it like an apron. This double-layered sac eventually forms the greater omentum. The ventral mesentery connecting the stomach (lesser curvature) to the ventral body wall is referred to as the ventral mesogastrium. The liver grows in it and divides it into lesser omentum (**D**, peritoneal fold that connects the liver to the stomach) and falciform ligament (**A**, peritoneal fold that connects the liver to the ventral body wall). Ligamentum venosum (**C**) and ligamentum teres hepatis (**B**) are embryological remnants of the ductus venosus and the left umbilical vein, respectively. These are not derived from mesentery.

40. Correct: Tricuspid stenosis (D)

Endocardial cushions contribute to septation of atria by fusing with the septum primum. Atrioventricular (tricuspid and mitral) valves also form from these cushions. Therefore, malformation of these cushions can lead to a variety of AV valve defects, including tricuspid stenosis.

The conotruncal cushions contribute to septate the outflow tracts of the ventricles (conus and truncus) and form the aorticopulmonary septum. Differential growth of tissue from these cushions also contributes to the formation of the semilunar (pulmonary and aortic) valves. Therefore, malformation of these cushions can lead to a variety of outflow tract septation or obstruction defects, including TGV (**A**), PTA (**B**), and aortic stenosis (**E**).

The muscular part of the ventricular septum (**C**) is formed by a mesenchymal growth from the primitive ventricular wall.

Index